The Health of Populations

Stephen J. Kunitz

The Health of Populations

General Theories
and Particular Realities

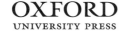

2007

OXFORD
UNIVERSITY PRESS

Oxford University Press, Inc., publishes works that further
Oxford University's objective of excellence
in research, scholarship, and education.

Oxford New York
Auckland   Cape Town   Dar es Salaam   Hong Kong   Karachi
Kuala Lumpur   Madrid   Melbourne   Mexico City   Nairobi
New Delhi   Shanghai   Taipei   Toronto

With offices in
Argentina   Austria   Brazil   Chile   Czech Republic   France   Greece
Guatemala   Hungary   Italy   Japan   Poland   Portugal   Singapore
South Korea   Switzerland   Thailand   Turkey   Ukraine   Vietnam

Copyright © 2007 by Oxford University Press, Inc.

Published by Oxford University Press, Inc.
198 Madison Avenue, New York, New York 10016

www.oup.com

Oxford is a registered trademark of Oxford University Press.

Library of Congress Cataloging-in-Publication Data

Kunitz, Stephen J.
The health of populations : general theories and particular realities / Stephen J. Kunitz.
    p.   cm.
Includes bibliographical references and index.
ISBN-13 978-0-19-530807-5
ISBN 0-19-530807-7
1. Public health—Economic aspects.   2. Public health—Social aspects.   3. Public health—History.
4. Industrialization—Health aspects.   5. Population—Health aspects.
[DNLM: 1. Epidemiology.   2. Culture.   3. Public Health.   4. Social Environment.
WA 105 K96h 2006]   I. Title.
RA427.K86   2006
362.1—dc22   2005035873

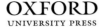
9 8 7 6 5 4 3 2 1

Printed in the United States of America
on acid-free paper

For Izzie, with love and gratitude

But if the while I think on thee (dear friend)
All losses are restored, and sorrows end.
—*W. Shakespeare, Sonnet 30*

And for Joseph.

Preface

The fox knows many things,
but the hedgehog knows one big thing.
—Archilochus (c. 710–676 BC)

In a famous essay, Isaiah Berlin used this brief fragment from an ancient Greek poet to characterize "[O]ne of the deepest differences which divide writers and thinkers, and, it may be, human beings in general." He continued,

> [T]here exists a great chasm between those, on one side, who relate everything to a single central vision, one system less or more coherent or articulate, in terms of which they understand, think and feel . . . and, on the other side, those who pursue many ends, often unrelated and even contradictory, connected, if at all, only in some *de facto* way . . . The first kind of intellectual and artistic personality belongs to the hedgehogs, the second to the foxes.[1]

Each way of knowing the world has advantages and disadvantages, but this book is a brief for foxes as guides to understanding the impact of social organization and culture on rates and patterns of disease and death in populations. The argument is that wherever one looks, there are exceptions to every generalization. Rather than ignore them, or force them into a Procrustean bed, they must be embraced. If the exceptions can be integrated into an existing explanation or theory, fine. If not, then the explanations must be modified or scrapped. There is another possibility, however, which I think more and more likely: that when considering the social determinants of the health of populations in the modern world, no overarching generalization—neither stress, nor income per capita, nor loss of community, nor inequality, nor globalization—is going to be possible. We must consider the possibility that the range and combination of determinants of health, and the various ways of reaching the same goal, are so great that they cannot be embraced by one explanation.

This book is meant to encourage people concerned with the health of populations, as a subject of study as well as of policy and practice, to think critically about the generalizations and abstractions they carry with them and to test them against their own research and experience. Alfred North Whitehead wrote, "You cannot think without abstractions; accordingly, it is of the utmost importance to be vigilant in critically revising your *modes* of abstraction."[2] I would like my readers to be vigilant, like a fox.

Acknowledgments

I have been thinking about this book for a long time, but its completion was made possible by a Health Policy Investigator Award from the Robert Wood Johnson Foundation. I am grateful to David Mechanic and Lynn Rogut, respectively director and assistant director of the program, for support, encouragement, and access to a circle of colleagues to whom I have been able to turn for help. The views expressed are my own and imply no endorsement by the Johnson Foundation.

Among the many friends and colleagues who have provided advice and help are Stanley Engerman, Larry Layne, David Leon, John Lynch, Irena Pesis-Katz, Ralph Sell, and George Davey Smith. I am grateful to Muriel Stanley and Eva Galambos for secretarial help. My editors at Oxford University Press, first Jeffrey House and then Carrie Pedersen, were efficient and encouraging. It has been a pleasure to work with them both. I also thank the three reviewers for the press for many helpful suggestions.

I have drawn upon several articles previously published elsewhere and am grateful to Oxford University Press and to the editors of the following journals for permission to use them here: the *American Journal of Public Health*, *Population and Development Review*, the *Milbank Quarterly*, and the *Journal of Health and Social Behavior*.

My greatest debt is to my wife, Isadora Derow Kunitz, for her love, encouragement and support, and good-humored forbearance.

Contents

Appendices

The Health of Populations

Introduction

Locke sank into a swoon;
The Garden died;
God took the spinning-jenny
Out of his side.
—W. B. Yeats, *The Tower*

This book is about three related issues. The first is the way inherited ideas about industrial growth, economic expansion, social change, and causes of disease have shaped explanations of the health of populations. The second has to do with the ways in which these inherited ideas have become assimilated to political ideologies that influence how epidemiologic and demographic data are understood, causal inferences made, anomalies ignored, and abstractions drawn. The third is about the importance of understanding the social context of the populations whose health we study and hope to improve—their history, culture, economy, and political institutions—for that often helps to explain the anomalous findings that are so frequent, and so frequently ignored.

Two revolutions have shaped the ways in which the health of populations is usually understood. The first, the industrial revolution in England, provoked a debate about the costs and benefits of industrial growth in particular and economic expansion more generally. What has been called the optimistic side claimed that the benefits far outweighed the costs and that, had industrialization not occurred, human existence would have been mired in misery. The pessimistic side argued that the working class paid an excessive and unfair price, and that when benefits were realized they were largely the result of working class activism and militancy.

The origin of this debate, known as the standard-of-living debate, was in England, for England was the first industrial nation and, in an important sense, the birthplace of the modern world. The issues raised about England in the first half of the nineteenth century, however, echo through later debates about inequality, about the role of the state, and about globalization, to take but three examples. More than that, the issues involve not only narrowly economic measures such as the standard of living and income per capita, for the industrial revolution (along with the contemporaneous French Revolution) raised deep concerns about the destruction of traditional communities and social relations, about alienating work, and about the psychological turmoil of anomie, concerns shared by people at all points on the political spectrum.[1]

The paired concepts of *gemeinschaft* (community) and *gesellschaft* (society), traditional and legal–rational authority, status and contract, and folk and urban society are all attempts to capture the social changes that dominated the experience of nineteenth-century Europeans. Many thought that the destruction of traditional communities and the emergence of the modern nation-state, unrestrained by countervailing power vested in traditional forms of aristocratic and religious authority, would result in mass society, a world of individuals without any organic connection to one another or to a particular place. The metaphor often used was of society as a dustheap. Conflicting beliefs about the benefits of modernization on the one hand and the costs of loss of community, social isolation, and inequality on the other, have permeated Western culture and have found their way into discussion of the social determinants of the health of populations. Describing how that has happened and the consequences is one of the major purposes of this book.

The second revolution with which this book deals was epistemological, caused by the development of bacteriology and the germ theory of disease in the late nineteenth century. The results were manifold. Ideas of causal necessity and disease specificity became dominant and shaped medical thought and training. No longer were diseases thought to change from one person to another, to result from several different causes, and to require knowledge of the particular patient. For if diseases were specific and the same from one person to another, then knowledge of disease at a deep biological level was of more value than knowledge of the unique individual who was sick. At the level of populations, the new knowledge legitimated a new role for scientific expertise while promising universally available preventive and curative interventions that would radically transform the health of individuals and populations.

Not everyone who accepted the validity of the new epistemology interpreted or used it in the same way. Some assimilated it to an older, religiously inspired ethic of individual responsibility. Others assimilated it to a then new notion of society as an important cause of individual and group behavior. Moreover, as in every revolution, there was more than one side. Not everyone at the time or later wholeheartedly accepted the new epistemology and its implications. Skeptics thought the approach reductionistic and oversimplified. Out of this reaction has emerged what in Chapter 2 is called a counterrevolution, in which susceptibility of the host rather than exposure to specific causes is considered of primary importance.

Part II explores the ways in which the key concepts described in Part I influence thinking about social factors and how they shape the health of populations. Each chapter is devoted to one of the concepts that have become especially prominent. They are the standard of living, inequality, community, and globalization. Because these concepts are so much a part of the culture, and because they evoke such passion, they are far more than useful ideas in highly specialized research. They are central to what we believe to be the essence of a good society, and they often shape the way empirical data are interpreted. More than that, they form the basis for generalizations about the social determinants of the health of populations that go well beyond the population or populations that have been the subject of a particular study.

This is inevitable, for induction is characteristic of science. But it carries a risk of committing what Alfred North Whitehead labeled the fallacy of misplaced concreteness.[2] This occurs when abstractions are based upon only a few cases and are not constantly checked against other cases. The risk is particularly great when the abstractions are shaped by deeply held values about the nature of society. The argument in each chapter in Part II is that that is precisely what has happened: there are discrepant results that make suspect generalizations about the role of income per capita, inequality, community and social support, and globalization and their impact upon the health of populations. A high or low standard of living, whether measured as income or as height, is not necessarily associated with better or worse mortality rates. High social status is not invariably associated with better health than is low social status. Differences in income inequality among societies are not invariably correlated with differences in life expectancy. Measures of community, whether civic or at a more intimate and personal level, have no necessary relationship with health. And globalization (measured as trade liberalization) is not necessarily associated with good or bad health.

In each instance, the larger context in which the populations being observed live and work contributes importantly to the causal associations that are reported. Repeatedly through the book governments are found to be among the most significant determinants of the context. Their ability to protect the health of their population is measurable, as are the consequences of their failures, as the experience of the Soviet Union and Yugoslavia demonstrate. To take one example by way of illustration, despite the common-sense assumption that high social status is always and everywhere associated with lower mortality than low social status, the expected pattern seems to be relatively new. For until the modern era, since, say, the late eighteenth century, for example, the differences in the mortality of segments of the population were often unrelated to status, wealth, or income but, rather, were associated with place of residence and with the culture of the group, including a culture of moderation. The widening gap between the mortality of rich and poor in the early nineteenth century and the narrowing that occurred beginning later in the century were associated with the provision first of public health services by local governments and later of personal services and income redistribution by national governments. Thus, patterns of mortality among social classes differ across historical periods, and much of the difference is accounted for by the role governments have played in shaping the physical and social environment.

That is, there are exceptions to every attempt at generalization, and to make sense of contradictory findings investigators need to understand and explain more completely than they do the particular societies, communities, and institutions in which the populations they observe are embedded. More than that, contradictory and anomalous findings need to be acknowledged and not ignored, as so often happens. To fail to do so may be no more than normal science, but it is self-defeating.[3] It happens not simply because scientists normally are wedded to their theories, but because—especially when considering the social roots of disease—deeply held preexisting values shape the interpretation of data and the abstractions inferred from them. Value commitments are no bad thing. They only become dangerous when they keep one from acknowledging, not to say searching for, contradictory findings that challenge one's generalizations. When that happens, one is engaged in a religious endeavor, not science.

It will become obvious that my own values drive much that I have written. These include egalitarianism and a belief that government has a central role to play in providing universally available health care; as well as a belief that markets and free trade have made possible a better standard of living and quality of life than other forms of economic organization, but, that left to their own devices, each can cause great inequalities and inequities that only states can control. Much of the data in the book support those notions, not all of them preconceived.

I

Epistemology, Ideology, and Epidemiology

1

Two Revolutions

Overwork! There's no such thing. I do the work of ten men. Am I
giddy? No. NO. If you're not well, you have a disease. It may be
a slight one; but it's a disease. And what is a disease? The lodg-
ment in the system of a pathogenic germ, and the multiplication
of that germ. What is the remedy? A very simple one. Find the germ
and kill it.
—G.B. Shaw, *The Doctor's Dilemma*[1]

The two revolutions of this chapter's title are the Industrial Revolution that began in England in the late eighteenth or early nineteenth centuries, and the
Epistemological Revolution that is conventionally attributed to the enunciation of the germ theory of disease by Louis Pasteur in France and by Robert
Koch in Germany in the last third of the nineteenth century. The former is the
source of what has been known to economic historians as the standard-of-
living debate, but which is part of a much larger set of concerns about the consequences of industrialization and urbanization, and which ramifies down to
our own period and informs many of the interpretations of the consequences
for the health of individuals and populations of economic change, inequality,
and globalization. The latter prompted a debate about the way diseases were to
be explained and defined, about reductionism versus holism, and about how
diseases in populations were to be understood and addressed. This chapter is
about some of the many ways in which these two revolutions have intertwined
and shaped thinking about the health of populations.

The Industrial Revolution and the Standard-of-Living Debate

Although the standard-of-living debate is as old as the Industrial Revolution
itself, it is convenient to begin with an article by Eric Hobsbawm published in
1957. Hobsbawm classified participants in the debate as optimists and pessimists. Optimists believed that the standard of living—conventionally measured as income per capita—had improved on average as well as for the

working class from the late eighteenth century to the mid 1840s. Pessimists believed that both absolutely and relatively the incomes and quality of life of the industrial working class had deteriorated during that period. Hobsbawm, himself a pessimist, wrote:

> This is not to deny that the increase in production, which greatly exceeded that of population, in the long run brought about an absolute improvement in material living standards. Whatever we may think of the relative position of labourers compared to other classes, and whatever our theory, no serious student denies that the bulk of people in Northwestern Europe were materially better off in 1900 than in 1800. But there is no reason why living standards should improve at all times. Whether they do, depends on the distribution of the additional resources produced among the population.[2]

Optimists argue that bad as life in industrial cities may have been during the early phases of the revolution, it would have been substantially worse had there been no revolution. Moreover, improved incomes, no matter how unequal their distribution, made possible all the improvements that even pessimists like Hobsbawm agree occurred in the long run. Pessimists argue that only working-class mobilization and active government intervention forced the business elite to accept improvements in working and living conditions that were, and would have remained, otherwise intolerable. These same positions are manifested in contemporary debates about the consequences of income inequality and globalization.

However important that debate may be, it is mainly about the economic well-being of the working class. It is not about the other consequences of the industrial revolution that also worried observers: alienation, anomie, and loss of community. Karl Polanyi argued that the cataclysm caused by industrialization and the urbanization that followed hard upon it was not only, or even primarily, about the standard of living. "Nothing so obscures our social vision," he wrote, "as effectively as the economistic prejudice."[3] It was "[N]ot economic exploitation, as often assumed, but the disintegration of the cultural environment of the victim" that was "the cause of the degradation."

> The economic process may, naturally, supply the vehicle of the destruction, and almost invariably economic inferiority will make the weaker yield, but the immediate cause of his undoing is not for that reason economic; it lies in the lethal injury to the institutions in which his social existence is embodied. The result is loss of self-respect and standards, whether the unit is a people or a class, whether the process springs from so-called "culture conflict" or from a change in the position of a class within the confines of a society.[4]

It was in this sense that the industrial revolution was a source of anxiety about the destruction of traditional communities and institutions, and the sense of fragmentation and alienation that followed,[5] to which holism and communitarianism have been responses.[6] In the period between the Civil War and World War I, many of these concerns became prominent in the United States as industrialization, urbanization, and immigration all occurred with explosive force. Simultaneously, a profound revolution in medicine and public health also took place.

The Epistemological Revolution

During the nineteenth century, a major transformation occurred in the way the causes of disease were understood in Western medicine; "Assumptions about disease shared by doctor and patient and oriented toward visibly altering the symptoms of sick individuals, began to be supplanted by strategies grounded in experimental science that objectified disease while minimizing the differences among patients."[7] No longer was the individual patient with his or her unique disease the physician's concern. Increasingly, it was the specific disease regardless of the peculiarities of the individual patient that was the concern of scientifically trained physicians.

Two reasons for this transformation are particularly important. One was the growth of physiological research based on assumptions nicely captured in the following remark by Claude Bernard, the great French physiologist, in his classic treatise *An Introduction to the Study of Experimental Medicine* (1865):

> [O]nly by basing itself on experimental determinism can [medicine] become a true science: i.e. a sure science. I think of this idea as the pivot of experimental medicine, and in this respect experimental physicians take a wholly different view from the so-called observing physicians . . . Most physicians seem to believe that, in medicine, laws are elastic and indefinite. These are false ideas which must disappear if we mean to found a scientific medicine.[8]

The other was the change in ideas of causal attribution that followed upon the elaboration of the germ theory in the 1880s. K. Codell Carter has shown that until that time, when Robert Koch enunciated the postulates that now bear his name, physicians explained diseases in terms of multiple weakly sufficient causes. [9] A sufficient cause is one that is followed by a particular effect. A weakly sufficient cause is one that is sometimes followed by the effect. Nineteenth-century physicians believed that diseases might be caused by a variety of factors, that a common cause could not be inferred from a common effect, and that diseases might blend into one another.

With the work of Koch and other bacteriologists, the idea of necessary cause of disease was introduced for the first time. A necessary cause is one without which an effect cannot occur. Without the tubercle bacillus there cannot be tuberculosis. The result was a subtle but far-reaching change. Many diseases could now be classified etiologically as well as anatomically or symptomatically. Disease specificity became increasingly possible, and with it the possibility of disease-specific interventions that would be applicable in all places and among all people, regardless of topography, climate or culture.[10]

This change in ideas of causal attribution made possible by exposure to German research methods, by major changes in medical education, and by the growing possibility of academic careers in medical research in the United States, all combined at the end of the nineteenth century to cause a major epistemological revolution. Diseases were now to be explained at a deep level, not simply described and classified. Increasingly, disease processes, not unique patients, became the focus of attention for the rising elite in medicine.

There were a number of responses to this revolution, for, like most revolutions, it was not uncontested. One of the most important responses, and the subject of the next chapter, was a growing concern with psychosomatic medicine on the part of a number of established academic physicians, called by Theodore Brown "the holistic elite."[11] These were men such as Lewellys Barker, Francis Weld Peabody, and G. Canby Robinson, who believed that concern with disease mechanisms was drawing attention away from the concern for the patient as a person—the title of an influential book by Robinson.[12] Another was the response of the public health profession.

The Germ Theory of Disease and the New Public Health

The rapid succession of striking discoveries in bacteriology,[13] all reinforcing the concept of causal necessity and of disease specificity, encouraged many influential public health workers to embrace the germ theory enthusiastically.[14] It underlay the Rockefeller Foundation's campaign during 1909–1914 against hookworm in the Southern United States;[15] it led to the creation of public health laboratories in state and city health departments; and it was incorporated by Charles Chapin, the influential health officer of Providence, Rhode Island, in his campaign to professionalize public health. Indeed, Chapin was so profoundly impressed with the force of the germ theory and of the idea of causal necessity and disease specificity that he offered a sardonic funeral oration over its predecessor:

> When our honored and lamented Reed went to Havana and discovered that yellow fever was transmitted by the bite of a mosquito, and Gorgas, by the most brilliant sanitary experiment ever made, put an end to this disease in its very stronghold, they drove the last nail in the coffin of the filth theory of disease. But it is feared that the devotees of this theory are loath to bury it, thus violating one of their cardinal principles. It seems to me it is the duty of the health officers of this country to see that this ceremony is properly performed.[16]

The germ theory, said Chapin, had made possible a more lucid, efficient, and economical attack on the causes of mortality. Specific diseases could now be directly targeted and directly defeated. Medicine, he said, had acquired a new precision. Depending on the situation, medical interventions would vary: they might require isolation of the infectious; they might require treatment with antitoxin; they might require measures to protect water and milk; and they might require health education. But, medicine could now focus directly on the fundamental cause of each disease and could conquer each with an effectiveness previously unknown.

Chapin also argued that necessary causation rendered irrelevant the activity of those he saw as misguided social reformers and politicians. Where an elegant precision in identifying the cause of disease was possible, there was no further need for the efforts at municipal cleanliness that had characterized the urban reform movement. He dismissed municipal cleanliness as uneconomical, unprofessional, and unscientific.[17]

Chapin sought to explain the striking decline of mortality in the nineteenth century in terms of the new causal concept of disease. He analyzed the decline of mortality in his own city, Providence, between 1856 and 1905 and sought to trace the reduction of deaths from specific diseases to specific interventions. He linked the decline in smallpox to vaccination; the decline in scarlet fever to isolation; the decline in diphtheria to antitoxin; and the decline in typhoid to the improvement of the water supply. Political, socioeconomic, and environmental conditions did not figure in his analysis.[18]

Chapin's influence was widespread. His work was popularized by Hibbert Winslow Hill, of the Minnesota Board of Health, in a series of newspaper articles later reprinted in a book. The book, *The New Public Health*, published in 1918, made the case for the greater economy and efficiency of the germ theory than of the miasmatic theory of disease. "To control tuberculosis, for example, it was not necessary to improve the living conditions of the 100 million people in the United States, only to prevent the 200,000 active tuberculosis cases from infecting others."[19] Hill wrote "The essential change is this: The old public health was concerned with the environment; the new is concerned with the individual. The old sought the sources of infectious disease in the surroundings of man; the new finds them in man himself."[20] He made clear that the "surroundings of man" was the physical environment:

> [D]irty clothes, bad smells, damp cellars, leaky plumbing, dust, foul
> air, rank vegetation, swamps, stagnant pools, certain soils, smoke,
> garbage, manure, dead animals, in fact everything physically,
> sensorially, esthetically, or psychically objectionable, were lumped
> together as "unsanitary."[21]

The germ theory, then, became a professional ideology for the new public health that was focused more on individuals than on the environment.[22] As Chapin wrote, "In recent times, since sewers have been constructed by the municipality and with engineering advice, details have been wisely left to the engineers,"[23] while bacteriology gave added legitimacy to other health department activities: the protection of milk supplies, reporting and isolation of patients with active tuberculosis, production of diphtheria antitoxin, monitoring of water quality, and so on. On the other hand, the day-to-day work of health departments did not change dramatically "during the transition from miasma to germ theory." [24]

Both theories left much room for alternative approaches to the problems facing urban departments of health. Even after widespread acceptance of the germ theory, for instance, there continued to be disagreements about the best way to protect milk supplies.[25] Although Chapin thought the germ theory had redefined the work of health departments, advocates of housing reform used it to strengthen their arguments for slum improvement.[26] And Nancy Tomes has pointed out with regard to tuberculosis prevention that, "[T]he code of individual protection was recast [by the garment workers' union] as a form of worker solidarity. The brochure emphasized that individual workers owed each other this carefulness, in order to do no harm to their workmates. Labor's version of tuberculosis religion also presented joining the union as the first and most important step of disease prevention."[27] She points out further that in Atlanta tuberculosis prevention became a vehicle for cooperation between whites and African Americans at a time of worsening racial prejudice.[28]

The point of these examples is to emphasize that there was nothing intrinsic to the germ theory that required the focus to be only on the individual to the exclusion of the social context. In this light, the observation of Elizabeth Fee and Dorothy Porter that "[T]he advent of bacteriology may have been even more important in helping weld a new professional, scientific identity for public health" in the United States than in Britain, assumes considerable significance.[29] The role of Medical Officer of Health in Britain had been established well before the enunciation of the germ theory, whereas in the United States, health officers were not nearly as well established until late in the nineteenth century, after the widespread acceptance of the theory. For American public health physicians, therefore, the germ theory became a lever with which to elevate their professional status. And status as expert professionals meant command of a body of knowledge that was above politics and was value free. The germ theory, as Chapin had argued, made it possible for public health to free itself from social reform and politics. One can sympathize with this impulse, for the politics in which public health officers were mired in the 1890s and early 1900s was often dominated by urban machines, bossism, and corruption. Moreover, while the germ theory was important for the advancement of public health as a profession, there is every reason to think that the diffusion of many of the innovations it made possible had beneficial consequences.

The Germ Theory and the Public

Much of public health and settlement house work and public education involved the education of immigrants and African Americans—usually women and school children—about cleanliness and about appropriate middle-class

domestic and public behavior. Norms of middle-class refinement were new in
the nineteenth century and were an adaptation to the increasing stratification
and inequality found in urban America. They required physical and emotional
control, the maintenance of distance, and respect for one's own and others'
privacy. "In public especially, but also in private, one sought particularly to sti-
fle all activities that might draw attention to the internal working of the body,
such as coughing, sneezing, yawning, scratching, tooth picking, throat clearing, and nose blowing. More intimate functions were generally beneath discussion."[30] Chewing tobacco and spitting were especially common and the
subject of criticism by European visitors and American authorities on etiquette. Wrote one, spit "is an excrement of the body, and should be disposed of
as privately and carefully as any other."[31]

Middle-class norms of restraint and refinement evolved well before the
germ theory had been articulated. They were diffused across the country by
the sale of millions of copies of many different etiquette books.[32] The germ
theory, however, gave added legitimacy to those norms. For example, hand-
shaking was regarded as a barbarity by mid-century etiquette authorities. The
obligation of political leaders "to shake the hands of all comers [was consid-
ered] as 'democratic intrusiveness.'"

> Nonetheless, the ritual continued from the days of Lafayette's
> American tour and Andrew Jackson's election in the 1820s throughout
> the nineteenth century, reaching a climax when on New Year's Day,
> 1907, President Theodore Roosevelt shook hands with an estimated
> 8,150 people. Yet secretly Roosevelt agreed with the ritual's critics.
> "Ugh! Ugh!" he grunted after a similar occasion. "Shaking hands, with
> a thousand people! What a lot of bugs I have on my hands, and how
> dirty, filthy I am!" He immediately washed himself thoroughly, and
> then announced, "Now I am clean. I always do this after a reception.
> You should remember it. It may save your life some time!"[33]

Kissing, too, was regarded as "a reprehensible custom," even between relatives or women when greeting one another. Late in the century, "writers seized
upon the germ theory to make hygienic appeals against promiscuous kissing:
'Disease may be introduced in this way that many years would fail to eradicate.'"[34]

Middle-class reformers attempted to inculcate these norms of refinement
in immigrants, both those from rural America and those from abroad. To be
clean was to be American, according to this gospel. The importance of protecting and preserving food, of using clean water, of bathing, of washing one's
hands after using the toilet, of keeping the home clean and airy, of screening
windows against flies,[35] and of not spitting were all subjects of health education activities whose legitimacy was enhanced by the germ theory. Until about
1910, it was reformers and public servants who were largely responsible for
persuading "the masses of the benefits of keeping clean." By 1920, marketing
by companies that manufactured soap, toothpaste, and all variety of cleaning

products became especially significant.[36] While it is impossible to determine the impact of the changes in personal behavior that were evoked by these educational and marketing activities, it seems likely that they were substantial. [37]

The Germ Theory and the New Social Medicine

A focus on the individual who harbored an infection was not the only way the germ theory could be understood. In the Progressive Era, however, the attempt to establish a profession that could be free of the undue influence of politics, and that would not challenge the interests of many of the major philanthropists who were an important source of financial support,[38] drove many in the field to avoid concerning themselves with the social context within which disease developed.[39]

Ironically, it was during this same period that conceptions of the environment expanded to include the social environment.[40] Thomas Haskell has written that in the period between the Civil War and World War I growing awareness of the interdependent nature of American society created a profound change in ideas of causal attribution of social and personal phenomena. No longer were they to be understood as caused by the individual actor, the local community, or God. Forces generated by a much larger society, though less remote than the Almighty, acted on individuals and communities. "The recession of causation and the consequent devitalization of island communities, individuals, and personal milieux gave a new concreteness and uniquely modern salience to the very idea of 'society' (or the 'polity,' or the 'economy') as an entity apart from particular people and concrete institutions."[41]

In contrast to the focus upon individuals that characterized the New Public Health, social forces such as ethnicity, income, and religion became important causal variables for the newly emerging social sciences and began to influence the way health and disease were understood. For example, in 1903, William H. Allen, a well-known reformer and, at the time, General Secretary of the New Jersey State Charities Association, wrote "[T]he limits to progress are not to be sought in sanitary science, but in social theories; not in the paucity of remedies, but in the unwillingness to justify them theoretically and to pay for their application."

> Perhaps we are about to argue that the study of sanitary problems
> will help us better to understand monopoly power? Is the standard of
> life dependent upon health and the means to protect it? Yes, perhaps
> we are about to argue that the study of sanitary problems will help us
> better to understand monopoly force; that sanitary conditions offer a
> criterion of the standard of life; that the health of a class depends
> upon its share of monopoly returns from industry; that man's hold
> upon life and vitality is intimately bound up with theories and
> methods of distribution; that sanitary progress depends upon right

theories of taxation; and that the saving of twenty thousand lives a
year in Pennsylvania alone waits upon public appreciation of the true
nature of monopoly and its earnings. . . . [B]ecause sanitary science
is a phase of social science rather than a branch of chemistry,
medicine, or biology.[42]

Voters, the courts, and administrators, he wrote, needed to understand
that health and disease resulted from institutional arrangements and social inequality. Doctors are concerned with pathology and disease and with dispensing
pills, not with public welfare. It was "state medicine, not laboratory medicine,
that has re-housed Britain's poor; it is the application of vaccine lymph and
the governmental utilization of antitoxin that have robbed smallpox and
diphtheria of their terrors."[43] "Sanitary administration," he concluded, "offers
a very direct and most efficacious means of reducing the inequality that even
the most conservative capitalist will concede to be incident on our present system of distribution."[44]

These observations were not especially original. Virchow, Engels, and early
nineteenth-century French public health specialists had written similarly.[45]
However, they assumed greater importance in the United States during the
Progressive Era than they had previously. The contrast between the New Public Health and the New Social Medicine corresponds broadly to the optimistic
and pessimistic sides respectively in the standard of living debate. For the New
Public Health devoted itself to changing the behavior of individuals, assuming
that the economy was largely beneficent. The New Social Medicine aimed to
reshape the environment. The distinction becomes clear when the difference
between the way hookworm and pellagra were understood in southern
cotton-mill villages in the early twentieth century are considered.

The Problem of the Cotton-Mill Villages

Cotton-mill villages developed in the post-Civil War years, primarily as the result of investment by southerners themselves, who aimed to compete with the
New England mills that had previously dominated the American textile industry. For their labor force they drew on poor whites from various regions of the
South. Most first-generation mill workers were farmers who had given up sub-
sistence farming for cash-crop farming of cotton, who had fallen into debt
from which they could not extricate themselves, and who saw work in the
mills as the only alternative. Mills usually employed several members of a
family, who found that the "family wage" was more than the same family unit
could earn as tenant farmers or as owners of marginal land.[46]

Mill villages were the southern equivalent of the slums of northern and
midwestern cities, which were populated by waves of immigrants from peasant societies in eastern and southern Europe. For middle-class southern
reformers, the problems were similar to those faced by their northern and
midwestern counterparts.[47] They included illiteracy and ignorance, which the

reformers feared would lead to social divisiveness, to the immigrants' susceptibility to the hollow promises of rural demagogues and urban bosses, and to
the newcomers' inability to function in the new occupations being created by
the new industrial order.

Mental and physical health were problems as well, for poor health would
make it impossible for the newcomers to benefit from the opportunities presented to them. It was feared that rather than becoming productive, contributing members of society, they would become a drain on society and a threat to
the middle classes now increasingly exposed to them.

Although progressive reformers might agree on the existence of these and
other problems, there was less agreement about causes and remedies. Some reformers thought that "cultural lag" was especially important. By this they
meant that the immigrants brought along their own traditional culture, which
was ill suited to the needs of the new society to which they had moved. Hence
education, both in schools and on the job, was important.

Others placed more emphasis on the significance of social institutions in
the new society, which were managed in an exploitative fashion. Although
such reformers did not deny the importance of education, they also believed
that reforms needed to be made in other social institutions, such as working
conditions in factories and access to services.

In this context, the living, working, and health conditions of southern textile workers became the subject of surveys of which the Progressives were so
fond. These included studies of both hookworm and pellagra. The approach
to the former was based largely on the assumption that cause and cure were
mainly matters of individual education and change. The approach to the latter
was primarily that cause and cure were both institutional. These differing approaches did not follow from the intrinsic nature of each disease but from the
values and ideology of the public health workers who investigated them.

Hookworm

Hookworm had been known in Europe for much of the nineteenth century
and by 1875 was "accepted as the cause of the severe anemia characteristically
found in warmer climates."[48] The ecology of the parasite had been determined
during the first decade of the twentieth century. The larva usually gains en-
trance to the human host through the tender skin between the toes of people
who go barefoot. It is carried in the blood to the lungs, where it crosses into
the respiratory tract, is coughed up, and then is swallowed. Then it fastens to
the wall of the duodenum, where it sucks blood from the host, matures, mates,
and lays eggs. The eggs are excreted and hatch in the soil, and the cycle begins
over again. Hookworm infestation is common in areas where the larvae can
survive in the ground, where human excrement is not disposed of safely, and
where people do not wear shoes.

The loss of blood causes iron-deficiency anemia as well as hypoalbumine-
mia; the major symptoms seem to be the result of the anemia. If the host has

low iron consumption and if the iron stores are not replaced, fewer worms will be required to cause anemia than if iron consumption is adequate.[49] It has also been suggested that an adequate diet is associated with increased resistance to the organism.[50] Thus, the interactions between host and parasite are complex and depend on factors in the physical environment, social status, customs, and nutritional status. Much of this was known by the 1910s.

The disease was recognized in the United States in the nineteenth century, but it was not until early in the twentieth century that a German-trained American parasitologist, Charles Wardell Stiles, first described an American type of hookworm, which almost certainly had been brought to the New World from Africa in the intestines of affected slaves. In 1902, during a survey in the American South, he discovered that hookworm was widespread and claimed that it might be responsible for some of the "proverbial laziness of the poorer classes of the white population."[51] Stiles also suggested that childrens' health improved when they moved from farms to mill villages, for the disposal of human waste was conducted under more sanitary conditions in the villages than on the farms. This observation earned Stiles the enmity of the reformers who were devoted to improving living and working conditions in the villages,[52] but he was almost certainly correct. Hookworm is a rural more than an urban disease.[53]

In a subsequent survey of cotton mill villages made as part of the *Report on Condition* (sic) *of Woman and Child Wage-Earners in the United States*, Stiles elaborated on this point. So-called cotton-mill anemia was the result of hookworm infestation, not of exposure to lint in the factory; it was widespread among mill hands, especially among those under 16 years of age; and it was more common among first- than second-generation mill workers. The anemia caused by hookworm was less severe and less prevalent in the mill workers than on farms. He wrote, "[W]e are here dealing with an easily recognizable disease which can be easily and satisfactorily treated in the vast majority of cases and which can be easily prevented by the simple means of a properly constructed, properly maintained, and properly used sanitary privy."[54]

Advocates of factory reform were displeased by Stiles's focus on hookworm to the exclusion of other problems, by his attribution of the bulk of health problems in the villages to hookworm, by his faith that easily administered treatment and improved sanitation were all that were required to solve the problems of children's health in the villages, and by his general support of the factory system. His views attracted more sympathetic attention from Frederick Gates, director of the then-new Rockefeller philanthropies, and in 1909 the Rockefeller Sanitary Commission for the Eradication of Hookworm was established.

The work of the Commission has been described elsewhere and need not be repeated here.[55] The important point is that the eradication campaign had many of the characteristics of a religious crusade. In accordance with its religious hue, the campaign was designed to rid the patient/sinner of his or her individual disease/sin, bypassing politics, society, economics, and culture.[56]

An older religious conception of sin, to which Gates, Rockefeller, and many others adhered, was assimilated to the conception of disease as advocated by The New Public Health. Just as the individual sinner was to be transformed and redeemed by his or her religious experience, so was the individual patient to be made whole by the ministrations of public health experts. Institutional and social changes were not a necessary part of the process.

Pellagra

Like hookworm disease, pellagra had been described in Europe before the twentieth century and before it had been recognized in the United States. By the early nineteenth century, its association with a diet of corn had been observed. Some researchers denied any causal association, while those who believed that such an association existed were divided between those who thought corn lacked a crucial nutrient and others who thought it was contaminated in some way.[57] By the turn of the twentieth century, after the germ theory had been articulated, an infectious agent of some sort, often associated with poor sanitary conditions, was also postulated.

The classic studies of the disease were carried out in several cotton-mill villages by Joseph Goldberger and his colleagues in the 1910s and 1920s. They demonstrated that contaminated corn was not a cause of pellagra, that the disease was not associated causally with poor sanitation, and that it was not infectious. The only difference between families in which pellagra occurred and those in which it did not was that protein consumption was much lower among the former than among the latter.[58]

If this had been the extent of their work, it would have been significant enough. There is little doubt that if Goldberger had lived just a little longer, he would have discovered that tryptophan was the missing dietary ingredient for which he was searching. It was soon found to be a precursor to the vitamin niacin, which is widely available in a variety of foodstuffs, including corn. However, niacin is not biologically available from corn unless it is soaked in an alkali such as lime, as was the case in Mexico and Central America (where pellagra was not a problem despite a high corn diet) but not in the American South (where it was a serious problem because of the high corn diet and inadequate availability of alternative sources of tryptophan, such as proteins).[59]

As it was, Goldberger discovered an animal model of the disease and was able to produce and cure it at will. By the new criteria of an adequate explanation, he and his colleagues had succeeded: they had all but discovered the *cause* of pellagra. They went further, however, for unlike the investigators of hookworm disease, they had assimilated another paradigm of causal attribution, one in which "society" had become an important independent variable. In a paper published in 1915, Edgar Sydenstricker, an economist who worked with Goldberger, wrote:

> It has . . . been observed that the disease is chiefly prevalent in the
> South and is especially prevalent in mill communities, and that it is

closely associated with conditions of poverty. Observation apparently tends to indicate a considerable increase in the prevalence of pellagra during the last seven or eight years.

Thus the possible relation of the incidence of pellagra to uncertain conditions of an economic character is at once suggested.[60]

In a 1920 article based on their intensive fieldwork in seven mill villages during 1916, Goldberger and his colleagues could be much more precise about the character of these economic and social conditions. They showed first that per capita family income was related inversely to the incidence of pellagra among families followed prospectively with biweekly visits for a year. This finding could have been due to bad hygiene and sanitation, differences in age–sex composition among income groups, or differences in diet. Only diet differed; the smaller the income, the smaller were the supplies of proteins that were purchased.[61]

The investigators moved next from the family to the village level of analysis, comparing a village with no pellagra to one with a very high incidence. The two villages did not differ in income and sanitation, but the village with a high incidence did not have access to meat markets or to local farmers who sold meat, eggs, or milk door-to-door. The village with a low incidence had both local markets and door-to-door vendors. Moreover, the village with a high incidence was in a region where local farmers had converted their land to cotton cultivation to the virtual exclusion of food crops. The village with no pellagra was in an area where the land was not conducive to growing cotton so the local farmers had continued to grow food crops and to engage in truck farming. Market conditions differed as well. The village with a high incidence of pellagra was adjacent to a small city, with which it competed for what local produce was available, and which also served as a distribution point for other markets. The village without pellagra was more isolated and did not compete with neighbors for food supplies. Goldberger and his colleagues concluded:

> Thus, of all the factors we have studied in relation to differences in pellagra incidence among our villages, the factor of food availability is the only one in connection with which significant evidence of such a relationship was found. The conclusion would, therefore, seem to be warranted that in this factor we have the explanation for the differences among villages studied in the incidence of the disease, so far as this incidence was a reflection of community conditions.[62]

Note that the explanations of the differing incidence rates were to be found in society, not in individual or family differences.

Finally, in respect of practical guides to action, Goldberger and his colleagues wrote: "The results of the present study clearly suggest fundamental lines along which efforts looking to the eradication of the disease should be directed, namely, (1) economic, by improvement of economic status (income), and (2) food availability, by improvement in availability of food supplies."[63]

Unlike the hookworm disease investigators, they had assimilated the new explanatory criterion of disease not to an old notion of individual responsibility but to a new notion of social responsibility. It is thus an entertaining irony that the solution to the pellagra problem turned out to be so relatively simple: to put niacin in bread. This was a magic bullet indeed, in contrast to the difficulties that stood in the way of the eradication of hookworm. The intrinsic nature of these two diseases did not lead the investigators inevitably to the solutions they urged.

Ideology and Explanations of Disease

The New Public Health and the New Social Medicine are entwined with and shape debates about health policy, the role of the state and social institutions, the significance of individual choice and responsibility, and the importance of economic growth and income distribution and redistribution—the standard-of-living debate—right through the twentieth century.[64] The pessimists in contemporary versions of the standard-of-living debate tend to see the poor as victims of the social environment, with little or no control over, or responsibility for, what befalls them. In this sense, they are determinists. They define disease broadly and share the view that diseases are caused by society and citizens are victimized by society.[65] The risk factors upon which they focus are such technological ones as toxic and carcinogenic chemical exposures from industry and agriculture; radiation from military, industrial, and medical sources; drugs and food additives; industrial and farm machinery; such implements of modern life as handguns, rifles, knives, and automobiles; such phenomena as the breakdown of social supports in the course of urbanization; the loss of autonomy by local communities; crowding, unemployment, and poverty; the competitive tensions of modern life; and, of course, differences in status and incomes—in short, an immense web of causation. To the degree that the poor are able to exercise choice, they are tightly constrained by the limits imposed upon them by poverty and social exclusion. Thus, in the context of capitalist industrial nations, pessimists confront every major social institution.

Pessimists are also egalitarians for whom inequality is unacceptable. That is why they prefer to use measures of relative rather than absolute differences in mortality. That is also why there is a strong implication that equality is the natural state of humankind, as typified by hunter–gatherer bands, the earliest form of human society. Richard Wilkinson has written that:

> [T]here are two basic forms of social organization among human
> and non-human primates: "agonistic" societies based on dominance
> hierarchies, and "hedonic" societies based on egalitarian cooperation
> (as typified among humans by hunter-gatherers). There is clearly a
> stark contrast between dominance hierarchies, or pecking orders, in

which power and coercion provide access to resources regardless of other's needs, and societies with more cooperative social relations, in which people's needs are recognized and mediated through the social obligations of sharing and reciprocity—as between friends.[66]

The optimists could not be more different. They are voluntarists who hold diametrically different positions on the central assumptions: society is not the first cause and thus, by implication, man is not inherently a victim; and inequality is not necessarily bad.[67] For the major causes of mortality, the locus of control is internal; it has to do with the individual's will and moral responsibility. Not irrelevantly, the optimists have different priorities and a different definition of disease, and they prefer to measure absolute rather than relative change and differences in mortality. Generally, they use the traditional physiological definition of diseases, and they claim to be concerned with the greatest good for the greatest number; the factors associated with reduction of the greatest number of deaths.

With the publication in 1976 of Thomas McKeown's two volumes, *The Modern Rise of Population* and *The Role of Medicine*,[68] the voluntarists became an identifiable group, for he had set their explanations of contemporary mortality patterns in industrial countries in a broad historical context. He argued that improvements in the standard of living, most especially in nutrition, had led to the decline of mortality in the nineteenth century, so that now individuals were freer than they had ever been before of exogenous forces affecting mortality, and that endogenous forces under the control of individuals themselves had become the major determinants of morbidity and mortality.

From all sides voices elaborated on these conclusions. John Farquhar declared *The American Way of Life Need Not Be Hazardous to Your Health*, the title of a book in which he advised readers how to alter their behavior to diminish their risks of heart disease.[69] Michael Shimkin stated, "Accidents, suicide, and homicide rank above all diseases. In older age groups, many of the diseases are self-induced . . . Our main threats to life are now based primarily on life-styles and habits."[70] Richard Doll claimed, "Relatively few causes of mortality . . . have become more common recently, and most of those that have are due to changes in behavior and not to the introduction of new toxic substances."[71] Lester Breslow said that the prevention of mortality had shifted from the identification of specific disease entities "toward the identification and reduction of the factors that lead to clinical disease."[72] The reduction of such risk factors was to be accomplished by educating the public to adhere to seven simple "health habits." And Robert Fogel wrote:

> From the standpoint of health equity, the most important issue today in rich nations is not the cleaning up of the environment, as it was a century ago, but the reformation of lifestyle. Practices that undermine the accumulation of physiological capital (such as bottle-feeding instead of breast-feeding infants) or that accelerate the depreciation of

physiological capital (such as recreational drugs, smoking, excessive alcohol consumption, and overeating) are more frequently practiced among the poor and the poorly educated than among the rich and the well-educated sectors of the population.[73]

An unmistakable theme of moral denunciation appropriate to the importance attributed to voluntary behavior emerges in many of these statements. Ernest Wynder said, "the leading causes of death today are the result of life style. The public must realize that the persons who are responsibly protecting their health are actually paying for the health care of those who behave irresponsibly."[74] Gio Gori, at the time director of the smoking and health program of the National Cancer Institute, declared, "Evidence accumulated during the last twenty years indicates that the most important of modern diseases are caused by a variety of factors, most significantly by reckless personal and social habits."[75] Robert Fogel wrote, "Food has become so cheap that corpulence is no longer a sign of opulence. It is instead a sign of weakness of will."[76]

And from one of the central institutional supporters of biomedical research came the voluntarist position complete with its philosophical and political implications. John Knowles, president of the Rockefeller Foundation, declared that "Cartesian rationalism, Baconian empiricism, and the results of the Industrial Revolution" had led the medical profession to hitch its wagon to the star of high technology. This orientation, he said, was strengthened by the development of the germ theory and the beguilingly simple notion of "one germ–one disease–one therapy." This, he continued, had resulted in very high-cost medical care and indifference to the moral responsibility of individuals for their own health.

> Prevention of disease means forsaking bad habits which many people enjoy—overeating, too much drinking, staying up at night, engaging in promiscuous sex, driving too fast, and smoking cigarettes—or, put another way, it means doing things which require special effort—exercising regularly, going to the dentist, practicing contraception, ensuring harmonious family life, submitting to screening examinations. The idea of individual responsibility flies in the face of American history which has seen a people steadfastly sanctifying individual freedom while progressively narrowing it through the development of the beneficent state.[77]

Politicians have found this message appealing. Donald Hodel, Secretary of the Interior in the Reagan administration recommended that the President not sign an international agreement to reduce chlorofluorocarbons in the atmosphere. It was believed that these chemicals were damaging the ozone layer, and that increased exposure to radiation would cause an increase in cancer. Instead, the Secretary recommended that people use "personal protection:" suntan lotion, hats, and sunglasses.[78] And Edwina Curry, a junior Health Minister in Margaret Thatcher's government explained to an audience in the north of England why health in the north was worse than in the south: "We have problems here of high smoking and alcoholism. Some of these problems are things we can tackle by impressing on people the need to look after themselves better. That is something which is taken more seriously down South. There is no reason why it cannot be taken seriously up here."[79]

The theme underlying all these statements is that individuals must assume responsibility for their own health, for to expect the beneficent state to do so would destroy the economic engine that has led to the improved well-being of all. For the optimists, human beings are the masters of their fate and responsible for what befalls them, with a few exceptions, such as epidemics. That is why it is so useful to call the noninfectious diseases "life-style" diseases and why the state is believed to have a minimal role, in terms of health services limited only to quarantine and other measures to control epidemics of infectious diseases. Richard Epstein has celebrated this as The Old Public Health,[80] what in the early twentieth century Hibbert Winslow Hill had called The New Public Health.[81]

Conclusion

Neither the nature of the germ theory nor the nature of particular diseases dictates necessary public health or policy consequences. They are rather like projective tests. They have been, and are, interpreted and used in ways that express values, ideological positions, and political and career considerations. The New Public Health was a way of assimilating a new theory of disease causation both to old values regarding the nature of individual responsibility and to new concerns about the establishment of a new kind of profession, one based upon scientific objectivity rather than social reform.

The New Social Medicine assimilated the same new way of understanding the deep causes of disease to a new way of thinking about society as a cause. Instead of place, climate, and the physical environment, it was the less tangible and less easily measured social environment that mattered most.

Just as the germ theory could be used in different ways, so can the way we understand and study the epidemiology of particular diseases be shaped as much by values and ideologies as by the nature of particular diseases. Indeed, what we consider a disease as contrasted with some other type of misfortune is also shaped by our values, beliefs, and occupational locations.[82] The fact that agreement may be unanimous in some cases does not make the statement any less true. The point is not to deny the reality of a broken leg but to assert that how it is labeled and explained is open to interpretation. Likewise, pellagra is real enough, but whether its cause was to be understood to be the uninformed choices made by mill hands or the ecological settings of the villages in which they happened to live and work was to a large degree determined by the values and beliefs of those who investigated it. That there is nothing intrinsic in the germ theory or in the epidemiology of various diseases that make their policy implications inevitable is what has allowed optimists and pessimists to use them in such different ways.

2

Counterrevolution

O chestnut-tree, great-rooted blossomer,
Are you the leaf, the blossom or the bole?
O body swayed to music, O brightening glance,
How can we know the dancer from the dance?
—W.B. Yeats, *Among School Children*[1]

In the previous chapter, a "holistic elite" of physicians was briefly mentioned, men who in the interwar years had reacted to the growing fascination with disease specificity and causal necessity by emphasizing instead concern for the whole patient and his/her ability to adapt effectively to the stresses and concerns of daily life. Holism was not uniquely limited to a small number of elite physicians, however, but was a much broader cultural phenomenon as well as an important element within physiology, medicine, and epidemiology.

Different definitions of holism have been offered over the years, but the most inclusive was set down in 1890: "the whole is greater than the sum of its parts,"[2] whether the unit of concern is an individual human being, or a biological or social system. At the individual level, holism means that the mind and the body are one. At the societal level, it means that communities are not simply aggregates of individuals but are greater than the sum of the individuals who comprise them.

The idea of holism emerged in the second half of the nineteenth century, but it became pervasive in Europe and North America between the two world wars. It implied, among other things, a concern with the adaptation of whole systems to change, whether environmental or social. It was in large measure a response to the disruptions in the late nineteenth and early twentieth centuries caused by industrialization; by the internal and international migration of millions of people to rapidly expanding cities from rural communities; and by World War I. All were developments that had led to a pervasive sense of both personal and social fragmentation.

The related quests for a sense of wholeness and of community were a common response. Many artists and writers sought them among the traditional Indian cultures of the American Southwest.[3] Social reformers sought to recreate a sense of community in the rapidly expanding slums of industrializing cities.[4] Industrial psychologists sought to create community in the workplace.[5] And sociologists and anthropologists found the sources of social pathologies in the breakdown of traditional communities.[6] The quest for community is the subject of another chapter. This chapter is concerned with the diffusion and use of the idea of holism in medicine, epidemiology, and public health.

Holism in Epidemiology and Medicine

Writing of the period before the epistemological revolution, Charles Rosenberg observed, "The model of the body and of health and disease . . . was all inclusive . . . capable of incorporating every aspect of man's life in explaining his physical condition. Just as man's body interacted continuously with his environment, so did his mind with his body, his morals with his health. The realm of causation in medicine was not distinguishable from the realm of meaning in society generally." Moreover, it was widely believed that diseases could change from one to another and that the distinctions among them were not fixed. "The idea of specific disease entities played a relatively small role in such a system."[7]

These older ideas were never entirely overthrown as enthusiasm for ideas of necessary cause and disease specificity became dominant, and inevitably there was resistance and reaction to these enthusiasms.[8] In his seminal address to medical students in 1927, Francis Weld Peabody concluded that, "One of the essential qualities of the clinician is interest in humanity, for the secret of the care of the patient is in caring for the patient."[9] Peabody had set aside acute infections in a separate category, implying that patients with these afflictions did not require the same "holistic" approach as patients with noninfectious conditions. This reflected a widely shared perception in the interwar years that infectious diseases were declining and that the new diseases confronting patients and their physicians would increasingly be the chronic diseases that would require the interpersonal and clinical skills of the experienced general physician.[10]

The shared concerns of the elite group of which Peabody was such an important member influenced their teaching of medical students and house staff,[11] their views of the way medical services ought to be organized in an age of specialization, and the research they undertook. Lewellys Barker, for instance, was a member of the Committee on the Costs of Medical Care and part of the majority that wrote an influential report recommending, among other things, that generalists be the ones to organize the care of patients, with specialists being called upon only as needed. "Under present conditions, the old-time relation with a family physician is often disturbed," they wrote. "The family physician should be restored to his place of responsibility and trust and his potentialities extended by substituting coordinated for uncoordinated relations with specialists and the other agencies which permit him to do his work effectively."[12]

Barker was, as well, one of many investigators who explored the constitutional bases of disease. He commented in 1922 that, "During the past fifty years . . . under the spell of bacterial and protozoan etiology, medical men have been so absorbed by studies of influences arising in the environment that they have, too often, forgotten to continue their investigation of influences of endogenous origin. . . . Recently, however, there has been a welcome revival of studies of constitution." For constitutionalists of the 1920s and 1930s like Barker, patients were "interconnected wholes, psychologically and physically," environment and heredity were viewed as equally important, and "[D]isease . . . was the individual's adaptive struggle with his or her social and/or physical environment."[13] That is to say, for constitutionalists as for holists more generally, healthy individuals were those who had adapted successfully to their environment, and their ability to adapt was a result of the characteristics of both their own constitution and of their social and physical environment.

Similar concerns were expressed in England, as the epigraph at the head of the previous chapter indicates. The English epidemiologist F.G. Crookshank criticized precisely the sort of reification of disease parodied by Shaw when he wrote:

> In modern Medicine this tyranny of names is no less pernicious
> than in the modern form of scholastic realism. Diagnosis, which, as
> Mr. Bernard Shaw has somewhere declared, should mean the finding
> out of all there is wrong with a particularly patient and why, too
> often means in practice the formal and unctuous pronunciation of a
> Name that is deemed appropriate and absolves from the necessity of
> further investigation. And, in the long run, an accurate appreciation
> of a patient's "present state" is often treated as ignorant *because* it is
> incompatible with the sincere use of one of the few verbal symbols
> available to us as Proper Names for Special Diseases.[14]

In physiological research, as well, an important body of thought emerged which was focused on the whole organism and the whole person, respectively. This work has more than a nodding acquaintance with, perhaps was even influenced by, the work of "the holistic elite." According to L.J. Henderson, professor of biological chemistry at Harvard, writing in 1927, "To-day, looking backward, we see how it was that bacteriological researchers for a long time took the first place which Claude Bernard believed to be already assured to those of his own science . . . In our time bacteriology grew into a fully developed science, perfected its methods, exploited its domain, and then, the most pressing work well done, resigned its leadership of the medical sciences." According to Henderson, bacteriology was merely technical; physiology required a deep knowledge of biology and medicine. Pasteur, he wrote, "always retained the chemist's outlook" whereas Bernard was as much a philosopher as a biologist, with an understanding of "the theory of organism" and of "the deeper problems of medicine."[15]

Henderson was himself an important physiologist who shared with his colleague, Walter B. Cannon (who coined the term "homeostasis"),[16] a belief that the entire organism was an open system that could only persist if it were able to adapt to changing conditions by maintaining a stable internal environment. According to John Parascandola, Henderson, whose early work was on the acid-base buffering mechanism of the blood, "believed that the concept of organization taught the biologist to recognize the wholeness of the organism and the interdependence of its parts and processes."[17] The important point is that both Henderson and Cannon took a holistic view, and understood living organisms to be open systems that had developed mechanisms to maintain the stability of their internal environments in the face of environmental change (what subsequently came to be called stress). These mechanisms were interactive and implicated in many different bodily functions. Failure of adaptation resulted in disease.

Henderson and Cannon each also discussed the relevance of his work to the practice of medicine and to society more generally. Indeed, physiology gave them each conceptual tools with which to address the economic and social crisis of the 1930s as well as the crisis they each perceived within medicine.[18] Henderson was by far the more influential in this regard. He moved on from physiology to the study of social systems and for a number of years in the 1930s taught an influential seminar on the sociology of Vilfredo Pareto and in the mid-1930s published a book on Pareto's sociology.[19] He drew the lesson that social equilibrium should not be interfered with by social engineering.

More important for present purposes, he also wrote about the doctor–patient relationship as a social system in several papers that influenced the sociologist Talcott Parsons and many later writers on the topic. "He urged physicians to return to a Hippocratic view of the patient as a human being living in a social as well as a physical environment . . . and to study the 'whole man'."[20]

Cannon, too, invoked Hippocratic ideas and the healing power of nature (the *vis medicatrix naturae*). He wrote that all he had done in his description of the "various protective and stabilizing devices of the body is to present a modern interpretation of the natural *vis medicatrix*."[21] And from his studies of physiological homeostasis he drew an analogy to the need for the central government to intervene to restore social equilibrium during the depression of the 1930s, a conclusion quite at odds with Henderson's and yet another illustration of the fact that scientific ideas can be employed in the service of very different ideological positions.

It was also Cannon's view of Hippocratic ideas that informed his position with regard to the doctor's role. In a speech to the Massachusetts Medical Society, he urged physicians to take an interest in the emotional lives of their patients because emotions had such profound physiological effects and because if physicians did not concern themselves with these aspects of care, patients would seek the ministrations of "cults, mental healers and the clergy. The doctor is properly concerned with the workings of the body and their disturbances, and he should have, therefore, a natural interest in the effects of emotional stress and in the modes of relieving it."[22]

This notion that disease had to be understood as a response of the individual to his or her environment was also reflected in an increasingly ecological approach to epidemiology. John Gordon, professor of epidemiology at Harvard, writing the history of his field, observed of the period following World War I:

> In the minds of many, realization took form that disease was no longer being studied, but rather the parts of disease; that too frequently the parts were considered the principal phenomenon; and that in pursuit of knowledge about infectious agents, the main objective was being lost.[23]

According to Gordon, these ideas crystallized in the years immediately following World War I as a result of the failure to explain and control the 1918 pandemic of influenza and outbreaks of polio, meningococcal meningitis, and encephalitis. Moreover, he wrote, the "changing social order" brought an increasing awareness that "cultural, economic, and social factors are important determinants of health and disease in groups of people." He continued:

> This movement did not originate precisely in 1920, nor in the years immediately following. Matters simply came to a head then. The return to a holistic interpretation of community diseases, its consideration as a unified and total process, had been under way for a number of years. Opinions solidified, to give general appreciation that there is no single cause of mass disease, that causation involves more than the agent directly giving rise to the process, that cause lies also in the characteristics of the population attacked and in the features of the environment in which both host population and agent find themselves. The result is the modern concept of epidemiology as medical ecology and of disease as an ecologic process.[24]

The studies of pellagra by Joseph Goldberger and his colleagues in the 1920s are a classic example of this ecological view.

Disease Specificity and General Susceptibility

In an important sense holism led in two different directions: toward disease specificity and toward general susceptibility. Constitutionalists tended to accept the notion of specificity, for they believed that people with different constitutions were susceptible to different clusters of diseases. For example, Franz

Alexander, the well- known psychoanalyst and psychosomaticist believed that certain diseases were influenced by the sympathetic nervous system and others by the parasympathetic system.[25]

On the other hand, the research of the endocrinologist Hans Selye from the 1930s to the 1970s has been an especially important source of ideas about general susceptibility. Like Alexander, he too acknowledged a major debt to Walter Cannon, dedicating an important publication "to the memory of that great Student of homeostasis, whose life and work have been the author's greatest inspiration,"[26] although he could never convince Cannon of the correctness of his theory.[27] Selye had coined the term *general adaptation syndrome* to describe the nonspecific response of the body to a wide variety of stressors. The response, mediated by the pituitary–adrenal axis, could include both inflammatory and antiinflammatory features. While specific stressors, for instance microorganisms or chemical toxins, can produce specific responses, there are general responses which, Selye argued, characterized all stressors. Moreover, there are diseases of adaptation; that is to say, diseases caused by "derangements of our adaptive mechanisms."[28]

He also argued that infectious organisms surround us and infest us all the time, but they do not always cause disease until we are stressed in some way.

> If a microbe is in or around us all the time and yet causes no disease until we are exposed to stress, what is the "cause" of our illness, the microbe or the stress? I think both are—and equally so. In most instances *disease is due neither to the germ as such, nor to our adaptive reactions as such, but to the inadequacy of our reactions against the germ.*[29]

A similar position was elaborated a decade later in a widely cited volume by Rene Dubos, who put the evolution of infectious diseases into the same historical context as had writers in the interwar years. He wrote:

> The sciences concerned with microbial diseases have developed almost exclusively from the study of acute or semi-acute infectious processes caused by virulent microorganisms acquired through exposure to an exogenous source of infection. In contrast, the microbial diseases most common in our communities today arise from the activities of microorganisms that are ubiquitous in the environment, persist in the body without causing any obvious harm under ordinary circumstances, and exert pathological effects only when the infected person is under conditions of physiological stress.[30]

This was not idle speculation, for by the 1950s research had shown that stressful life events in families were associated with an increased risk of streptococcal infections.[31]

The quotation from Dubos illustrates two related points. First, there had been a major transformation in the prevailing epidemiological regime. And second, the ever-changing epidemiological regime was best understood in evolutionary terms, and disease was best understood as a failure to adapt to evolutionary change. This was a widely shared view, particularly in psychosomatic medicine. For example, John Romano and George Engel defined health and disease, as "phases of life, dependent at any time on the balance maintained by devices, genically and experimentally determined, intent on fulfilling needs and on adapting to and mastering stresses as they may arise from within the organism or from without," where health represents a successful adjustment and disease a failure.[32] In an evolutionary context, this meant "that biological and psychological devices are to a considerable degree mutually interchangeable, a phenomenon which is phylogenetically and ontogenetically determined. The mental apparatus uses for expression and defences somatic systems which had been so used in the phylogenetic or ontogenetic past of the individual. The behavior of the organ or system so used is limited by its structure and function. Thus, the stomach may respond in the same way to a poison, foreign body or carcinoma as to a distasteful idea; it may manifest the same physiological response to a need for love as for a need for food. . . . It is probable that every system of the body participates in such reactions."[33] Like Selye's conception of the general adaptation syndrome, Engel's formulation was a way to describe general susceptibility to disease.[34] It is the opposite of disease specificity, for it means that many different causes may have the same effect. Moreover, this evolutionary understanding of human development and disease is implicitly holistic, for it is understood as the way to integrate the psychological and the biological, the mind and the body, and it resulted ultimately in what Engel and subsequently others called the biopsychosocial model.[35]

Romano was a psychiatrist and Engel was a specialist in internal medicine who also had had psychoanalytic training, thus exemplifying the importance of the relationship between clinical medicine and psychiatry in the endeavor to create a more holistic medicine. Indeed, the influence of psychiatry was profound. A number of elite physicians had studied psychiatry, for instance. Among the most influential was Harold Wolff, who had worked with Stanley Cobb at Harvard, Adolf Meyer at Johns Hopkins, Pavlov in Moscow, and Otto Leowi in Austria, before moving to Cornell in the 1930s, where he became chief of neurology and a well-known psychosomaticist.[36] Like his contemporaries, he too argued that disease was evidence of maladaptation to stress, but he also argued that not only could different stresses cause the same response, but the same stress could provoke different responses, even in the same individual under different circumstances.[37] For example, in population studies, he and his colleagues had observed that ill health was not spread evenly but that a relatively small proportion of the people accounted for most of the illness, and the illnesses were of various sorts. "Indeed, it was rare to find an individual with much illness who had disease confined to one category."[38]

Wolff was a remarkably productive investigator and prolific writer, and he led an extremely prolific group at Cornell. Not only did they publish original studies on gastric function and the response of the mucus membranes to various stimuli, and on hypertension and headache,[39] but they also developed a series of instruments for assessing physiological and emotional systems that ultimately resulted in the Cornell Medical Index (CMI),[40] as well as the Berle Index, a measure of psychosocial assets.[41] These and other instruments were used in a variety of important population-based and community studies as well.

In his book *Stress and Disease* Wolff wrote that:

> [T]he stress accruing from a situation is based on (*sic*) large part
> on the way the affected subject perceives it; perception depends
> upon a multiplicity of factors, including the genetic equipment, ba-
> sic individual needs and longings, earlier conditioning influences,
> and a host of life experiences and cultural pressures. . . .
>
> The characteristics of a situation acting as a stimulus may activate,
> but do not determine the nature of the response. The response will
> depend upon the state of the organism at the time of stimulation
> and on the organism's genetic equipment and other inherent charac-
> teristics. Thus, a precisely similar situation may have entirely different
> effects on two individuals or on the same individual at different
> times.[42]

This is a very different way of thinking about causality than that made possible by the germ theory of disease. For Wolff was saying that the same effect is not always preceded by the same cause, and that the same cause may have different effects, depending upon the condition of the individual affected. Indeed, toward the end of his book, Wolff addressed this issue directly. He commented that the idea of a single cause of a disease was misleading, for "newer concepts of disease hold that illness and incapacity arise from efforts on the part of the body to deal with adverse forces in the environment more frequently than they do from the direct effect or intrinsic nature of the adverse stimulus itself. In a sense, disease is a reaction to rather than an effect of noxious forces."[43]

According to Thomas Holmes, a trainee and colleague of Wolff's and one of the developers of the Schedule of Recent Events (SRE) and the Social Readjustment Rating Scale (SRRS), one of the important influences on Wolff, and through him on Holmes himself, was the *life chart* first developed by the psychiatrist Adolf Meyer.

> Information is provided by the patient and is arranged by year and
> the patient's corresponding age. The entries on the life chart describe
> life situations—experiences having to do with growth, development,
> maturation, and senescence—as well as the patient's emotional re-
> sponses to those situations. Certain life experiences that we arbitrar-
> ily call "disease" are listed in a separate column. In this approach to
> patients and their problems, the word "disease" applies to change in

health status and includes a broad spectrum of medical, surgical, and psychiatric disorders. The life chart thus allows us to take into account not only the occurrence of disease, but also the setting in which it occurs.[44]

Holmes wrote that the life chart "opened the way for all the studies of Wolff et al. because it gave us a way to document the relationship of life situations, emotions, and disease." While originally used with individuals to capture the uniqueness of the circumstances surrounding their illnesses, the life chart was adapted by Holmes and his colleagues for use with populations, first using the SRE in the mid-1950s and then the SRRS 8 years later.[45] Studies using these instruments generally found that the magnitude and frequency of life events were positively associated with the onset, severity, and duration of illnesses of a variety of sorts. However, Holmes observed, "Despite the fact that life change magnitude is related to seriousness of illness, and that *seriousness* of illness establishes a continuum along which individual diseases are distributed, the life change concept does not contribute much to an understanding of specificity of disease type."[46] That is, the diseases resulting from stressful life events could be of many different sorts.

But life events were not the same for everyone. The response depended largely upon how serious they were perceived to be by the affected individual. Other factors were also important, however. For example, in studies of patients with asthma and others with tuberculosis, it was observed that life events were associated with illness among people with few psychosocial assets, as measured by the Berle Index.[47] Psychosocial assets included "strong family ties, steady employment, adequate income and job satisfaction, regular recreation, frequent social participation, flexibility and reliability, realistic goals, and adequate or good [job] performance."[48] People with many psychosocial assets tended not to become sick in the face of major life changes.

Population-based studies by Lawrence E. Hinkle, another of Wolff's colleagues, supported the finding that illness was not randomly distributed in populations. Hinkle observed that 25% of the individuals studied in any of several settings accounted for about 50% of the illnesses, and the illnesses were of different types.[49] The inferences that Hinkle, Wolff, and their colleagues drew were: (1) diseases of different organ systems occurred in the same individual either consecutively or concurrently during times of stress, when the individual was attempting to adapt to what he/she perceived to be a threatening situation; (2) such episodes tended to occur in clusters lasting a year or more and often separated by several years; (3) not all individuals reacted similarly, some having many such episodes, others few; and (4) the differences between the people with many and few episodes were probably due to both constitutional and acquired differences in susceptibility.[50]

In a subsequent intensive study of Chinese immigrants to the United States, Hinkle, Wolff, and their colleagues observed that those who reported the most sickness of all sorts seemed to be people who held themselves to extremely high standards whereas those who reported less sickness were people who seemed to be more self-centered and less concerned about doing their duty and meeting high standards they had set for themselves.[51] Thus, psychological attributes of individuals seemed to be associated with general susceptibility to diseases of all sorts.

In a series of studies widely cited in the literature on psychosocial epidemiology, Stewart Wolf, another of Harold Wolff's trainees and junior colleagues, investigated the incidence of ischemic heart disease in a small community in Pennsylvania. The community, known as Roseto, was chosen because of the perception of one of the local physicians that people living there had much lower rates of heart disease than people in surrounding communities.[52] The argument made by Wolf and his colleagues was that (1) the unusually egalitarian nature of the community and the close bonds among family members were protective against the development of coronary heart disease, and (2) as the population became less traditionally Italian and less egalitarian, and as the social fabric was disrupted by modernization, coronary heart disease became more frequent. The Roseto study is considered further in Chapter 5. For the moment it suffices to say that it, like the pellagra studies, was an attempt to understand the changing incidence of disease in its ecological context, understanding ecology to include the social and cultural environment.

Susceptibility in Epidemiology

The body of work described above has been important in several ways. Arguably, Thomas McKeown's thesis that nutritional deprivation resulted in susceptibility to a variety of diseases derived from this tradition, perhaps through his early research experience with Hans Selye.[53] More directly, it has contributed significantly to the idea that (1) in economically advanced societies characterized by chronic noninfectious and mild rather than virulent infectious diseases, individual susceptibility (the *host* in the host–agent–environment equation) is more important than specific exposures as a cause of morbidity and mortality, and (2) the social environment could exert more or less protective effects on individuals experiencing stressful situations. It is in the writings of John Cassel that the clearest and most coherent applications of these ideas in epidemiology are to be found.

Cassel was a South African who had worked with Sidney Kark, a well-known social medicine physician, before emigrating to the United States in the 1950s.[54] He had done a number of important empirical studies, but his major contribution was to synthesize more explicitly than anyone else ideas about the social environment and general susceptibility and put them into an historical context.

In an early paper, he and his colleagues outlined a program of research that drew upon conceptions already common in the social sciences and psychiatry.[55] They were critical of epidemiology for being too descriptive and insufficiently analytical. "[T]oo many current epidemiological studies content themselves with describing incidence and prevalence data by selected demographic variables and drawing few if any inferences." This raised for them "a more fundamental issue. What is the nature of the inferences that can be derived through epidemiological investigation? Specifically, has epidemiological analysis a contribution to make in identifying etiological factors, or is this the prerogative of clinical and laboratory investigation?" "The answer to this question," they wrote, "is dependent upon the nature of the model of health subscribed to and the nature of the phenomena included in the concept of etiology. Dating from the discovery of bacteria, medical thinking has until recently favored a closed-system mechanistic model of illness and health. This model ascribes a single specific cause to each disease which, if present, would ideally always cause the disease. Conversely any disease would always be due to a specific cause." They went on to point out that even when ideas of multiple causation developed, the closed-system model of disease meant that multiple causes "are regarded as causes under all circumstances." This might have been appropriate for infectious disease, but it was not appropriate for "the diseases of contemporary industrialized society," for which "a more useful model would appear to be the open-system model . . . suggested by von Bertalanffy." "One of the cardinal features of such a model is that any specific stimulus may lead to a variety of reactions, depending upon the circumstances. Conversely any specific reaction may have as its antecedents a variety of stimuli," just as the work of Engel, Wolff, and others had suggested. They also drew on work by these same investigators to suggest that the "adaptive capacity of the individual to resist noxious stimuli" shaped the disease experience, and that "pathological end states, other than those included under specific categories . . . could be regarded as appropriate indices" of ill health in epidemiological studies.

In 1974 he wrote that, "In human populations the circumstances in which increased susceptibility to disease would occur would be those in which there is some evidence of social disorganization." However, "[N]ot all members of a population are equally susceptible to the effects of [social disorganization]. Dominant members are less susceptible than subordinate members. Both biological and social processes are protective. Chief among [the latter] are the nature and strength of the group supports provided to an individual." "[S]uch variations in group relations, rather than having a specific etiological role, would enhance susceptibility to disease in general."

The importance of these group factors would be diminished "in preindustrial societies, living in small, tightly organized communities, [where] the exposure to highly potent disease agents may account for the major part of disease causation. Under these circumstances variations in susceptibility due to social processes may be of relatively little importance. With increasing culture contact, populations become increasingly protected from such disease agents but simultaneously exposed to the social processes discussed above. Variations in susceptibility now assume greater importance in the etiological picture and the concomitant changes in such factors as diet, physical activity, and cigarette smoking will facilitate the emergence of new manifestations of such susceptibility."[56]

In the Wade Hampton Frost Lecture delivered in 1975, Cassel cited several studies, including some by Wolff, Hinkle, and Holmes, that together, he argued, supported the claim that general susceptibility to a wide variety of exposures (toxic, infectious, psychologically stressful) resulted when individuals (1) lacked appropriate feedback from others in their environment, and (2) received inadequate social support. Under such circumstances, individuals were likely to fall ill from any of a number of causes, depending upon what noxious agents happened to be present in the environment.

Cassel was clear that under the prevailing epidemiological regimes characteristic of rich countries, susceptibility mattered more than specific exposures. He was critical of the view that he said was held by many investigators, that "stressors are invariant, affecting all people in a similar manner,"[57] and he cited Hinkle[58] approvingly, who had taken a position similar to his. It was, Cassel believed, the way situations were perceived and the psychosocial environment that determined susceptibility. Causal necessity and disease specificity had no significant role.

General Susceptibility

The theory explicated by Cassel, and subsequently by others,[59] is compelling. The question is, how much does it explain and how useful is it? Broadly, there are two levels of response to this question, the clinical and the epidemiological. With respect to the former, it is significant that many of the original ideas emerged from the perceptions and values of clinicians and from the research of clinical investigators. Caring for patients in a "holistic" way has often been understood to be quite different from simply treating the disease.[60] The unique experience of each patient, for whom the existential questions "why me?" and "why now?"[61] are of major concern, is not adequately dealt with when the focus is on the disease as an entity with an existence separate from the patient's, what has been called the ontologic view of disease, and when the physician hasn't the skills to elicit the information required to render adequate care.[62]

It was concern with the patient rather than the disease that characterized the inter-war generation of psychosomatic physicians, and that has persisted under the rubric of the biopsychosocial approach to the patient. Recent evidence suggests that such a focus results in better care and better results for patients than simply treating the disease.[63] One reason for its effectiveness is that when physicians listen to and know their patients as unique human beings and understand their strengths, vulnerabilities and social circumstances, they are likely to be able to provide appropriate guidance and treatment, to intervene sensitively in stressful circumstances, and to cooperate with their patients effectively. Thus, the impulse that led physicians to advocate a holistic approach to patients has—to the extent it has had an impact on medical education, training, and care—very likely had beneficial consequences for individual patients.

Another more contentious possibility is that many presumptively stress-related diseases may be ameliorated by personal contact with a caring and compassionate physician. The magnitude and clinical significance of the impact of psychoneuroimmunological responses to stress is still far from clear.[64] Ideas regarding general susceptibility have undergone major challenges and changes in recent years,[65] numerous different pathways from stressful experiences to adaptive and maladaptive responses have been identified,[66] and current thinking suggests that the response to stressful experiences is not general, as Selye believed, but highly specific and highly variable, thus explaining "the low correlations obtained between stressful experience and disease."[67] Even if the psychoneuroimmunological and endocrine responses turn out to be of minimal clinical significance in some or all instances, however, the fact that clinical care and outcomes are improved is in itself a significant contribution of this approach to patients.

Similar uncertainties emerge when the focus is expanded from clinical encounters with individual patients to entire populations. Two questions arise. First, do psychosocial factors have an impact on all, some, or no causes of morbidity and mortality? That is, do stressful events and circumstances increase susceptibility generally or only to selected agents? Second, if there is an effect, how important is it?

Here are a few examples of studies that have made a definitive answer to the first question difficult: (1) Some cancers do not follow the socioeconomic gradient that would be expected if dominant members of a group invariably had lower levels of morbidity and mortality than subordinate members;[68] (2) Likewise, heart disease mortality is higher among high than low social strata in southern Europe, just the reverse of the northern European pattern and of what would be expected if superordinatation were universally protective;[69] (3) There is no difference in mortality from heart disease or all-cause mortality between white and blue collar workers in Honolulu, when the major risk factors for heart disease were controlled;[70] (4) On the other hand, numerous studies have shown that psychosocial variables such as depression, hostility, and lack of support are associated with increased risk of heart disease;[71] (5) The same or similar measures of social support that predicted reduced mortality in several studies failed to do so in a study of Japanese Americans in Hawaii,[72] among rural African Americans,[73] and among French women (but not men);[74] and (6) Psychoneuroimmunological research to date has produced inconsistent results regarding the impact of stress on the onset and progression of AIDS and cancer, although the association of stress with regard to minor infections is consistent and convincing.[75]

These results suggest that the argument for general susceptibility is not convincing, although psychosocial factors clearly have a role to play in certain conditions, perhaps most notably a variety of minor infections and coronary heart disease. The question is, how much of a role? The measure most commonly used to determine whether a cause, or risk factor, is significantly associated with a particular outcome is relative risk. That is, if a group characterized by a particular attribute, such as heavy tobacco use, has a higher rate of lung cancer than a group that doesn't use tobacco at all, or than a group that uses it moderately, then the relative risk is higher among heavy smokers than moderate smokers, and higher among moderate smokers than nonsmokers.

But this does not say how much of the lung cancer is actually caused by smoking. For this, another measure, population-attributable risk percent (PAR%), is used. This is a measure of how much of the lung cancer in the population can be attributed to tobacco use. It turns out to be extremely high: perhaps 95% of lung cancer is attributable to smoking.[76]

A risk factor may be very significant with respect to relative risk and not very important with respect to how much of the condition it causes in the population. For example, in a study of alcohol dependence among Navajo Indians, we found that conduct disorder in childhood was a significant risk factor for alcohol dependence in adulthood. People whose childhood behavior had been consistent with a diagnosis of conduct disorder were likely to have become alcohol dependent in adulthood. However, conduct disorder accounted for only about 5% of alcohol dependence.[77] A high proportion of people with conduct disorder became alcohol dependent, but a small proportion of people who were alcohol dependent had manifested conduct disorder as children.

This is the sort of measure that is required to determine the significance of a risk factor for any particular population, but for reasons about which one can only speculate, it is not often calculated. Perhaps finding a statistically significant relative risk is so exciting that investigators are reluctant to dilute the pleasure by reckoning how truly insignificant the risk factor they have discovered may be in reality. Whatever the reason, the population-attributable risk percent is an important and too infrequently calculated measure, but it has been calculated in a number of studies of coronary heart disease. A review by Magnus and Beaglehole[78] suggested that at least 75% of coronary disease could be accounted for by the so-called traditional modifiable risk factors: high serum cholesterol, high blood pressure, and cigarette smoking. Several more recent studies have come to similar conclusions.[79]

On the other hand, Emberson and his colleagues have calculated the population-attributable risk percent accounted for by social class in the United Kingdom.[80] After adjusting for a variety of traditional risk factors, the PAR% was between 10% and 22% of coronary disease accounted for by social class. This is not insignificant by any stretch of the imagination, but it does not match the contribution of the more traditional risk factors. Moreover, it is still not clear what the mechanism is by which social stratification is associated with increased risk of coronary heart disease when traditional risk factors are controlled, whether it is autonomy or some other characteristics associated with stratification. Whatever it is, some of the studies cited above suggest that it is not universal. For in Hawaii there is no association between occupational stratification and coronary heart disease, and in southern Europe it is the reverse of the pattern in northern Europe.

Conclusion

Virtually all who have written on and advocated the concept of holism have described themselves as responding to three interrelated transformations, one epistemological, another epidemiological, and the third sociological. The epistemological transformation was wrought by the germ theory of disease, which introduced for the first time the idea of causal necessity in medicine, as well as the idea of disease specificity.

The second great transformation was of the prevailing epidemiological regime: the decline of infectious and rise of chronic noninfectious diseases. Many observers have been impressed with the fact that the idea of causal necessity that had made possible specific preventive and therapeutic interventions in infectious diseases was less salient when it came to the newly important noninfectious diseases, for which multiple weakly sufficient causes appeared to provide more adequate explanations.[81] The recession of epidemic infectious diseases also meant that the newly important diseases were thought to be caused by factors of a psychosocial nature and were a manifestation of susceptibility and the breakdown of adaptive capacity.

The third transformation is the one described at the outset: the change from "traditional" communities to "modern" societies. It was the perception of that transformation that created the context in which the quest for wholeness occurred; for it was understood to mean that a sense of community had been lost and that isolated individuals were more likely to suffer psychological and physical distress.

These transformations both shaped the principles first clearly enunciated by Cassel and comprised a paradigm that has guided a considerable body of research during the past several decades. Its intellectual coherence; its integration of many widely shared assumptions about the nature of social organization and disorganization, the nature of community, and the consequences of social change; and the alternative it provides to reductionist modes of explanation, have made the paradigm attractive to people searching for a unifying explanation of seemingly diverse conditions. As such, it represents an important continuing epistemological tradition in medicine, one that stands in opposition to the dominant paradigm of the past 100 years.[82]

The two revolutions described in Chapter 1 and the counterrevolution described in this chapter are the sources of ideas about how social organization and the economy shape the health of populations. Inevitably, the reality to be explained is complex and the results of studies often ambiguous, as well as highly charged ideologically. Consequently, explanations of the relationship between socioeconomic measures and diseases often function as projective tests of the values and beliefs of investigators. The chapters in Part II describe the ways in which the ideas whose histories have been briefly traced in this and the previous chapter shape debates about some of the major social determinants of the health of populations.

The Social Determinants of
Mortality and Morbidity

3

The Standard of Living

I wander thro' each dirty street,
Near where the dirty Thames does flow,
And mark in every face I meet
Marks of weakness, marks of woe.

In every cry of every man,
In every infant's cry of fear,
In every voice, in every ban,
The mind forg'd manacles I hear.
—W. Blake, *London*[1]

This chapter addresses explanations that have been offered for the decline of mortality in both the nineteenth and twentieth centuries and makes the argument that while it would be foolish to reject the importance of a rising standard of living, too often the role of purposeful intervention has been denigrated. The two are not necessarily incompatible of course. The first attributes the improvement to a rising standard of living due to economic expansion, generally understood to mean industrial development and improved agricultural productivity. This translated into higher wages, improved nutrition, and better housing, and thus better health as measured by declining mortality. The second explains the decline as the result of purposeful human agency: the application of a variety of public health interventions to the problems of water, food, and airborne infectious diseases. A third less-common explanation invokes the biological selection and adaptation of human hosts and/or microorganisms. The first two explanations are manifestations of the optimistic and pessimistic sides of the standard-of-living debate.

The Standard of Living and the Decline of Mortality in England in the Eighteenth and Nineteenth Centuries

Thomas McKeown had argued that it was improved nutrition, the result of rising living standards, that primarily explained the decline of mortality in the late eighteenth and nineteenth centuries.[2] Economic and demographic historians found his work important because it addressed the standard-of-living

45

debate and gave support to the optimists.[3] McKeown argued that nutrition was the only possible explanation of most of the mortality decline after he had eliminated, to his satisfaction, other possibilities. This was in a sense a negative argument. Economic historians approached the problem more positively, by using adult height as a measure of nutritional status over the life course. Height was first used as a proxy for income, the usual measure of the standard of living, in populations such as slaves for whom there were no income data. Subsequently it has been used as a measure of the standard of living in populations for which estimates of real income were more or less uncertain.

Height has the advantage of being an output—a reflection of the standard of living—rather than simply an input as income is. This is indeed an advantage, but it is also a disadvantage. For height is responsive to both nutritional intake as well as to the so-called claims on nutrition. Thus, the growth of infants and children exposed to frequent bouts of gastroenteritis and respiratory diseases may falter and, depending upon subsequent nutrition and disease experience, the lost growth may or may not be made up subsequently. Height is therefore not simply a reflection of food availability but of the disease experience of infants and children and their ability to absorb nutrients, and this is often a reflection of the cleanliness and crowding of their environment.

Of course, the ability to withstand diarrhea and pneumonia in infancy and early childhood is also a result of, among other things, the child's nutritional status. Thus, as has often been observed, malnutrition and disease in infancy are synergistic and their association often hard to disentangle. For this reason, height does not allow one to distinguish as clearly as might be wished between nutritional status as a reflection of the standard of living and the sanitary environment of the population.

Even recognizing these problems, height and subsequently weight have proven to be interesting and useful complements to other measures of well-being.[4] Summarizing much of the research through the early 1990s, Robert Fogel wrote that:

> The available anthropometric data tend to confirm the basic results of the analysis based on energy cost accounting: chronic malnutrition was widespread in Europe during the eighteenth and nineteenth centuries. Furthermore, such malnutrition seems to have been responsible for much of the very high mortality rates during this period. Moreover, nearly all the decline in mortality rates in England and France between 1750 and 1875 appears to be explained by the marked improvement in anthropometric measures of malnutrition.[5]

He went on to say:

> [I]n the U.S. case reductions in exposure to disease were probably more important than improvements in the diet, accounting for perhaps half the nutritional effect on mortality. Applied to the European case, this proportion would imply that improvements in the diet

per se may have accounted for 35 to 45 percent of the mortality decline before 1875 but only for about 25 to 30 percent of the mortality decline after 1875.[6]

A large study of height and health in the United Kingdom by Roderick Floud, Kenneth Wachter, and Annabel Gregory[7] is particularly useful because

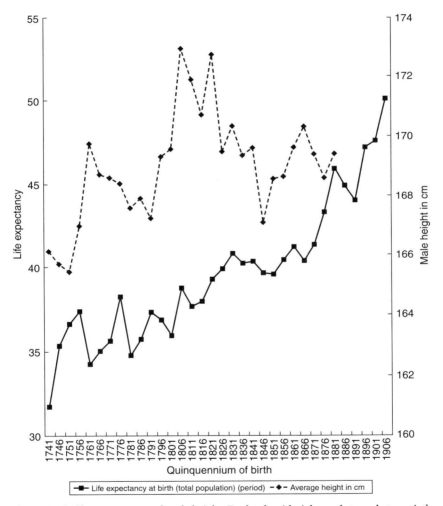

Figure 3-1. Life expectancy and male height, England, mid-eighteenth to early twentieth centuries. (Data from R. Floud, K. Wachter, and A. Gregory, *Height, Health and History: Nutritional Status in the United Kingdom, 1750–1980.* Cambridge: Cambridge University Press, 1990; E.A. Wrigley, R.S. Davies, J.E. Oeppen, and R.S. Schofield, *English Population from Family Reconstitution.* Cambridge: Cambridge University Press, 1997; and *Human Mortality Database.* University of California, Berkeley [USA], and Max Planck Institute for Demographic Research [Germany], available at www.mortality.org.)

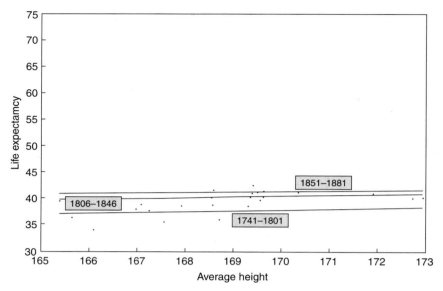

Figure 3-2. Life expectancy regressed on male height (in cm), England, 1741–1801, 1806–1846, 1851–1881.

it deals with the same place and most of the same period as McKeown did and clearly attempts to assess the impact of social change on nutrition. According to their data, which are displayed in Figure 3-1, the height of men fluctuated but generally increased from the 1740s to the 1760s; decreased from the 1760s to the 1790s; increased from the 1790s to the early 1800s; stagnated from 1806 to 1821; declined to the mid-1840s; and fluctuated but generally increased until the early 1880s, when the series ends. Other studies show a continuing increase from the late nineteenth century through the twentieth century.[8]

We may compare the height data with life expectancy at birth in the same years.[9] The results also appear in Figure 3-1. Life expectancy fluctuated but generally increased from the 1740s to the 1820s, although the amplitude of the fluctuations diminished. Thereafter, life expectancy declined from the 1830s through the 1850s and then began a rapid increase, with only a small reversal in the late 1870s and 1880s.[10] It is striking that there appears to be no consistent relationship between height and life expectancy over the 160 years.

Figure 3-2 displays the association between life expectancy and height for three periods: 1741–1801, 1806–1846, and 1851–1881. These periods were chosen to examine specifically the association between height and mortality during the early nineteenth century in the period of earliest industrialization and urbanization. None of the associations is significant, which is itself significant. For it suggests that if early childhood nutrition is truly reflected in adult stature, then there was no association between childhood nutrition and life expectancy. A potential complication of the analyses above is that the height data are for birth cohorts whereas the life expectancies are for periods. This is considered in Appendix 1: it appears that the use of period life expectancies is not a problem.

These findings do not eliminate the importance of short stature as a risk factor for premature death. The association has been demonstrated in the twentieth century both ecologically[11] and at the individual level in prospective cohort studies.[12] Not all causes of death are related to short stature, however. Respiratory and cardiovascular diseases are more common among short people, whereas a variety of cancers are more likely among tall people. George Davey Smith and colleagues have suggested that:

> Height in Britain has continued to increase through the second half of the 20th century. The causes of death that are inversely associated with height are those that tend to be decreasing, such as stroke, stomach cancer and respiratory disease mortality. The causes of death that show a positive association with height are those showing less favorable trends, such as prostate cancer, lymphoma, and colorectal cancer. The factors that underlie the secular trend of increasing height in the population may also be influencing the cause specific mortality rates.[13]

This is important because it means that some chronic diseases are positively, and other negatively, associated with height. Unfortunately, this and other cohort studies were all done when infectious diseases had waned in significance. It is therefore unclear whether there are associations between height and risk of death from infectious diseases, although tuberculosis is more common in tall than short people (see Appendix 2). This is a problem because historical anthropometric research assumes that what is true of the impact of height on life expectancy in the late twentieth century was also true of the impact of height on life expectancy under an entirely different epidemiological regime, that is, when the spectrum of prevalent diseases was different. Indeed, the same relative risks calculated for height as it affects mortality in Norwegians in the late twentieth century and among middle-aged American Civil War veterans in the early twentieth century have been applied to American and European data from a century or more earlier.[14]

It appears that in severely malnourished infants the immune response may be permanently compromised, and this may lead to increased susceptibility to infectious diseases in later life. The degree and type of early malnutrition necessary for this to occur, however, is unknown but is evidently severe.[15] Severe malnutrition in adulthood is also a risk factor for premature death, but again the malnutrition must be extreme. Furthermore, as already noted, short stature is not associated with general susceptibility to all chronic diseases. Hence, the relative risks will vary over time as certain diseases wane and others wax. For all these reasons, it is problematic to apply relative risk figures from one population to others that lived under an entirely different epidemiological regime.

This simply serves to emphasize the striking fact that the same height is associated with different life expectancies historically in the United Kingdom as well as cross nationally.[16] For example, as Figure 3-1 illustrates, men born in the 1780s and 1840s achieved the same average height, 167 cm, but life expectancy was 35 in the first period and 39 in the second. And this means both that context matters, especially the prevailing epidemiological regime,[17] and that attempts to investigate the importance of McKeown's nutrition hypothesis provide a spurious accuracy with respect to the proportion of the mortality decline attributable to improved nutrition. The same is true when body mass index (BMI) is considered rather than height (see Appendix 3).

The Public Health Contribution to Mortality Decline in England

There have been many critiques of McKeown's work and of the nutritional hypothesis more broadly.[18] Some are driven by a wish to recapture a central role for public health in particular and purposeful human and social intervention more generally in the decline of mortality in the United Kingdom and elsewhere. It is meant to reassert the importance of both national and local government: the visible hand of human agency as contrasted with the invisible hand of the market. Among the most polemical, most articulate, and most sustained of these is Simon Szreter's.[19]

McKeown had argued that respiratory diseases, including especially pulmonary tuberculosis, were particularly important in accounting for the mortality decline in England and Wales. And as respiratory diseases had begun to decline in the mid-nineteenth century, well before any preventive measures were available, only host resistance, not decreased exposure, could be given the credit. Szreter pointed out that only tuberculosis had declined, whereas other respiratory diseases had actually increased through the second half of the nineteenth century; tuberculosis had actually begun to decline later than McKeown had said; and it wasn't significant in the mortality decline anyway. He argued further that it was the gastroenteric diseases that had declined from 1870 on, as a result of public health measures brought about by national and especially local governments responding to an expansion of the electorate in the late 1860s to include a large number of working class men.[20] Tuberculosis then declined because its victims were less and less likely to be weakened by other diseases.

Szreter provides suggestive evidence[21] of the many ways in which government medical officers used growing epidemiological knowledge to improve the quality of water and the safety of sewers. In addition, as Anne Hardy has demonstrated, much public health was not focused on large construction projects but was instead devoted to health education, isolation of contagious cases, inspection of homes and work places, and lobbying for various pieces of public health legislation.[22] Thus, expenditures on public works are not a sufficient index of the importance of public health interventions.[23] Taken together, both make a compelling case for the substantial role that health officers played in improving especially urban health in the late nineteenth century.

Moreover, Robert Woods has shown that tuberculosis did not contribute as much to the decline of mortality between 1861–1870 and 1891–1900 as McKeown had suggested (35% instead of 44%). The largest share of the decline of mortality in that period, about 57%, was in the combined categories of typhus/diarrhea (typhus and typhoid not having been distinguished in the 1860s).[24] Thus, Woods accepts Szreter's and Hardy's general argument that public health interventions were far more important than McKeown had allowed. He has also shown, however, that tuberculosis was more significant than Szreter seemed to allow and that its decline was more or less the same across the country, in contrast to the gastroenteric diseases, which declined primarily in the large cities. (For a more extensive discussion of the decline of tuberculosis, see Appendix 2.)

George Davey Smith and John Lynch have argued that conditions for children improved after 1850 as fewer entered work at young ages, food consumption and housing conditions improved, and fertility declined.[25] They claim that these improvements occurred well before the public health movement was galvanized by previously disenfranchised working men who got the vote later in the century, as Szreter has shown. These claims have, of course, not gone uncontested.[26]

There is no doubt that successive cohorts of English men and women died at lower rates than those who preceded them, as Figure A-1 in Appendix 1 indicates. With the important exception of the period 1831 to 1851 and some earlier times when life expectancy declined transiently, there was a general improvement from the mid-eighteenth century right through the nineteenth century. Improvement accelerated in the second half of that century, but improvement had been going on for 100 years by that time. The deterioration that occurred in the 1830s and 1840s is important because it is a reflection at the national level of the severe living and working conditions to which the urban working class was exposed.

Szreter and Mooney have estimated life expectancy in large English cities and have shown that in the first half of the nineteenth century urban life expectancy was 6 to 7 years less than the national figure. They summarize the pattern of urban change as follows: "[A] sharp deterioration when the decade of the 1830s is compared with the 1820s and no significant recovery in the 1840s; a substantial recovery in the 1850s but not enough to make good the losses of the previous two decades; no further improvement in the 1860s; finally, a trajectory of sustained improvement from the 1870s through the 1890s (and beyond, of course)."[27]

Thus, while sustained improvement in life expectancy nationally seems to have begun in the late 1840s and 1850s, in large industrial cities, improvement began at about the same time but was less dramatic, proceeded in fits and starts, and did not become sustained until the 1870s. These data suggest that the early improvement in life expectancy may well have been the result of the changes suggested by Davey Smith and Lynch, whereas sustained improvement in large cities had to await the major public health improvements of the 1870s.

The evidence shows that life expectancy fluctuated but generally improved from the mid-eighteenth century; that there was a downward deflection in the 1830s and 1840s, corresponding with the worst excesses of industrialization and urbanization; that the early improvements do not seem to have been associated with increased height, used as a measure of the standard of living; and that the dramatic acceleration of life expectancy after 1870 is associated with improvements in public health. That height and life expectancy are not impressively correlated does not necessarily mean that the standard of living was unimportant but, rather, that height imperfectly reflects the standard of living.

These data are all from England and Wales, not simply because the best records are to be found there, but because the standard-of-living debate was originally about England's industrial revolution. Tracing England's population history has thus been central to any resolution. But economic expansion and improvements in life expectancy were not only an English phenomenon, and the debate looks different when placed in a broader perspective.

Mortality and the Standard of Living in Comparative Perspective

There are models of industrial and economic expansion and their impact on health other than England's. For example, Jorge Vogele has shown that in the period 1870 to 1913, mortality in the 10 largest cities in England and in Germany followed somewhat different paths. He writes:

> In Germany, the mortality rates of the 1870s were significantly higher than in England and Wales, with respect to both urban rates and nationwide, but due to the rapid decline in German urban mortality in the following decades the ten largest towns in both countries registered similar death rates after the turn of the century. By contrast, national figures still reveal better health conditions in England and Wales when compared with Prussia.[28]

There were several reasons for the more rapid decline of urban mortality in German than in English cities. One was political. England had been a leader in public health legislation and in sanitary engineering. German cities were able to rapidly adopt these innovations without the time, trouble, and expense they had cost the English. Cities had "strong financial powers, a corps of trained bureaucrats, and far-reaching police rights that enabled them to intervene in private property rights and to regulate municipal building policies."[29] Vogele goes on to suggest that municipal electoral power in Germany was in the hands of a small minority who "very probably gained the most substantial economic benefits" from sanitary improvements.[30] Improvements may have also been made for the same reasons Bismarck developed social insurance in the early 1880s: to pull the teeth of the Social Democrats.

In contrast, there was more resistance in England. In English cities, middle-class rate payers often blocked sanitary reform to keep their taxes low until the electoral reforms of the late 1860s that increased the number of working class men who could vote.[31] Moreover, as Anne Hardy has noted, the English idea that a man's home is his castle, dating at least from the sixteenth century, was reinforced by "the growth of a middle-class culture in the later eighteenth and early nineteenth centuries" when "the notions of liberty became involved with refinement of social distinctions and the search for privacy."[32] She suggests that these impediments to sanitary reform began to erode in the last decades of the nineteenth century.

In addition, gastroenteric diseases were more significant than respiratory diseases in German than in English cities. These were just the conditions that were responsive to improvements in the provision of pure water and the safe disposal of sewage. The result was that even with per capita incomes well below the English,[33] and with a narrower electoral base, German cities were able to reduce their mortality rates to the same level as those in English cities of comparable size.

There were, of course, differences among German cities and states, even after unification. Cities in the less-developed eastern part of the country had higher mortality than cities in the more developed West, for instance. And some states, especially in southern Germany, were active in improving water supplies in small towns and rural areas whereas Prussia was not. Thus, Prussia had not only higher death rates from gastroenteric disease than South German states, but the death rate was inversely correlated with community size in Prussia, unlike the pattern in the South. Similarly, some states were active in promoting smallpox vaccination whereas others were not. Differential mortality was the result.[34] And Hamburg's political and economic structure was in many ways unique, with profound consequences for its experience of the 1892 cholera epidemic.[35]

Regional differences in mortality were strikingly important up until 1890. In contrast, standard socioeconomic variables (e.g., income per capita) were not especially important. By 1910 to 1925, the pattern had reversed. Region was far less important and measures such as per capita income and urbanization had become far more important.[36] This suggests that regional differences in government policies, cultures, and breast-feeding practices had diminished in response to the growing integration of the German state.

A final example comes from a comparison of Swedish and English height and mortality data.[37] Figure 3-3 displays height and life expectancy at birth from 1820 to 1965 in Sweden. Sandberg and Steckel have described these data and their socioeconomic and political context in some detail. Here only a few observations are necessary.

First, Sweden's industrialization began about 1870, well after England's. Unlike England, however, there was no downturn in either height or life expectancy at that time. The earlier short and severe decline was due to an increase in child mortality resulting from a relatively brief period of serious malnutrition coupled with the spread of infectious diseases. The spread of infectious diseases followed upon (a) a large amount of internal migration, and (b) the passage and implementation of legislation requiring universal primary school attendance.

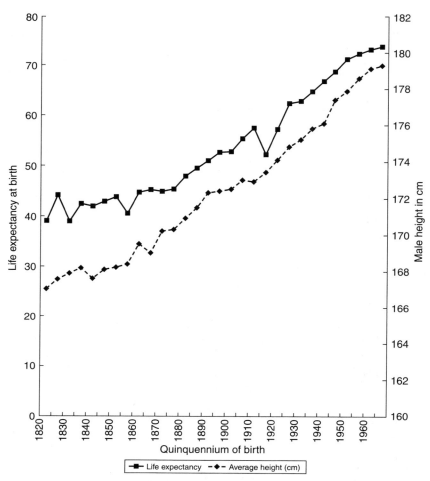

Figure 3-3. Life expectancy and height of men, Sweden, 1820–1965.

Sandberg and Steckel write that the usual explanation for the increase in life expectancy during the pre-1870 period is not an increase in income, which, in fact, had stagnated. It was due rather to the introduction of the potato, to peace, and to public health measures including, but going beyond, smallpox vaccination. Among the measures that were introduced "were marked improvements in sanitation, hygiene, and child care."

Much of this was accomplished through government propaganda in favor of breast-feeding and general improvements in sanitation. The church and, even more so, the system of compulsory schools were effectively used to spread official views on these subjects. The fact that Sweden was a highly literate country with a long tradition of bureaucratic and church control over the individual's private life meant that these campaigns were a good deal more successful than would have been the case in countries, such as England or the United States, where much more emphasis was put on individual freedom and autonomy.[38]

The period of rapid industrialization from 1870 was remarkable for the sustained increases in height and life expectancy that accompanied it. As already observed, this is all the more remarkable when compared to the experience of England during its period of industrial expansion. Part of the explanation has to do with factors already noted as important in the earlier period: improvements in public health measures, adequate nutrition, and peace. Another important factor has to do with the fact that Swedish industrial development was not accompanied by nearly the same degree of urbanization as had occurred in England. Much industrial growth took place in towns, some of them small, as well as rural areas. There was, moreover, large-scale emigration from Sweden to the United States in these years, which contributed to a reduction in poverty among those who remained.

The importance of the Swedish and German examples is that they demonstrate that England's experience of industrial growth and the responses to it was far from universal. First, countries that industrialized later benefited by being able to import English inventions and engineers to build their urban water supplies and sewer systems.[39] Second, political culture proved important as well. Local and/or national governments in Germany and Sweden had far more police power than national and local governments in England and were able to implement public health policies with less difficulty. Thus, they accomplished dramatic reductions in mortality at income levels that were less than half those of England (Table 3-1).[40]

The construction of protected water supplies and adequate sewage disposal systems clearly reduced exposure to enteric pathogens, but it may have had another beneficial effect as well by causing a diminution in the virulence of enteric pathogens. Paul Ewald has argued that the virulence of pathogens is shaped to a large degree by their mode of transmission.[41] A highly virulent microorganism that reduces the mobility of its host to such a degree that the host cannot transmit the pathogen to another host will soon reach a dead end.

Table 3-1
GNP per Capita (in 1985 U.S. $)

Year	United Kingdom	Germany	Sweden
1850	1943	835	871
1900	3792	1743	1895

Source: R.H. Steckel and R. Floud, eds., *Health and Welfare During Industrialization.* Chicago: University of Chicago Press, 1997, p. 424.

Vector-borne pathogens such as malaria and yellow fever do not become less virulent because, even though the host may be immobilized, mosquito vectors are still available to transmit the pathogens. Enteric pathogens that cause diarrheal diseases may not lose virulence as long as they can be efficiently transmitted by water, by flies, by human hands, and by other means. However, when water purification systems are developed, there is no selective advantage to virulence. Indeed, the selective advantage would be towards reduced virulence so that the sick host would be less immobile and would thus be a more efficient transmitter of the pathogenic organisms. And indeed, as Ewald points out, this is precisely what happened as water systems were purified in India in the 1950s. This may be part of the explanation of the reduction of mortality due to diarrheal diseases in the 1- to 4-years age group in the second half of the nineteenth century in England. Thus, human intervention may create selective pressures toward reduced virulence, just as it has produced selective pressures towards increased virulence of some microorganisms with the profligate use of antibiotics more recently.

The Personal Physician and the Decline of Mortality

McKeown's work attracted such interest among policy makers and analysts in the 1970s and subsequently, not because they were persuaded by the argument favoring nutrition and its acceptance by neoclassical economic historians. They were attracted because it discredited claims by the medical profession to have had a significant impact on health in the past and by implication in the present as well. And this in turn was understood to legitimate contemporary efforts at cost containment, as well as a more generalized attack on the welfare state,[42] at a time when costs were escalating at a high and increasing rate.

There is no doubt that many members of the medical profession had believed that declining mortality in the nineteenth and early twentieth centuries could be attributed in large measure to the care provided by personal physicians to their individual patients.[43] Before the 1880s, such a claim would have been dubious, except perhaps under special circumstances such as long sea voyages.[44] On the other hand, the passage of sickness insurance in various European countries, beginning with Germany in the early 1880s (Table 3-2), at the same time as the discovery of the infectious origins of many of the most important causes of mortality and morbidity, may well have had a beneficial effect. Sickness insurance broadened exposure of the working classes to physicians at a time when knowledge of the causes of infectious diseases was expanding rapidly.[45]

The political origins of state support for health care in the modern era are widely recognized. The first program of social insurance began in Germany in the 1880s and was understood by Bismarck to be a means of assuring the loyalty of the working class to the state.[46] Details of the organization, administration and financing of accident, sickness, and old age insurance programs in

Table 3-2
Dates of the Introduction of Compulsory Health Insurance in Europe

Year	Country
1883	Germany
1888	Austria & Hungary
1901	Luxemburg
1909	Norway
1910	Serbia
1911	Great Britain
	Russia
	Switzerland (several cantons)
	Irish Free State
	France (Alsace-Lorraine)
1912	Roumania
	Esthonia
1918	Bulgaria
1919	Czechoslovakia
	Portugal
1920	Poland
1921	Austria
1922	Kingdom of the Serbs, Croats, and Slovenes
	Greece
	Soviet Union
	Latvia
1925	Lithuania
	Italy (new provinces)

Source: International Labour Office, *Compulsory Sickness Insurance.* Studies and Reports, Series M (Social Insurance) No. 6. Geneva, 1927, p. 11.

Europe varied widely.[47] Some programs were compulsory, others voluntary. Financing was from the state, from workers, and/or from employers. The extent of coverage varied greatly although it increased over time, generally starting with adult male workers. Despite these differences, there is suggestive evidence that increased availability of health care from the late 1870s to 1913 was associated with an acceleration in the decline of mortality.[48] The greater the coverage in the five continental countries analyzed by C.R. Winegarden and John Murray, the more rapid the decline, even taking into account real per capita GDP and several other covariates.

Although surgical techniques and safety were improving in the late nineteenth and early twentieth centuries, there was not much that physicians had to offer individual patients in terms of curative interventions for most diseases that would have had a major impact on mortality rates. Nonetheless, in the context of increasing knowledge regarding the causes of infectious diseases, broadening health care coverage and sickness benefits may have (1) increased the likelihood that sufferers with tuberculosis would be able to rest in hospitals and sanatoria, (2) reduced the risk of pauperization of the family when the breadwinner was sick, and (3) made advice about appropriate child care increasingly accessible. All this may have been beneficial, especially for tuberculosis.[49] For example, in his 1912 study of social insurance in Germany, Lord Dawson, a leading English expert on Germany at the time,[50] described the changes in tuberculosis death rates that he thought were attributable to social insurance.

> It is not without significance that from 1876 to 1885, prior to the insurance era, the rate of mortality . . . for German towns, stood still; from 1885 forward from that time there was a steady fall from 3.1 to 2.2 per 1,000 in 1897; from that time the normal influence of the three Insurance Laws [Sickness, Invalidity and Old Age, and Accident], all now in full operation, was reinforced by the anticonsumption crusade of the Pension Boards, and there was simultaneously a further fall in the mortality rate to a figure which in 1908 was little less than that of the United Kingdom.[51]

More generally, he thought that the work of the insurance system in Germany was unique in its preventive activities, including inspection of dwellings and lectures and literature on questions of personal health and sanitation. In fact, he continued, programs "do their utmost to discourage amongst the working classes personal habits prejudicial to health."[52] Quoting a German physician, he wrote:

> "As is the case with insurance in general," writes Dr. Zahn, "the German social insurance legislation educates the working classes in providence, self-control, and prudence, and it is well known that the social causes of poverty are specially operative where these qualities are lacking, for wholesale poverty is due not merely to faulty organisation of production, but to the absence of education and foresight on the part of the workman. . . . The moral influence of industrial insurance must not be overlooked. To a large extent the self-help of the workers is promoted by the insurance institutions; the sense of frugality, prudence, and self-control is extended, and voluntary benevolence is vitalised and stimulated to a degree which would have been inconceivable without the Insurance Laws."[53]

As another contemporary German medical professor had written:

> It must be regarded as a happy dispensation for the crusade against tuberculosis that at the very time Koch pointed the way to the prevention of this disease the German Insurance Legislation came into

operation, giving to the less favoured sections of the population, which are the special victims of this disease, a legal claim to treatment in the event of sickness.[54]

Thus, while the personal physician system cannot explain most of the decline in European mortality in the late nineteenth and early twentieth centuries, the evidence suggests that its contribution was more significant than McKeown had claimed,[55] and that it varied depending upon the extent to which populations were protected by social insurance. More generally, the European pattern of mortality decline indicates that the causes were not everywhere the same and that the mix of government intervention and economic expansion varied from place to place.

The discussion of mortality and life expectancy in the nineteenth century should have made clear that (1) historically, measurement of the standard of living is no mean feat; and (2) when countries are compared, mortality rates and life expectancy vary in ways that cannot readily be explained by differences in the standard of living, even when reasonably adequate comparative income estimates have been constructed by economic historians. In the second part of this chapter, the same case is pursued using comparative data from the late twentieth century. The argument is that mortality patterns reflect many more variables than can be captured in a single measure such as income per capita.

The Discovery of Income in Public Health

As observed previously, economic position had been used in the nineteenth century to account for differences in the health of populations. In the United States, however, the use of this measure occurred later. In 1920 Edgar Sydenstricker described the method used in the pellagra studies for classifying families according to income. He wrote:

> In studies of disease prevalence and incidence, emphasis is being laid nowadays upon the possible influence of environmental conditions that formerly were given no more than cursory consideration. This tendency undoubtedly is in line with the realization that the occurrence of most diseases, especially those which are of the non-infectious type, is more or less intimately dependent, not upon a single condition or set of conditions, but upon the mass of interrelated conditions under which a population lives.[56]

The problem, he continued, was that so many conditions were implicated in the cause of disease that it was impossible to deal with all of them effectively. Therefore a general expression—"an index of living conditions"—was required, and "for purposes of accuracy and convenience [it] should be expressed in *numerical* form."

The desired index must then be both specific and commensurable, and the only single index yet discovered which meets these requirements and which also conveniently and accurately approximates the whole complex of conditions under which a family lives is family income. The reason for this is obvious. Whether or not nutritious diet, sanitary housing, adequate clothing, proper facilities for the care of children, opportunity for wholesome recreation, and sanitary neighborhood conditions can be enjoyed is determined mainly by the family's financial status.[57]

Thirteen years later he wrote, "Environment is not merely the physical world upon which we live. . . . Nor does it include also only the physical changes that man has accomplished in adapting his physical habitat to himself. . . . Our 'social heritage,' as Graham Wallas put it, is also a very important part of human environment." The environment was to a large degree the *social* environment: occupations, social class, economic status, "tradition, superstition, and mores; modes of living, fads, and fashions; standardization of ideas and attitudes by the press, movies, radio, and schools; cultural factors, such as the esthetic idea of posture or a religious regimen of diet or of personal cleanliness."[58]

Income was meant to capture the whole range of conditions that affected the health of individuals. Increasingly in the 1920s and 1930s it was used to powerful effect to explain regional mortality differences,[59] to chart the impact of the Depression on the health of the population,[60] and to discredit climatologic explanations of the distribution of disease.[61] It is not too much to say that the use of income in these ways represents the domestication of nature and a repudiation, perhaps premature, of the importance in western epidemiology of the Hippocratic concern with Airs, Waters, and Places. Indeed, its use has become second nature. In England, the use of occupation as a measure of social class occurred slightly earlier than income was used in the United States, but for much the same reason. In each case, these measures of stratification had become the most salient as well as the most convenient for measuring social distinctions. But to expect one numerical measure to adequately represent all the elements of the social environment that are relevant to health is unrealistic, for many of the relevant dimensions may on occasion act independently of income.

Mortality Decline in the Twentieth Century

The nineteenth-century European evidence suggests that reductions in mortality were achieved by populations at very different economic levels. Something similar happened in the twentieth century when many poor countries began to achieve life expectancies equal to those of countries with much higher incomes. For example, Samuel Preston[62] compared the association

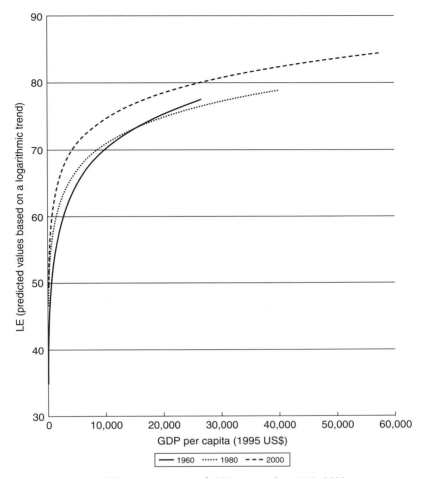

Figure 3-4. National life expectancies and GDP per capita, 1960–2000.

between life expectancy and per capita income using data from a large number of countries over a period of several decades and demonstrated that at the same income per capita, life expectancy was higher in more recent than in more distant years. He interpreted this to mean that something other than GNP per capita explained the increase in life expectancy, and he argued that this factor was imported public health technologies in developing countries.

Figure 3-4 displays data comparable to those Preston analyzed, but for the years between 1960 and 2000. They demonstrate, first, that life expectancy and per capita income are positively associated, thus supporting the strong relationship between the two. Second, however, the data indicate that at the highest income levels the association weakens, though it does not entirely disappear. And third, though the patterns were essentially the same in 1960 and 1980, by

2000 the same per capita income (in 1995 U.S. $) was associated with higher life expectancy than in the more distant periods of observation.

The problem is that the explanation offered by Preston of the importance of imported public health interventions suffers from the same deficiency as Mc-Keown's: it is not based upon the observation of a positive association between public and personal health care interventions on the one hand and reduced mortality on the other. A cause is inferred in the absence of more persuasive explanations. Thus, while suggestive, to deal with that problem a more refined analysis of the impact of different health care systems on mortality is required.

Causes of Death Amenable to Health Care Interventions. There are several types of evidence pointing to an important role for health services in the reduction of mortality in the contemporary era. None by itself is definitive, but taken together they support the proposition that there has been a discernible and important effect. In the 1970s, perhaps responding to the same influences that had made Thomas McKeown's work so influential at the same time, a Working Group on Preventable and Manageable Diseases first proposed a way of measuring the quality of medical care available to populations. "*Medical care*," the Working Party wrote,

> [I]s used in its broadest sense. Included are the application of all relevant medical knowledge, the basic and applied research to increase that knowledge and make it more precise, the services of all medical and allied health personnel, institutions and laboratories, the resources of governmental, voluntary, and social agencies, and the co-operative responsibilities of the individual himself. *Quality* is the effect of care on the health of the individual and of the population. Improvement in the quality of care should be reflected in better health. But quality must be differentiated from the *efficiency* of medical care. Both are important, but they must not be confused. Whereas quality is the output of the medical-care machine in the form of better health, efficiency has to do with how well the parts of the machine work, how well they work together, and at what cost. In a word, quality is concerned with outcome, and efficiency is related to the process of care.[63]

The Working Party proposed a method for "establishing quantitative negative indexes of health. Cases of unnecessary disease, and unnecessary disability, and unnecessary untimely deaths can be counted. Their occurrence is a warning signal, a sentinel health event, that the quality of care may need to be improved."[64] Sentinel events, they continued, are like airline crashes: they need to be investigated to determine where the health care system failed in its ability to prevent and manage the occurrence.

The lists of events classified by the Working Party need not detain us here (see, however, Table 3-3 for a more recent example that is the basis for subsequent analyses). Inclusion was based upon consensus. Their occurrence was to be used to determine whether any particular health care system was dealing appropriately

Table 3-3
Selected Avoidable Causes of Mortality

Cause	ICDA 9th Revision Code	Age Group	Responsible Health Care Sector	Other Potential Factors Contributing to Excess Mortality
Maternal mortality	630–676	All ages	Primary care **Hospital**	
Perinatal	All causes	<1 wk and stillbirths, >28 wks gestation	Primary care **Hospital**	Prevalence of premature births
Chronic rheumatic heart disease	393–398	5–44 yr	**Primary care** Hospital	
All respiratory diseases	460–519	1–14 yr	**Primary care** Hospital	
Hodgkin's disease	201	15–64 yr	Primary care **Hospital**	
Cervical cancer	180	15–64 yr	Public health **Primary care** Hospital	Sexual habits, coding error
Breast cancer	174	25–64 yr	**Screening programs** Public health Primary care Hospital	Risk factors affecting incidence: obesity, family history
Tuberculosis	010–018, 137	5–64 yr	**Public health** Primary care Hospital	Ethnic group (immigration) Noncompliance with treatment
Asthma	493	5–44 yr	**Primary care**	Prevalence of disease
Appendicitis, cholelithiasis, cholecystitis, abdominal hernia	540–543 574–575.1 576.1, 550–553	5–64 yr	Primary care **Hospital**	Coding error
Ischemic heart disease	410–414, 429.2	35–64 yr	**Public health** **Primary care** Hospital	Coding error Health behavior affecting incidence: smoking, weight, nutrition
Hypertension and cerebrovascular disease	401–405, 430–438	35–64 yr	Public health **Primary care** Hospital	Coding error Health behavior affecting incidence: smoking, weight, nutrition

(continued)

Table 3-3
Continued

Cause	ICDA 9th Revision Code	Age Group	Responsible Health Care Sector	Other Potential Factors Contributing to Excess Mortality
Peptic ulcers	531–534	25–64 yr	Primary care **Hospital**	Drug use, alcohol, smoking
Diabetes	250	All ages	Public health Primary care Hospital	Diet, obesity
HIV/AIDS	042–044	All ages	Public health Primary care Hospital	Drug use, sexual behavior

Boldface emphasizes the most important sector.
Sources: Adapted from D.G. Manuel and Y. Mao, "Avoidable mortality in the United States and Canada, 1980–1996." *American Journal of Public Health* 92: 1481–1484, 2002 and from EC Working Group on Health Services and "Avoidable Deaths," *European Community Atlas of "Avoidable Death"* 1985–89. Oxford: Oxford University Press, 1997. HIV/AIDs and diabetes do not appear in either publication.

with the problems confronting it, including primary, secondary, and tertiary prevention. Primary prevention refers to prevention of the condition entirely. Secondary refers to early detection and treatment. Tertiary refers to treatment of the full-blown condition and prevention of disability and/or death. Hence the occurrence of vaccine-preventable diseases such as polio and measles represents a failure of primary prevention. Death from cervical cancer represents a failure of adequate screening (secondary prevention). Deaths from myocardial infarction represent a failure of tertiary prevention. The method is particularly valuable for comparative purposes. For if the beneficiaries of one health care system have higher death rates from a condition than the beneficiaries of another system, that should be cause for investigation of possible deficiencies in the former system.[65]

The lists of avoidable events have been modified and expanded over time, and they have been used not simply for comparative purposes but to chart the decline of mortality. In general, such studies show that causes of death defined as amenable to interventions by health care systems have declined more rapidly than causes of death not considered amenable to such intervention.[66] The inference has been that health care has been the ingredient most responsible for the difference. However, rarely have studies shown a significant correlation between indicators of health care availability, such as physicians per 1000 population or percent of GDP spent on health services, with differences in rates of occurrence or decline of these different categories of causes.[67] On the other hand, studies that include temporal trends before and after the introduction of specific types of interventions have often shown a downward deflection in mortality, as when the rapidity of the rate of decline of tuberculosis accelerated after the introduction of antibiotic treatment.

The study of avoidable deaths has been expanded to include the study of avoidable hospitalizations, that is, hospitalizations that could be avoided were adequate primary care available.[68] The results indicate that poor people have higher rates of preventable hospitalizations than those who are more affluent, and again the inference is that inadequate access to primary services is the major cause. And although not generally treated as part of the same literature on avoidable deaths, a substantial number of publications in the 1980s showed that increased mortality from a variety of causes was associated with the loss of health care benefits.[69]

On the other hand, there have been a number of studies showing little or no effect of health services on mortality. For example, although the rate of hospitalization of Medicare beneficiaries was much higher in Boston than New Haven, mortality rates were virtually identical in the two cities.[70] And the RAND Health Insurance study found inconsequential differences in the health of people randomly assigned to fee-for-service and prepaid health care, though the latter had much lower rates of hospitalization than the former.[71]

The discrepant findings may result from the fact that poor people are especially vulnerable to the loss of health care benefits, and they tend to be swamped in studies that are concerned with total populations. For example, the RAND Health Insurance Experiment found that the poor benefited more than the nonpoor from the availability of free care with respect to the treatment of hypertension.[72] Thus it is ironic that investigators on the political left[73] who have taken up McKeown's work with enthusiasm as a way of debunking the claims of the medical profession may have contributed in some small way in the 1980s to loss by the poor of what benefits they had.

There have been studies of a variety of specific conditions that have attempted to determine the share of the decline in mortality that may be accounted for by specific interventions.[74] To take but one example, in a study of the decline of stroke mortality in a defined population over approximately 20 years,[75] it was observed that the incidence of stroke remained the same over the period but the severity declined significantly and, as a result, case-fatality rates and overall stroke mortality also declined. It is possible that more effective treatment of hypertension may have reduced the severity of strokes even though the incidence had remained unchanged.[76]

All of these various studies point to the utility of considering the impact of health services on mortality, primarily for purposes of comparing health care systems, but also to consider how health services may have influenced changes in mortality over recent decades. The United States and Canada are an apt pair for comparison because they are neighbors with access to the same health care technologies. Both are English-speaking, liberal democracies, although there are important political and cultural differences. Most significant for present purposes, until the early 1970s, Canada had a health care system similar to the one in the United States. Since then, all Canadians have been covered by national health insurance, whereas a substantial proportion of the United States population has not had health insurance. In addition, over the

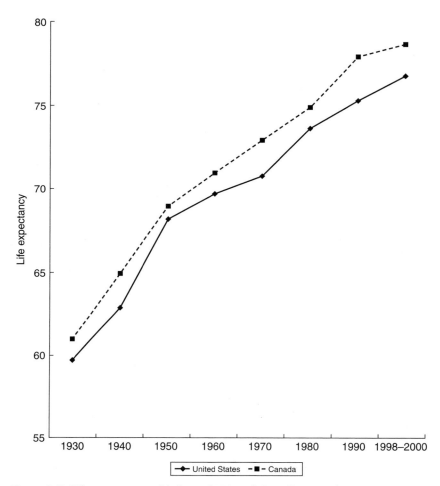

Figure 3-5. Life expectancy at birth, total U.S. and Canadian populations, 1930–2000. (*Source*: M.R. Haines and R.H. Steckel, Eds. *A Population History of North America.* Cambridge: Cambridge University Press, 2000, pp. 697–698.)

same period, Canadian per capita income has been 70% to 73% of per capita income in the United States.[77]

Comparisons Among and Within Two National Populations. It has been widely recognized that white and African American citizens have long had very different mortality experiences.[78] Perhaps somewhat less well-known is the fact that the populations of the United States and Canada have also had different rates of mortality. Figure 3-5 indicates that for most of the twentieth century Canada has had a small but significant advantage with regard to life expectancy.

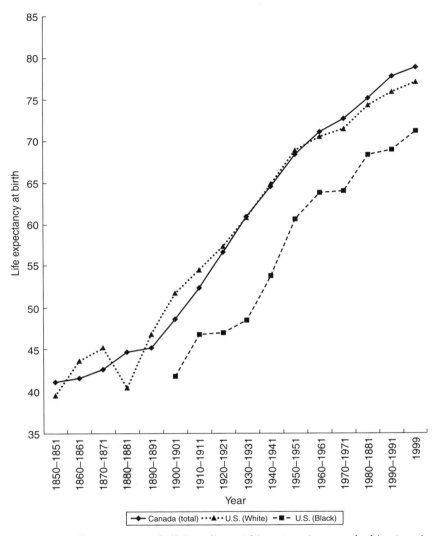

Figure 3-6. Life expectancy of all Canadians, African Americans, and white Americans, 1850–2000. (*Source*: M.R. Haines and R.H. Steckel, Eds. *A Population History of North America*. Cambridge: Cambridge University Press, 2000, pp. 697–698.)

Figure 3-6 provides more detail and shows that white American life expectancy was the same as, or better than, that of all Canadians for most of the period from 1850 to 1950.[79] Only in the 1970s did the Canadian figures rise above those of white Americans. Life expectancy of African Americans was substantially below that of white Americans and of Canadians for the entire twentieth century. That is primarily what accounts for the Canadian advantage until 1970. After that date, both whites and African Americans have had lower life expectancy than Canadians.

Disparities Due to Avoidable Conditions. Amenable causes of death among whites and African Americans have been examined in several studies to consider the differential effects of access to health services.[80] The EC consensus conference observed that "An excessive number of such unnecessary events serves as a *warning signal* of possible shortcomings in the health care system, and should be investigated further."[81] "Warning signal" is emphasized because it is not claimed that all the disparities are attributable only to unequal access to, and utilization of, health services even broadly understood. But disparities in causes of death widely regarded as amenable to intervention by the health care system should not simply be dismissed. At the very least, differences in rates of death from avoidable causes between populations should be cause for concern that a health care system is not functioning adequately.

Conditions considered amenable to intervention by the health care system are listed in Table 3-3. Among them are several that account for much of the difference between white and African American life expectancy, most notably cardiovascular diseases and hypertension.[82] Figure 3-7 displays curves of the rates of death due to several of these causes from 1980 to 1984 through 1995 to 1998 in the broad age groups displayed in Table 3-3, and then age adjusted within each age group to the 2000 standard U.S. population.[83] Among the causes accounting for the greatest disparity in life expectancy of African Americans and whites are ischemic heart disease, and hypertension and cerebrovascular disease. Although there has been a decline in both causes of death among African Americans, a decline that began as early as the 1950s but was generally more rapid for whites,[84] there is still a substantial difference in the rates in the two populations. Some of the difference is due to lower rates of vascular surgery among African Americans than among whites.[85]

One sees similar substantial differences between the two populations in the other causes of death amenable to interventions by the health care system. In a few, there have been dramatic declines (Hodgkin's disease, cervical cancer, peptic ulcer, and tuberculosis). Indeed, the decline of tuberculosis began for each group early in the century, before effective therapy was available.[86] In a few there has been little or no change (breast cancer, appendectomy, cholecystectomy and hernia, and maternal mortality). Of these, breast cancer has been of particular concern. There is reasonably persuasive evidence that mammography has had a beneficial impact upon death rates due to this condition.[87] However, African American women have benefited less than white women because they tend to be screened less frequently, to have lower rates of repeat mammography, and to have lower rates of follow-up of abnormal examinations. Factors such as breast density and obesity, which are more common among African American than white women, may also reduce the efficacy of mammography when it is used. Thus, the story is complicated, but the evidence

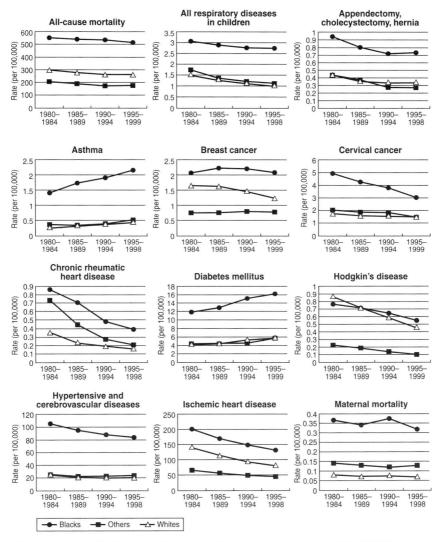

Figure 3-7. Avoidable mortality in the United States by race, 1980–1998/9. (Age-adjusted mortality rates using U.S. 2000 standard population.) *Continued on p. 70.*

suggests that programs specially targeted to African American women do increase the use of mammography and may well be beneficial.[88]

Unlike the preceding conditions, there has been a substantial increase in asthma among both African Americans and whites, although greater in the former than the latter. Hospital admissions for acute asthmatic attacks are much more common among African American than white youngsters and are much more common from inner city than other urban or suburban neighborhoods.

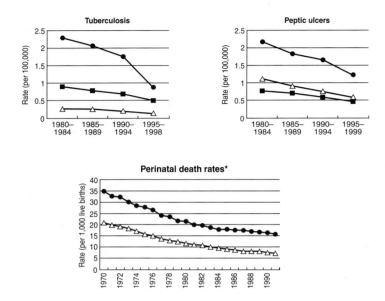

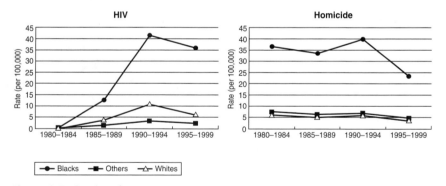

*Includes fetal deaths (stillbirths of 28 or more weeks' gestation and infant deaths under 1 week [7 days] of age).

Figure 3-7. *Continued.*

It has been suggested that both adverse environmental conditions and lower quality primary care are responsible for the differences.[89]

Two of the causes of death that account for much of the difference between white and African American life expectancy are not mentioned by the European Community consensus conference: HIV/AIDS and diabetes.[90] Nonetheless, there is reason to believe that the health care system has a great deal to offer in each case, both with regard to advice about prevention and with regard to treatment. In both cases, there has been an increase since 1980, more dramatic for African Americans than whites. In the case of HIV/AIDS, however, there has been a sharp decline since the 1990s, the result of both preventive and therapeutic interventions.[91] This sharp decline parallels the dramatic acceleration in the decline of the death rate from tuberculosis in the same period, suggesting that the two are associated. In the case of diabetes, there has been no such decline. Indeed, there has been a much greater increase of the diabetes death rate among African Americans than whites, and the evidence suggests that the former are admitted to hospital with advanced disease requiring amputation more frequently than the latter.[92]

It is difficult to say with certainty how much of the disparity in death rates from conditions amenable to health care interventions is the result of unequal access to, and use of, the full range of public and personal preventive, therapeutic, and rehabilitation services, and how much is due to circumstances beyond the reasonable reach of health care systems. Nonetheless, such consistent differences lead to the conclusion that a great deal is indeed due to unequal access.

In addition, there is evidence that (1) the quality of primary care physicians who treat African Americans may not be as good as the quality of other primary care physicians,[93] and (2) even when whites and African Americans have similar types of health care coverage (for example, Medicare) and are admitted to hospital, the care they receive differs. Notwithstanding the importance of Medicare as an integrative force in health care,[94] the fact remains that studies of Medicare fee-for-service and managed care programs reveal "differences in care patterns . . . for cancer treatment, treatment after acute myocardial infarction, use of surgical procedures, hospice use, and preventive care."[95]

As David Barton Smith[96] has shown, this is largely the result of lax enforcement of requirements for equal treatment in facilities receiving federal monies, though differences in Medigap coverage may also play a role. After a brief burst of enthusiasm for civil rights following the passage of Medicare, the federal enforcement of equal treatment in hospitals declined. There are a number of reasons why this occurred, according to Smith. Among them were a diminished commitment to civil rights enforcement in the Executive Branch, growing preoccupation with cost containment and shrinking the federal bureaucracy, and organizational changes within DHHS. The result has been continuing disparities in the treatment of African Americans and whites.

Mortality of Canadians and White Americans. Figure 3-6 shows that the differences between the life expectancy of Canadians and white Americans emerged in the 1970s and have widened since then. Significantly, the differences between social insurance coverage in the two countries emerged in the 1950s, when Canada developed broader protection than the United States. Both countries by then had industrial accident, pension, and unemployment insurance, but, in addition, in 1944 Canada had developed a system of family allowances. The gap in social insurance opened much wider after Canada implemented a universal health insurance program in 1972,[97] in contrast to the far from universal programs, Medicare and Medicaid, created in the United States in 1965.

Additionally, Canada's social insurance programs are more redistributive than America's, and the result has been much greater income equality in the former than the latter country. Although between 1974 and 1985 income inequality widened in both Canada and the United States, the trend in Canada reversed in the following decade while it persisted in the United States. In the period 1985 to 1997, Canadian patterns of income taxation and transfer payments were far more redistributive than those in the United States.[98]

After the implementation of universal health insurance in Canada, a number of studies were done of the consequences regarding health care utilization. The results were mixed. Some studies showed inequalities in utilization and health status to have persisted,[99] but for the most part utilization has increased, especially among the poor.[100] Although waiting times for elective and semiurgent procedures have lengthened since the 1970s, the degree to which the increase has reduced life expectancy, as contrasted with quality of life, is not significant.[101] Moreover, the differences among socioeconomic groups with respect to avoidable hospitalizations are far greater in American than Canadian cities;[102] the risk of inadequate prenatal care is greater for poor American women than for poor Canadian women;[103] survival from some heavily technology-dependent conditions, e.g., end-stage renal disease, is better in Canada than in the United States;[104] and among hospitalized victims of myocardial infarction, Americans have more technologically intense interventions than Canadians, but the same 1-year survival.[105] On the other hand, survival from hip fractures is worse in Manitoba than in New England,[106] though comparisons with adjacent U.S. states may have been more appropriate. In general, however, most causes of death as well as mortality differences among income groups have declined since the 1970s.[107] Furthermore, the use of U.S. services by Canadians is too miniscule to have a measurable impact on cause-specific mortality or life expectancy.[108]

Several comparative studies[109] of the association between income and survival rates from various cancers in American and Canadian cities reveal that:

1. There were few if any differences in survival of different income groups in Canada but substantial differences in the United States.
2. People with cancer who came from poor populations in the United States had worse survival than equally poor people in Canada. This was as true for poor whites as it was for poor African Americans.
3. Survival among the wealthiest groups in Honolulu was better than for the wealthy in Toronto, but, for the most part, differences between upper income groups in the two countries are neither statistically nor substantively significantly different.
4. Cancer survival patterns in Honolulu were more nearly like survival in Toronto than was any other American city. Because Hawaii is the one

American state that has attempted, though with only partial success, to implement universal medical insurance, the evidence suggests that the differences in cancer survival documented in these studies are primarily the result of differences in access to health services.

Similarly suggestive evidence of the importance of universal coverage comes from a comparison of changing Canadian and American mortality rates from 1980 to 1984 to 1995 to 1996, from causes of death amenable to intervention by the health care system. Douglas Manuel and Yang Mao[110] have shown the following:

1. Breast cancer, Hodgkin's disease, and peptic ulcer declined equally and were essentially indistinguishable in each country.
2. Asthma deaths increased in the United States and declined in Canada.
3. Death rates from cervical cancer, hypertension/cerebrovascular disease, ischemic heart disease, tuberculosis, and appendectomy, cholecystectomy and hernia declined in each country, but more rapidly and to lower levels in Canada than the United States.

These observations, too, suggest that the Canadian system of comprehensive care, free of charge at the point of service, and with a greater emphasis than in the United States on primary care, may be generally more effective than the American system for the total population. In light of the great inequalities between whites and African Americans, however, the question is whether the differences between the two countries are accounted for by the high rates of death among African Americans, or whether these differences affect white Americans as well? The lower life expectancy of white Americans than Canadians since the 1970s and the results of the analyses of cancer survival both suggest that there should be differences in most of the causes of death amenable to intervention by the health care system.

The data displayed in Figure 3-8 are comparisons of age-adjusted death rates of Canadians[111] and white Americans from the same causes as those described previously when African American and white rates were compared. In virtually every case, Canadians have lower rates than white Americans. The exceptions are breast cancer, all respiratory diseases in children, and peptic ulcer, where the rates are very similar or the same. Moreover, among conditions in which the rates are declining, they tend to be declining more rapidly among Canadians. These are hypertension and cerebrovascular disease, Hodgkin's disease, appendectomy, cholecystectomy and hernia, cervical cancer, and chronic rheumatic heart disease. Ischemic heart disease has declined at about the same rate in each population. HIV/AIDS increased more rapidly and to higher levels among white Americans than Canadians, and in the 1990s fell more rapidly. Nonetheless, the rates are still higher in the United States. Diabetes is increasing in both populations as well, but far more rapidly among white Americans than among Canadians.

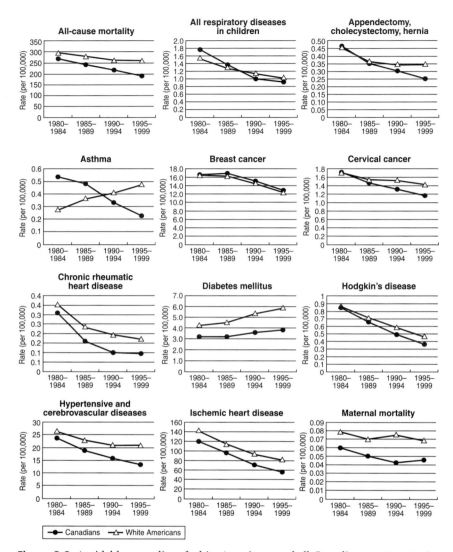

Figure 3-8. Avoidable mortality of white Americans and all Canadians, 1980–1998/9. (Age-adjusted mortality rates using U.S. standard population.)

These comparisons strongly suggest that the Canadian health care system, though not without serious problems,[112] serves the interests of Canadians better than the U.S. health care system serves the interests of white Americans, not to mention African Americans. Not only has Canadian per capita income been 70% to 73% of U.S. income since 1970, but Canadian per capita health expenditures are less than half those of the United States.[113] In current U.S. dollars in 1999, per capita health expenditures in Canada were U.S.$1939

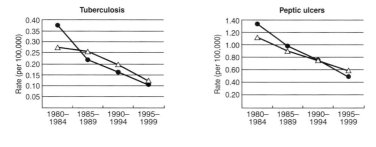

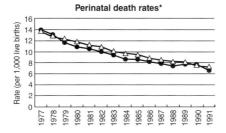

*Includes fetal deaths (stillbirths of 28 or more weeks' gestation) and infant deaths under 1 week (7 days) of age.

Other selected causes of death in the United States and Canada, 1980–1998/9

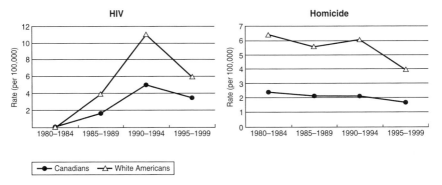

Figure 3-8. *Continued.*

compared to U.S.\$4271 in the United States.[114] Thus, both efficiency and quality as defined by the Working Group on Preventable and Manageable Diseases in the 1970s are greater in Canada than in the United States.

Conclusion

The historical and contemporary evidence indicates that the standard of living, whether measured as height or as income, is not invariably positively associated with life expectancy. This is because the health of populations is responsive to many more factors—including personal and public health services—than are summarized by the measures conventionally used. Much depends upon the context, epidemiological, sociopolitical, as well as economic. For example, height is inversely associated with some causes of death (respiratory and cardiovascular) and positively associated with others (some forms of cancer and, as shown in Appendix 2, tuberculosis). Thus, the prevailing epidemiological regime will shape the relationship between this measure of the standard of living and overall mortality, even as the overall standard of living may help shape the prevailing epidemiological regime.

Similarly, while only a wealthy society, such as England was in the nineteenth century, may have been able to make the initial investments necessary to develop and install clean water supplies and sewer systems, once the technology and trained engineers were available, poorer populations could adopt those innovations at much lower cost. This appears to be what happened within Europe and the United States in the nineteenth century and more broadly internationally in the twentieth century.

Finally, political culture and institutions have a profound effect that may well be more significant than the standard of living as measured by income per capita. This is the lesson to be drawn from the comparison of mortality rates in the United States and Canada. Given the existing technologies, the ability to make services universally accessible can have a measurably beneficial impact upon the health of the population.

The standard-of-living debate has been too narrowly conceived. It is based upon the assumption that if income rises for everyone, even if unequally, everyone will benefit. For some purposes this may be true, and, indeed, income has proven itself over and over again to be a useful indicator of social status and social difference. When considering the health of populations, however, it may also be seriously misleading for, as Edgar Sydenstricker pointed out when he first advocated the use of income as a measure of the adequacy of the social environment in public health, the social environment included "tradition, superstition, and mores; modes of living, fads, and fashions; standardization of ideas and attitudes by the press, movies, radio, and schools; cultural factors, such as the esthetic idea of posture or a religious regimen of diet or of personal cleanliness."[115] As we will see in the next chapter, it is a lot to ask of any single indicator that it adequately reflect the impact of all of these on the health of populations.

4

Inequality

In short, whoever you may be,
To this conclusion you'll agree,
When everyone is somebodee,
Then no one's anybody.
—W.S. Gilbert, *The Gondoliers*[1]

Optimists and pessimists disagree strongly on the extent and severity of inequality resulting from industrialization and economic advance. Optimists argue that it is far less than what would have prevailed had industrialization not happened, and that everyone has benefited, even if unequally. Their focus is upon absolute improvements in the standard of living. Pessimists claim that industrialization worsened inequality, and even if everyone is now better off than in past times, it is the growth of relative differences that is of most significance. Both positions have informed debate about the health consequences of inequality, which is the subject of this chapter.

Two related issues are examined: (1) the association between inequality and measures of health is shown to be not the same everywhere but is dependent upon the historical and sociocultural context; and (2) the association of the degree of income inequality in a society and life expectancy in that same society is also shown to be context specific. It is argued that the health and mortality of populations are shaped by so many factors that, as in the case of income per capita, so in the case of income inequality, no universally true generalizations are available. To understand the association, or its absence, between inequality and mortality, it is crucial to understand the epidemiological, sociocultural, political, and economic context of the population being observed.

The Changing Relationship of Mortality and Inequality

Despite assertions to the contrary, for instance, that "*Throughout history*, socioeconomic status has been linked to health,"[2] that "Life expectancy has *always* differed according to status in society, with a higher mortality among those of lower social status,"[3] and that "high socioeconomic status has allowed people to live much longer lives—*over the centuries and around the world*,"[4] the association between inequality and mortality has not been a universal truth in human history. In the West, it appears to have become a pervasive fact of life only in the nineteenth century, and even then differences in income and wealth could not account for all disparities among strata and classes. Despite some classic nineteenth century examples—Villerme's study of early nineteenth century Paris,[5] Engels' description of the working class of Manchester,[6] and Virchow's description of a typhus epidemic in Silesia[7]—in the past, *place* of residence has often been more significantly associated with mortality than has social status.[8] To take but a few examples, (1) infant and child mortality rates of the offspring of agricultural workers in England in the late nineteenth and early twentieth centuries were similar to those of urban professionals with much higher incomes, and this in an extraordinarily unequal and stratified society;[9] (2) even as late as the early twentieth century, people of different income and wealth levels living in the same central city neighborhoods of Holyoke and Northampton, Massachusetts had mortality rates that were indistinguishable from one another;[10] (3) similar effects are observed with respect to infant mortality in England at about the same time;[11] and (4) in nineteenth-century France, male and female life expectancy at age 40 was 29.7 and 28.2 respectively for men and women of the nobility and bourgeoisie (noblesse, industriel bourgeois) and 30.6 and 31.2 respectively for men and women among fermiers (farmers), laboureurs (laborers), and proprietaires (property owners). The latter lived in more isolated areas where infectious diseases were less common.[12]

Aaron Antonovsky seems to have been the first to suggest that differences among social strata in mortality were not observable when mortality rates were high because until the seventeenth century, epidemics killed rich and poor alike. Differences among social strata emerged and widened as economic expansion during the industrial revolution exacerbated inequality, caused an increase in urban population size and density, worsened conditions for the working class, and resulted in medical and sanitary improvements that benefited people unequally. It is noteworthy that the three classic studies noted above, by Villerme, Engels, and Virchow, all date from the period of the industrial revolution. Antonovsky claimed that differences diminished in the late nineteenth and early twentieth centuries as welfare states developed.[13]

In addition to the data used by Antonovsky to argue his case, there is more recent evidence that provides some support for, but also complicates, his findings. For example, when the life expectancy of British peers and peeresses is compared with that of the British population, it does indeed reveal such a pattern, as indicated by Figure 4-1. The gap between the peerage and the total population began to widen substantially around the mid-eighteenth century and then began to narrow by the end of the nineteenth century.[14]

Several explanations are possible. I have suggested elsewhere that the recession of epidemics in the eighteenth century benefited the peerage more

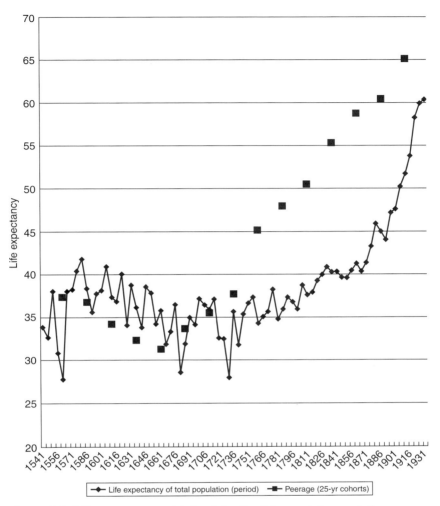

Figure 4-1. Life expectancy at birth of the English population and the peerage. (*Sources*: Hollingsworth, *Demography of the English Peerage*; Wrigley & Schofield, *Population History of England*; *Human Mortality Database*.)

than common folk because, once epidemics had receded, the better living conditions and nutritional status of peers were able to express themselves in improved life expectancy.[15]

Sheila Ryan Johansson has argued that the reason for the rapid improvement of mortality among the peerage through the eighteenth century was that peers and peeresses were better able to afford the expensive and increasingly effective medical innovations that were becoming available at the time.[16] These included safer deliveries as a result of the use of "man-midwives"; the use of expensive cinchona bark to treat fevers and malaria; an increase in

Table 4-1
Life Expectancy of Men at Age 20, Fourteenth–Nineteenth Centuries

Approximate Birth Cohort	European Rulers	British Dukes	French Dukes & Peers	Families of British Peers	English Gentry	Genevan Bourgeoisie	Milanese Patricians	Scottish Advocates
1350–1399		31.5						
1400–1449		31.5						
1450–1499		31						
1500–1549	27.7	30.5			43			31.7
1550–1599	27.7	30.5		31.1	43	35.8		31.7
1600–1649	27.1	30.5		29.3	44	36	37	33
1650–1699	27.1	32.8	34.5	30	36	40.3	43.5	38.1
1700–1749	35.8	37.1	34.5	35.5	42	40.3	43.5	41.8
1750–1799	35.8	42.7	34.5	39.2	49	40.8	40	41.9
1800–1849	39.3	43		41.2	46	41.3	39	
1850–1899		45.7		43.4		45	44.5	

Source: R. Woods and N. Williams, "Must the gap widen before it can be narrowed?" *Continuity and Change* 10: 105–137, 1995.

breast-feeding and bringing wet-nurses into the home where they could be more thoroughly supervised; and so on.

Jim Oeppen has reanalyzed the peerage data and compared adult life expectancy of ever-married peers and peeresses to that of the population of non-metropolitan England, excluding violent deaths among peers. Selecting in this way, he finds that life expectancy is remarkably similar among the peerage and the general nonmetropolitan population, increasing gradually from 1700 and then more rapidly in the late nineteenth and twentieth centuries. Considering only peers, Oeppen finds that "unmarried men had the lowest life-expectancy, followed by ever-married females, then ever-married males, and finally unmarried females."[17] He suggests that unmarried men were younger sons who could not afford to marry and who led dissolute lives and died prematurely, even excepting violent causes. Married women seem to have died at higher rates than unmarried women due to the complications of childbearing, presumably including greater interference in the birth process by elite physicians.

However, there is also evidence that does not support the sequence outlined by Antonovsky. Alfred Perrenoud has shown that in preindustrial seventeenth-century Geneva, there was the expected gradient of mortality from the upper class to the middle class to the working class.[18] Life expectancy at birth for the two sexes combined was respectively 35.9, 24.7, and 18.3 years.

Also in contrast to Antonovsky's hypothesis, Robert Woods and Naomi Williams[19] have summarized data from the fourteenth to the late nineteenth centuries, showing that there were substantial differences in male life expectancy at age 20 among categories of individuals. Their data are displayed in Table 4-1 and show that life expectancy differed among several groups, but the differences were not associated with differences in wealth.

If we consider only people living in the United Kingdom, we see that life expectancy at age 20 for men of the gentry was substantially higher than that of dukes and the families of peers from the sixteenth through the end of the nineteenth centuries, although the differences had diminished dramatically by the end of the period. Similarly, Scottish advocates had greater life expectancy than British dukes or the families of peers from the early sixteenth century to the late eighteenth century.

Table 4-2, compiled by Sheila Ryan Johansson, displays male and female life expectancies at age 25, to which I have added estimates of male and female Quaker life expectancy at age 25 to 29. The estimates of Quaker life expectancy are for ages slightly older than 25 and are therefore not precisely comparable to the other figures, but they too suggest that this group, made up disproportionately of middle- and upper-middle-class tradesmen and professionals, had life expectancies similar to those of men of much greater income and wealth, especially if they lived in rural rather than urban places.[20] Indeed, as Table 4-3 indicates, life expectancy at birth of Quaker males and females in Bristol and Norwich in the second half of the seventeenth century was essentially the same as that of upper-class Genevois at about the same time, whereas

Table 4-2
Life Expectancy at Age 25, British Elites and the General Population, Seventeenth–Nineteenth Centuries

Birth Cohort	British Peers	Tontines	Barristers (England)	Members of Parliament	Scottish Advocates	Reconstituted Families		Quakers							
								Urban		So. England		Ireland		No. Britain	
						M	F	M	F	M	F	M	F	M	F
1600–1649	25		30		29	30	31.2								
1650–1699	27	28		26	31	32	30	31	29.4	32.2	29.2	33.5	32.7	35.8	33.7
1700–1749	32	34		31	38	33.5	33	29.6	28.8	34.1	31.9	35.8	36.3	35	32.8
1750–1799	36	36		37	38	36.3	34.5	33.6	32.2	36.7	35.0	35.3	31.3	34.4	33.4
1800–1849								30.5	35.2	36	35.1	N.A.	33.3	35.9	32.6
1850–1899															

Sources: S.R. Johansson, *Death and the Doctors*, p. 21. R.T. Vann and D. Eversley, *Friends in Life and Death*, p. 230.

Table 4-3

Life Expectancy at Birth of British and Irish Quakers and Genevan Social Classes, Seventeenth–Nineteenth Centuries

| Period | Quakers | | | | | | | | | | Genevan Upper Class | | Genevan Middle Class | | Genevan Working Class | |
| | Irish Quakers | | So. England | | No. Britain | | Bristol & Norwich | | London | | | | | | | |
	M	F	M	F	M	F	M	F	M	F	M	F	M	F	M	F
1650–1699	47.0	50.0	46.4	50.4	52.3	57.6	36.6	38.9	26.0	26.4	36.9	38.0	25.5	26.7	18.9	20.3
1700–1749	41.3	45.8	45.8	49.8	49.4	54.2	30.1	34.8	29.1	31.4						
1750–1799	44.1	47.9	49.0	50.3	53.5	55.6	38.2	46.8	44.0	43.5						
1800–1849	58.3	59.4	54.4	57.0	59.1	63.1	53.1	51.1	45.3	57.0						
1850–1899					63.2	66.6										

Sources: R.T. Vann and D. Eversley, *Friends in Life and Death*, p. 228. A. Perrenoud, "L'Inegalite sociale devant la mort," p. 236.

the life expectancy of London Quakers was substantially lower, and of Irish and rural English Quakers substantially higher.

These data suggest that it was something besides wealth, income, and social status that frequently influenced differences in mortality. Part of the difference is explained by urban and rural differences, and part is explained by cultural differences. Richard Vann and David Eversley write of the Quakers:

> We can hardly accept volumes of evidence about Quaker pre-eminence in medicine, science, and industrial innovation, and a mass of literature about their belief in a certain lifestyle (or "testimonies") with its attendant valuation of the human individual, and at the same time suppose that these abundantly documented practices and ideas are not in any way reflected in their experience of sickness and death. Their mortality should have been below that of the population in general, and also below that of Britain's usually dissolute and occasionally vicious aristocracy.[21]

The abstemiousness and self-control of the Quakers was presumably similar to that of the Calvinist *haute bourgeoisie* of Geneva. And while the English gentry may have been as dissolute and even as vicious as the aristocracy, no doubt living in rural places was of considerable benefit. The point is not that all these variations in mortality are readily explainable but, rather, that some of them were the result of a culture of moderation and some the result of living in salubrious places, and that these factors were more important in reducing mortality than high rank, great wealth, or income.

The groups with life expectancies that compared favorably with those of the nobility were generally of at least moderate means. They were not representative of the entire population. Thus, income and wealth must have made some contribution to their well-being, over and above their moderate style of life. We may consider the matter further, however, by examining infant and child mortality data from another population. Jews have long been known to have more favorable mortality rates than their equally poor (or affluent) non-Jewish neighbors. In almost 200 comparisons of Jewish and non-Jewish infant mortality rates from Europe and North America from 1819 to the 1960s, Jews had higher rates in fewer than 10 instances. The same was true of early childhood mortality.[22] In the few instances in which figures were reported by income and social class, Jews continued to have lower mortality rates. For example, in a study in Baltimore in 1915, Jewish immigrants with an income below $650 had lower infant mortality rates than non-Jews with higher incomes.[23] Other studies from the United States before 1920 that adjust for income and occupation, as well as for feeding practices, give similar results.[24] In every instance, Jews had substantially lower infant mortality rates than non-Jews of the same socioeconomic status.

Not much information is available from Jewish communities in Asia and North Africa, but what data there are suggest that mortality under 5 years of age was similar in the mid-twentieth century to that prevailing in late nineteenth century eastern and central European communities.[25] In Tunis in the 1940s and 1950s, Jewish infant mortality rates were less than half the Muslim rates but higher than the rates of Europeans resident in the city.[26]

The reasons for these patterns are complex and have never been fully explicated. The general level of social and economic development is important, for eastern European Jews had higher infant mortality rates than western European Jews in the nineteenth century, and North African and Asian Jews in the mid-twentieth century had rates that were similar to those prevailing in Europe in the previous century. But something about Jewish culture was also important. Observation of dietary laws has been suggested, but that is to confuse ritual with biological purity, as anyone who has inspected a kosher slaughter house will confirm. Jews have generally had lower fertility than their neighbors, although Jewish infant mortality rates were lower even when it was possible to adjust for the number of prior births. But the overwhelming concern of Jewish mothers for the well-being of their offspring that has entered North American and European humor and folklore has a basis in reality, as anyone with a Jewish mother can attest. And alcoholism, illegitimacy, and venereal diseases have all been less frequent among Jews than non-Jews. Indeed, moderation and even abstemiousness is something that Jews share with Quakers and with the Genevan *haute bourgeoisie*.

To take but one more example, Jan Sundin cites Swedish data showing that (1) in the second half of the eighteenth century, the infants of unskilled foundry workers died at lower rates than those of well-to-do crofters living in rural areas, and (2) in the first half of the nineteenth century, infant mortality was lower "among relatively poor crofters than among more well-to-do farmers."[27] These differences could not be ascribed to the income or wealth of the groups but seem instead to have been caused by feeding and child-care practices. Similar differences have been noted in other historical studies.[28] All these examples demonstrate that mortality has not always and everywhere followed the social gradient that has been claimed to be universal.

Disparities in Mortality Since the Late Nineteenth Century

The narrowing mortality gap between social strata toward the end of the nineteenth century that was first identified by Antonovsky has never been closed completely. Indeed, whether as absolute or relative difference, change during the twentieth century has been uneven. In general, it is fair to say that in all the developed countries of Western Europe and the Americas north of Mexico, mortality in all classes has declined, but very unevenly. Generally, the more privileged have experienced earlier and more rapid declines than the poor. That was true at the turn of the twentieth century and continues to be true 100 years later.

Robert Woods and Naomi Williams point out that in the late nineteenth and early twentieth centuries as mortality declined, there were what they call

Table 4-4

Age-Adjusted Mortality Rates and Standardized Mortality Ratios for White Women and Men, Chicago, 1930–1960

	1929–1931	1940	1950	1960
White Men				
City, age-adjusted mortality rate:	14.4	12.6	11.4	11.0
SE1 (low)	1.3	1.3	1.32	1.45
SE2	1.07	1.06	1.01	1.02
SE3	0.94	0.91	0.85	0.92
SE4	0.86	0.85	0.82	0.83
SE5 (high)	0.80	0.87	0.76	0.87
Suburbs	—	—	(0.79)	(0.76)
White Women				
City, age-adjusted mortality rate:	11.6	9.4	7.5	6.7
SE1 (low)	1.25	1.29	1.26	1.34
SE2	1.07	1.07	1.04	1.04
SE3	0.97	0.96	0.93	0.92
SE4	0.90	0.88	0.88	0.86
SE5 (high)	0.77	0.81	0.80	0.88
Suburbs	—	—	(0.85)	(0.82)

Source: Calculated from E.M. Kitagawa and P.M. Hauser, *Differential Mortality in the United States.* Cambridge: Harvard University Press, 1973, p. 53.

"trailing occupations," those especially in the dangerous trades in which mortality rates declined more slowly than in others, or even increased in some instances.[29] Analyzing similar data, Michael Haines has shown that from 1890 to 1911, childhood mortality declined in all classes but more rapidly among the privileged.[30]

In Sweden, a similar pattern was observed between 1885 and 1910: childhood mortality rates declined in all social classes, but the relative differences increased between the upper and middle class on the one hand and artisans and workers on the other.[31] Likewise, in the United States between 1895 and 1924, there was a far more rapid decline of mortality among children of professionals than among children of clerical or manual workers.[32]

In Chicago from 1930 through 1960, the mortality rate declined in every neighborhood, regardless of the socioeconomic class of the residents. However, as Table 4-4 indicates, the relative differences increased, again demonstrating a more rapid decline among the affluent than the poor.

Inequality has persisted. Data from Paris from 1817 to 1946 reveal a general decline in overall mortality and a narrowing of the gap between wealthy and poor districts, but at no time was equality attained.[33] In England from the 1920s to the 1940s, there was a decline in absolute and relative class differences in male and female age-adjusted mortality, but an increase in the differences from 1951 to the end of the century. Absolute differences in infant mortality declined from the 1920s through 1970, while relative differences declined to 1940 and widened after 1951. This was puzzling because the National Health Service had been established in the late 1940s, and the assumption was it would further reduce inequalities. Instead, differences increased.[34] Across Western Europe in the 1980s and 1990s, mortality declined at different rates within the manual and nonmanual classes, leading to increasing relative inequality.[35]

Some Causes of Continuing Disparities in Mortality

The persistent differences described above are due to both structural and cultural factors, though it is often difficult to disentangle the two. For example, David Mechanic has made the point that interventions that do not depend upon changes in individual behavior—chlorination and fluoridation of water, improved highway engineering and air quality—may benefit all equally.[36] Other interventions requiring behavioral change may be adopted at unequal rates because people in higher status positions are better placed to take advantage of new knowledge and new technologies, both because they value the advice of experts even when they do not understand the content and basis of the experts' knowledge, and because they have better access to new technologies and services, and to opportunities to engage in health-promoting behaviors. Curative, preventive, and behavioral interventions, then, may result in improvements in health that are shared unequally, even if everyone benefits to some degree. Indeed, this is the basis upon which Jo Phelan and Bruce Link have argued that social class is a fundamental cause of disparities in health, for no matter what the condition, unequal access to, and use of, preventive and curative interventions invariably differentially benefits the well-to-do.[37]

Subcultures and Disparities in Death. Clearly, access to decent housing and nutrition, to a safe work environment, and to adequate medical care are all enormously important in explaining differences in mortality. This is so well known and so widely accepted that it is not necessary to pursue it further at the moment. What I should like to consider instead is some of the ways in which the culture and values of different social classes may influence health. When subculture is invoked as an explanation, it is generally with respect to the feckless and reckless behavior of the poor. For a refreshing change, consider Pierre Bourdieu's description of the dining preferences of different segments and strata of the French population. He points out that,

> The art of eating and drinking remains one of the few areas in which
> the working classes explicitly challenge the legitimate art of living.
> In the face of the new ethic of sobriety for the sake of slimness,

which is most recognized at the highest levels of the social hierarchy, peasants and especially industrial workers maintain an ethic of convivial indulgence. A bon vivant is not just someone who enjoys eating and drinking; he is someone capable of entering into the generous and familiar—that is, both simple and free–relationship that is encouraged and symbolized by eating and drinking together, in a conviviality which sweeps away restraints and reticence.[38]

The calculation that it is better to indulge in present conviviality rather than defer gratification for the sake of improved beauty and health "is the only philosophy conceivable to those who 'have no future' and, in any case, little to expect from the future." It is an expression of solidarity with others in the same situation and the reason "why the sobriety of the petit bourgeois is felt as a break: in abstaining from having a good time and from having it with others, the would-be petit bourgeois betrays his ambition of escaping from the common present."[39]

In contrast, consider his description of bourgeois culture. "In opposition to the free-and-easy working-class meal, the bourgeoisie is concerned to eat with all due form. Form is first of all a matter of rhythm, which implies expectations, pauses, restraints; waiting until the last person served has started to eat, taking modest helpings, not appearing over-eager . . . [T]his whole commitment to stylization tends to shift the emphasis from substance and function to form and manner, and so to deny the crudely material reality of the act of eating and of the things consumed, or, which amounts to the same thing, the basely material vulgarity of those who indulge in the immediate satisfactions of food and drink."[40]

What is true of dining practices is also true of the distinctions among classes with respect to their choice of favored sports: "[P]hysical culture and all the strictly health-oriented practices such as walking and jogging are . . . linked . . . to the dispositions of the culturally richest fractions of the middle classes and the dominant class . . . they presuppose a rational faith in the deferred, often intangible profits they offer (such as protection against ageing or the accidents linked to age, an abstract, negative gain)."

It is therefore understandable that they should find the conditions for their performance in the ascetic dispositions of upwardly mobile individuals who are prepared to find satisfaction in effort itself and to take the deferred gratifications of their present sacrifice at face value. But also, because they can be performed in solitude, at times and in places beyond the reach of the many, off the beaten track, and so exclude all competition (that is one of the differences between running and jogging), they have a natural place among the ethical and aesthetic choices which define the aristocratic asceticism of the dominated fractions of the dominant class.[41]

What is missing, then, from many discussions of health inequalities is the way in which the social organization and values of segments of the population are shaped by social and economic forces on the one hand, and, on the other hand, the way social organization and values operate to make individuals conform to the standards of the group. Studies of social disparities in health are often written as if behavior and culture are simply what happens when people don't have enough money or are not well enough educated to make rational choices regarding their health. They miss the ways in which communities at all income, educational, and occupational levels shape behavior, assuming instead that choices are an individual matter constrained (or made possible) only by income and education (or their absence).

Fashion and Disparities in Health. Health-related behaviors are not necessarily stable. There are many reasons why change occurs, and occurs unevenly.[42] One of the most important has to do with what is considered fashionable. From Simmel[43] to Elias[44] and more recent authors, the literature on diffusion of innovation and fashion suggests that different social strata adopt fashions, including clothing, manners, and a wide variety of practices to distinguish themselves from, as well as to mimic, others. The elite use dress and other badges of distinctiveness to set themselves apart from their inferiors, but their inferiors readily copy the fashions of the elite, so the elite then adopts new styles to set itself apart once again.[45] This explains the dynamic by which fashions change. Sumptuary laws were an ultimately vain attempt to prohibit such mimicry.

Herbert Blumer claimed that Simmel's thesis was correct for patterns of dress in seventeenth-, eighteenth-, and nineteenth-century Europe, but that it did not operate in the contemporary world with its "many diverse fields and its emphasis on modernity."[46] It certainly does not operate in the world of clothing fashion at present. If it did, affluent suburban youth wouldn't be wearing their baseball hats backwards and their expensive running shoes without laces.[47] Blumer also argued that fashion "is not guided by utilitarian or rational considerations."[48] Where one model can be objectively shown to be better than another, he wrote, fashion cannot operate. This assertion is problematic, but even if it were true, it would not vitiate the claim that many health-related behaviors are best understood as fashion. Dietary preferences, the popularity of psychoanalysis among certain urban groups in the 1940s and 1950s,[49] whether or not to exercise, the preferred type of exercise, child rearing practices—all are largely matters of fashion, for the *best* model of each of them is not known.

Even cigarette smoking, however, which is now known incontrovertibly to be damaging to health and a cause of lung cancer and ischemic heart disease (IHD), is best thought of as a fashion, and the practice diffused, just as Simmel would have predicted. For it was first adopted by high-status people (especially physicians) in several different countries, and then spread down the social hierarchy. Like many other fashions, by the time the lowest strata had adopted the practice, high-status people had largely given it up, often for health-related as well as moral[50] and esthetic reasons, and perhaps also to continue to differentiate themselves from their social inferiors who were mimicking their behavior.[51]

The epidemiology of IHD has followed a similar path. In England, upperclass men had higher mortality from IHD than lower-class men until some time in the 1950s, although upper-class women had had lower mortality than lower-class women during the period 1931 to 1971. The change among men paralleled reduced consumption of sugar and cigarettes and increased consumption of whole-meal bread among the upper as compared with the lower classes over the same period.[52]

In the United States "[T]he pattern of onset of decline [of IHD]— metropolitan to non-metropolitan and centers of the Pacific West and Northeast to the South and mid-sections of the country—is similar to cultural diffusion . . . This phenomenon includes not only aspects of popular consumer culture such as diet and recreation, but also shifts in productive economic activities from manufacturing and extractive industry to high technology industry and the service economy."[53] The regions in which the start of the decline lagged had comparatively low levels of income, education, and occupation (proportion of population engaged in white-collar occupations). These community characteristics provide "the context in which positive changes in diet, exercise, smoking, stress and medical care are possible."[54] More generally, the rise of cardiovascular disease (including IHD) in the course of the epidemiological transition occurred first among the upper classes in industrialized countries, and the decline in these countries, beginning in the 1960s, has also occurred first among these classes. The same sequence is now being observed in South America and Asia, where cardiovascular disease is found disproportionately among the upper classes.[55]

Part of the reason this sequence has occurred is that diets, smoking, exercise patterns, and standards of beauty and attractiveness have changed, following the trajectory of fashion suggested by Simmel. This is because, while in many instances one model may not be demonstrably better than another, it is generally endorsed by an authoritative figure, a "scientific" expert. Because upper-class people on average have higher educational attainments than others, they value expertise even if they cannot understand the science on which its claims rest.[56] That is why behavior that is fashionable can also seem, and also occasionally be, rationally utilitarian.[57]

Fashions do not change simply as a result of mimicry and passive diffusion. They change as a result of purposeful interventions. If Jane Austen is to be believed, ladies of the gentry intruded into the affairs of their social inferiors in early nineteenth-century England. In Sweden, urban bourgeois reformers worked to transform peasant communities.

> During the nineteenth century, people in the countryside were exposed
> to a systematic barrage of propaganda aiming to teach them better
> morals and hygiene, to bring them up to be citizens pure in word,

thought, and deed. This message came from the schools, the social organizations, and the mass media.[58]

The introduction of social insurance in European nations accelerated these changes, for along with universal primary education, it was in large measure an extension under government auspices of changes that had been under way through much of the nineteenth century. It is part of what Norbert Elias called "the civilizing process."[59] According to Elias, manners evolved and became increasingly refined as a result of the growth of courtly societies and ultimately of the growth of absolute states in which the nobility and haute bourgeoisie were dependent upon the monarch for advancement and preferment.[60] As the bourgeoisie was incorporated into the elite, style and manners diffused down the social ladder. Thus, "politeness" became "civilized behavior" as it spread to the working class. Elias's emphasis upon the importance of courtly society and the state in this process has been criticized.[61] Nonetheless, his insistence upon the growth of self-control, restraint, and the suppression of physical and emotional displays as hallmarks of civilized behavior is of great significance, for much of the behavior inculcated in the working class— such as not spitting, maintaining cleanliness in food preparation, and bathing regularly—had important consequences for improved health.

Psychosocial Explanations of Disparities in Mortality

So far the emphasis has been on material and cultural differences that contribute to disparities in the health and mortality rates among social strata. There are also psychological, or what are more generally called psychosocial, explanations. The experience of stress is said to activate the neuroendocrine and immune systems, leading to increased morbidity and mortality from many causes (what has been called general susceptibility) among those whose subordinate position constrains their autonomy and self-realization. This is the explanation offered for the observation that in contemporary affluent societies there is a socioeconomic gradient in both mortality and self-reported morbidity even among people who cannot be considered poor, what Michael Marmot has called the Status Syndrome.[62] For example, in the Whitehall study, "Executive grade civil servants are not poor by any absolute standard yet they have higher mortality rates than administrators."[63]

Indeed, Marmot observed that the same inverse correlation between health and the precisely differentiated ranks within the British civil service are also found more nearly universally in economically advanced societies. Analyzing data from three studies, one in the United Kingdom and two in the United States, he and his colleagues showed that people of lower status, whether measured as grade within the civil service, occupational status using a status ranking of jobs, or educational attainment, report worse health than those of higher status.[64] It is reasonable to ask, however, whether the inverse association between finely graded distinctions in status on the one hand and morbidity and mortality on the other is found universally in economically advanced societies?

In the United States, male life expectancy at age 45 differs by social class in the expected fashion in urban and suburban places. In cities and suburbs, men of the highest social class have life expectancy at age 45 of 31.4 and 31.8 years respectively, whereas the poorest survive 28.1 and 27.9 years respectively. The situation is different in rural places, however, where the figures for the lowest and highest socioeconomic classes are 30.6 and 30.5 respectively.[65]

Or consider an international example. Melvin Kohn and his colleagues showed in a comparative study of the United States, Japan, and Poland that both social stratification (measured by income, occupational status, and education) and social class (control over resources and/or the labor of others) were significantly associated with psychological functioning. While stratification and class overlapped, they were not perfectly aligned. In each case, though, people at the top of the hierarchy within each of the three countries were more likely than those lower in the hierarchy to value self-direction in their children, ideational flexibility, and autonomy in their own work. Kohn and his colleagues found that occupational autonomy was the crucial link between values of flexibility and standing in the stratification and class systems, for high-ranking men had more opportunity for self-direction in their work, and that shaped their values with regard to flexibility, conformity, and childrearing.

Strikingly, however, there were no consistent cross-national associations between stratification and class on the one hand and psychological distress on the other. Distress was reflected in, among other attributes, anxiety and distrust.[66] "In the United States, managers have a strong sense of well-being, and manual workers are distressed; in Poland, just the opposite; in Japan, managers have a strong sense of well-being, but it is the non-manual workers, not the manual workers, who are most distressed."[67]

Kohn and his colleagues were not able to explain the surprising differences they discovered, and it is not necessary for present purposes to pursue their speculations except to say they thought that in some national settings other work-related conditions were at odds with the effects of self-direction. Whatever the reason, the fact is that psychological distress among men in different work settings in these three very different countries did not follow a consistent pattern, although other aspects of psychological functioning, most notably the valued placed on occupational self-direction, did. Because psychological distress is said to be associated with increased risk of morbidity and even mortality, one might reasonably ask whether status and role within work settings, both white and blue collar, have the same health effects everywhere. The answer appears to be that control over one's work—occupational self-direction—is associated with low levels of distress, and presumably with health-promoting effects in some work settings and not in others. Once again, this points to the need to examine particular settings in historical and social context rather than to assume that the effects of social inequality, even when limited only to economically advanced societies, are everywhere the same.

Consider two more examples. In the Whitehall studies of British civil servants, grade in the bureaucracy is associated with a variety of measures of morbidity, including coronary artery disease, even adjusting for a large number of risk factors upon enrollment in the study.[68] On the other hand, in a study of blue- and white-collar workers in Hawaii, neither deaths due to coronary heart disease nor all-cause mortality differed between the two groups.[69] And in a study of coronary artery disease among 270,000 men employed by Bell Telephone System in the United States, education and other background factors (e.g. dietary history) were found to be more significant than either occupational mobility or grade within the company in predicting first coronary events and all coronary events.[70] The American private corporation and the British civil service may have been very different kinds of bureaucracies. We may speculate, for instance, that mobility was greater in the former than the latter, and that a relatively open opportunity structure may have reduced the stratification of risk for heart disease and made background factors more significant. This would be consistent with observations of populations of monkeys, in which dominant animals in stable hierarchies are less likely to show stress responses than subordinate animals, but in which dominant animals in unstable hierarchies experience no such advantage.[71]

Potentially, however, there is even more going on. The Whitehall and Bell System studies, like most large epidemiological studies, are based upon individuals as the units of analysis. The work group is rarely considered, although studies as far back as those at the Hawthorn General Electric plant showed that the work group was in fact important in a variety of ways.[72] Thus, in an ethnographic study of a manufacturing plant, Craig Janes and Genevieve Ames reported that average morbidity was higher in certain groups than in others. At the root of the problem of high morbidity rates was the seniority system that had been disrupted by the closure of other plants owned by the same corporation, the movement of workers to the plant being studied, the loss of seniority by many workers, and the creation within certain parts of the plant of occupational subcultures, often based upon the misuse of alcohol and other substances, that were implicated in increased morbidity and use of health services.[73]

The point is that in most studies of the health of people in organizations or in communities, the organization or community is not itself a subject of study. The subjects are the people who happen to work or live in the same place. However, both the context in which organizations exist and social processes within organizations shape the health of individuals. Stratification is clearly an important part of the lived experience of individuals in communities and workplaces, but to infer that it is always overwhelmingly significant and that stress is invariably caused by inequality, or even by lack of self-direction in work, is not supported by the evidence.

Income Inequality and the Level of Mortality Among Countries and Regions

The persistence of relative differences in mortality among social classes and racial groups prompted Richard Wilkinson to argue that when societies have attained "the threshold level of living standards marked by the epidemiological transition," a fundamental change occurs between economic growth and the benefits it has to offer in respect of improved health and reduced mortality. At the point when infectious diseases give way to the noninfectious diseases, "what matters within societies is not so much the direct health effects of absolute living standards as the effects of social relativities." He continues:

> The crucial evidence on this comes from the discovery of a strong international relationship between income distribution and national mortality rates. In the developed world it is not the richest countries which have the best health, but the most egalitarian . . .
>
> Looking at a number of different examples of healthy egalitarian societies, an important characteristic they all seem to share is their social cohesion. They have strong community life. Instead of social life stopping outside the front door, public space remains a social space. The individualism and the values of the market are restrained by a social morality. . . . These societies have more of what has been called "social capital" which lubricates the workings of the whole society and economy.[74]

Social capital is dealt with in the following chapter. For the moment, two points are important. First, Wilkinson has argued that hunter–gatherer bands, the most of egalitarian of societies, are characterized by "more cooperative social relations, in which people's needs are recognized and mediated through the social obligations of sharing and reciprocity—as between friends."[75] This assertion does not withstand scrutiny. In a study of homicide among various American Indian tribes in the late nineteenth century, Jerrold Levy and I showed that there was a remarkable range, with band-level egalitarian hunting groups ranking much higher than hierarchical sedentary agriculturalists such as the Pueblo Indians in New Mexico and Arizona.[76] Joel Savishinsky has observed high rates of violence and unwillingness to intervene in conflicts between spouses among hunter–gatherers in Canada, and Peter Sutton has noted a similar phenomenon among Aborigines in Australia.[77]

That these are not new phenomena to be explained simply as the consequences of European dominance is demonstrated by (1) the observations of Aborigines made by the first English soldiers and settlers in Australia. One wrote "of the pitiable condition of women, who are accustomed to bear on their heads the traces of the superiority of males, with which they dignify them almost as soon as they find strength in the arm to imprint the mark." He described some women with "more scars upon their shorn heads, cut in every direction, than could well be distinguished and counted."[78] (2) The extraordinarily high prevalence of fractures, especially of the skull, found in aboriginal female skeletal remains from thousands of years before contact with Europeans, the result of severe beatings.[79] These examples all suggest that egalitarian societies are not, and were not in the past, necessarily characterized by harmonious social relationships, though no doubt some were (and are). Generalizing from the experience of tribal peoples does not necessarily point to the benefits of egalitarianism and suggests yet again that it is often more useful to examine particular situations in their own context rather than grasp prematurely for universal truths.

Second, consider the assertion that the greater the income inequality in rich societies, the greater the average death rate of the entire population. This has been the subject of numerous studies, many of which have been reviewed by John Lynch and his colleagues.[80] They point out that while some of the association between income inequality and mortality is a statistical artifact, this cannot explain all of the positive findings. More problematic are the following examples:

1. *The original international comparisons that led to the claim that inequality and mortality were associated have not held up when other advanced countries have been added to the analysis.* Table 4-5 displays the correlations of

Table 4-5
Correlation of Infant Mortality, Life Expectancy, Income Inequality, and GDP Per Capita in 15 European Union Countries

	Life Expectancy	Gini	P90/P10	GDP/capita
Life Expectancy, 2000	—			
Gini, 1994	−0.29	—		
P90/P10, 1994	−0.30*	0.96	—	
GDP Per Capita, U.S.$, 2000	−0.14	−0.20	−0.27	—
Infant Mortality Rate Per 1000 Live Births, 2000	−0.49**	0.65***	0.62***	0.05

*p = 0.27
**p = 0.06
***p < 0.01

P90/P10 is the ratio of the income of the richest 10% of the population to the poorest 10% of the population.

Countries: Belgium, Denmark, Germany, Greece, France, Ireland, Italy, Luxemburg, Netherlands, Austria, Portugal, Finland, Sweden, United Kingdom, Spain.

The results are essentially the same when Gini coefficients from the Luxembourg Income Survey are used for the 13 countries for which comparable data are available (Portugal and Greece are not included in the LIS). The correlation between Gini coefficient in the two series is 0.79 (p = .0013).

Sources: Gini coefficients and P90/P10 from J.P. Mackenbach, M.J. Bakker, A.E. Kunst, and F. Diderichsen, "Socioeconomic inequalities in health in Europe." In J.P. Mackenbach and M. Bakker, eds., *Reducing Inequalities in Health: A European Perspective.* London: Routledge, 2002. Infant mortality rate, life expectancy, and GDP per capita from World Development Indicators CD-ROM, Washington, D.C.: The World Bank, 2002.

Table 4-6

Political Context, Life Expectancy, and Infant Mortality 1960–2000

A. Life Expectancy at Birth

Country Name	Political Context	1960	1965	1970	1975	1980	1985	1990	1995	2000
Austria	Social Democracy	68.7	69.6	70.3	71.4	72.6	74.3	75.7	76.7	78.2
Sweden	Social Democracy	73	73.9	74.6	74.9	75.7	76.7	77.5	78.7	79.6
Denmark	Social Democracy	72.2	72.7	73.3	74	74.3	74.6	74.7	75.2	76.4
Norway	Social Democracy	73.4	73.7	74.2	75	75.7	76.1	76.5	77.7	78.6
Finland	Social Democracy	68.5	69.3	70.3	71.6	73.2	74.3	75	76.4	77.5
Belgium	Christian Democracy	70.4	70.9	71.2	71.9	73.3	75.1	76	77.2	78.2
Germany	Christian Democracy	69.5	70.2	70.5	71.4	72.6	74.2	75.1	76.2	77.4
Netherlands	Christian Democracy	73.4	73.6	73.6	74.5	75.7	76.3	76.9	77.4	77.9
France	Christian Democracy	70.2	71	72	72.8	74.2	75.3	76.7	77.8	78.9
Italy	Christian Democracy	69.7	70.4	71.9	72.6	74	75.5	77.2	77.8	78.7
Switzerland	Christian Democracy	71.3	72	73.2	74.7	75.8	76.8	77.3	78.4	79.7
United Kingdom	Liberal	70.8	71.1	71.7	72.4	73.8	74.6	75.6	76.6	77.3
Ireland	Liberal	69.7	70.8	71.1	71.7	72.7	73.5	74.6	75.8	76.3
United States	Liberal	69.8	70.2	70.9	72.6	73.7	74.6	75.2	75.6	77.1
Canada	Liberal	71.1	71.8	72.5	73.4	74.7	76.3	77.2	78.2	78.9
Spain	Ex-fascist	69.2	71.1	72.3	73.2	75.5	75.9	76.7	77.1	78.2
Portugal	Ex-fascist	63.4	65.3	67.4	69.3	71.4	73.4	73.7	74.9	75.6
Greece	Ex-fascist	68.9	70.4	71.8	73.2	74.4	75.0	76.9	77.5	77.9

B. Infant Mortality[a]

Austria	Social Democracy	37.5	28.3	25.9	20.5	14.3	11.2	7.8	5.4	4.8
Sweden	Social Democracy	16.6	13.3	11	8.6	6.9	6.8	6	4	3.4
Denmark	Social Democracy	21.5	18.7	14.2	10.4	8.4	7.9	7.5	5.3	4.3
Norway	Social Democracy	18.9	16.8	12.7	11	8	8.5	6.9	4.1	3.9
Finland	Social Democracy	21.4	16.6	13.2	9.5	7.6	6.3	5.6	3.9	4.2
Belgium	Christian Democracy	31.2	23.7	21.1	16.1	12.1	9.8	7.9	6.1	5.3
Germany	Christian Democracy	35	24.1	22.5	18.9	12.4	9.1	7	5.3	4.5
Netherlands	Christian Democracy	17.9	14.4	12.7	10.6	8.6	8	7.1	5.5	4.9
France	Christian Democracy	27.4	21.9	18.2	13.8	10	8.3	7.3	4.9	4.4
Italy	Christian Democracy	43.9	36	29.6	21.2	14.6	10.5	8.2	6.3	5.3
Switzerland	Christian Democracy	21.1	17.8	15.4	10.7	9.1	6.9	6.8	5	3.7
United Kingdom	Liberal	22.5	19.6	18.5	16	12.1	9.3	7.9	6.2	5.6
Ireland	Liberal	29.3	25.2	19.5	17.5	11.1	8.8	8.2	5.7	5.9
United States	Liberal	26	24.7	20	16.1	12.6	10.5	9.4	7.5	7.1
Canada	Liberal	27.3	23.6	18.8	14.2	10.4	7.9	6.8	6.1	5.2
Spain	Ex-fascist	43.7	37.8	28.1	18.9	12.3	8.9	7.6	5.6	3.9
Portugal	Ex-fascist	77.5	64.9	55.5	38.9	24.3	17.8	10.9	7.4	5.5
Greece	Ex-fascist	40.1	34.3	29.6	24	17.9	14.1	9.7	8.2	5.4

[a]per 1,000 live births

Sources: V. Navarro and L. Shi, "The political context of social inequalities and health." *Social Science and Medicine* 52: 481–491, 2001. World Bank, *World Development Report* 2002, CD-ROM.

measures of income inequality, GDP per capita, infant mortality, and life expectancy at birth in 15 European Union countries. None of the associations with life expectancy is significant.[81] On the other hand, infant mortality is strongly associated with income inequality but not with per capita income. The greater the inequality, the higher the infant mortality rate.

Vicente Navarro and Leiyu Shi have made the important point that income inequality is the product of political institutions.[82] They have classified 18 western nations according to sociopolitical context and argued that in those that have been led by the Social Democrats, equality is greatest. Those that have been led by the Christian Democrats are somewhat less equal. And the liberal Anglo-Saxon political economies and the ex-fascist countries are the most unequal. In fact, using World Bank estimates from the early 1990s, the average Gini coefficients were as follows: Social Democrats, 26.6; Christian Democrats, 30.8; ex-fascist states, 34.0; and Liberal states, 36.7.[83] They show that mean infant mortality in 1996 was lowest in the social democratic countries (4.5/1000); next lowest in the Christian Democratic ones (5.3/1000); and the same in the liberal and ex-fascist countries (6.4/1000). The story is actually somewhat more complicated, however. To illustrate, Table 4-6 displays life expectancy at birth (Panel A) and infant mortality (Panel B) from 1960 through 2000 for the countries analyzed by Navarro and Shi.

In 1960, there was an almost significant ($p = 0.07$) difference in life expectancy among the four groups of countries, with the ex-fascist countries having substantially lower life expectancies than the others. By 2000, there were no significant differences among the four types of countries. However, in both 1960 and 2000, there were significant differences among the groups of countries in respect of infant mortality. In 1960, the ex-fascist countries had an average infant mortality rate of 53.7 per 1000 live births, whereas the three other groups of countries had infant mortality rates ranging from 23.2 (Social Democrats) to 29.4 (Christian Democrats) ($p = 0.0089$). In 2000, the Liberal countries had an average infant mortality rate of 5.9 compared to 4.1 for the Social Democracies, 4.7 for the Christian Democracies, and 4.9 for the ex-fascist states ($p = 0.0118$).

The results displayed in Tables 4-5 and 4-6 suggest that political context and income equality are strongly associated and are especially significant for infant mortality but play lesser roles with respect to mortality at older ages, presumably because mortality at older ages is less immediately responsive to changes in policies and programs than is infant mortality. But they also suggest that the patterns are not stable over time. For example, the ex-fascist countries have evidently pursued policies that have led to rapid improvement compared to other types of countries, presumably the result of reforms required for membership in the European Union.

2. *Studies within countries have not shown consistent associations between income inequality and mortality*[84] *(or self-reported health) when provinces/states or cities have been the units of analysis, with the striking exception of the United States, and perhaps Great Britain.*[85] And in the United States, the association

has not been observed in all age-sex groups. Moreover, high income inequality in U.S. counties with large concentrations of African Americans is associated with lower mortality than in counties with low income inequality and high concentrations of African Americans, suggesting the possibility that a relatively affluent African American middle class may be able to exercise sufficient political influence to obtain good services.[86]

3. *Virtually all of the studies have been cross-sectional, not longitudinal.* The studies of temporal change have not shown any compellingly significant results. For instance, Neal Pearce and George Davey Smith have published data from New Zealand during much of the twentieth century showing no association between the trends in income inequality and mortality. Similar evidence is reported from Israel.[87] And Lynch et al show there is no temporal association between income inequality and all-cause and cause-specific mortality in the total U.S. population and in different regional U.S. populations.[88]

Richard Wilkinson has described as a "travesty" the review by Lynch and his colleagues because "it made no distinction between data based on larger or smaller areas, even though the importance of the issue has been pointed out several times . . . and an earlier review of studies on violence and inequality drew attention to exactly the same tendency for studies in smaller areas to produce weaker relationships."[89] Leaving aside the appropriateness of the description, the question of size of the sampling unit is an important one that has been addressed by Angus Forbes and Steven Wainwright. They write:

> How is social status psychologically referenced—what are its spatial
> dynamics? . . . Is it a keeping up with the Joneses phenomenon, i.e.
> local? Or do we refer ourselves to the national or international
> levels—perhaps as communicated by the media.[90]

The answers that have been suggested are not compelling, for psychosocial explanations (e.g., stress) would seem to be most in evidence at the level of neighborhood and workplace. But there is a more serious problem that, to my uncertain knowledge, has not been addressed in any of the ecological studies of inequality and mortality. That is the problem that ecologists and geographers call spatial autocorrelation (see Appendix 4). This is a type of confounding that is caused by the fact that geographic units near to one another may be very similar for any of a variety of reasons. The consequence is that the units of analysis are not independent of one another as conventional statistical analyses require. Moreover, the problem of spatial autocorrelation may worsen as the level of aggregation increases because average values tend to converge as the units increase in size. This might, then, explain both the positive associations that have been reported and the increasing proportion of significant findings as the level of aggregation increases.

The problem is not insurmountable, for measures exist that can be used to analyze how much of a significant ecological correlation is explained by the variable of interest (e.g., income inequality) and how much by some other unmeasured latent variable.[91] Appendix 4 contains preliminary analyses of data from U.S. counties and states. The results demonstrate a very strong effect. Uncorrected for spatial autocorrelation, the association between the Gini coefficient on the one hand and age-adjusted and infant mortality on the other strengthens, as does the measure of spatial autocorrelation (Moran's I). However, when adjusted for spatial autocorrelation, the association weakens substantially—though it does not disappear entirely—from the county through the state level of aggregation. The analyses in Appendix 4 show further that the nationwide association is completely determined by the South, which has particularly high mortality and inequality. In the rest of the country there is no association. Thus, sociocultural and economic factors in the South drive the positive results for the entire country.

These preliminary analyses therefore support the possibility that spatial autocorrelation may explain many, if not all, of the positive associations that have been reported, as well as the increasing proportion of positive associations at higher levels of aggregation. The story is complicated and has not yet been fully examined, but until spatial autocorrelation is taken into account, positive results should be regarded with some skepticism.

Homicide and Inequality

Of all causes of death, homicide is widely believed to be the one most directly associated with income inequality as well as poverty. In a study of the United States, state homicide rates were significantly correlated with income inequality, even adjusting for median income.[92] It is also the cause of death that should be consistently responsive to inequality and poverty whatever the prevailing disease regime happens to be, for it is the product of social and psychological forces that would not be expected to change as infectious diseases wane and noninfectious diseases wax. Although an association has been reported in cross-sectional analyses, there has been no temporal association in the United States, as Figure 4-2 indicates, except perhaps when both inequality and homicides rates were increasing from the early 1980s to the mid-1990s. The data in Figure 4-2 are for the entire United States. However, regional differences reported by Lynch et al[93] show that changes in income inequality were entirely unrelated to changes in homicide rates between 1968 and 1998. Nonetheless, it is worth considering the existing cross-sectional data as they are based upon cities, states and other smaller geographic units and thus may allow us to consider the impact of size of the sampling unit as it influences the context for assaults and homicides.

Homicide rates are higher in urban than rural areas, higher among African Americans than whites, and higher in the southern United States than elsewhere in the country. Both the high rates among urban African Americans and the high southern rates have been the subject of the same debate that has run through much of the discussion of differences and trends in mortality in general: how much is due to structural factors and how much to culture, in this case, a culture of violence?

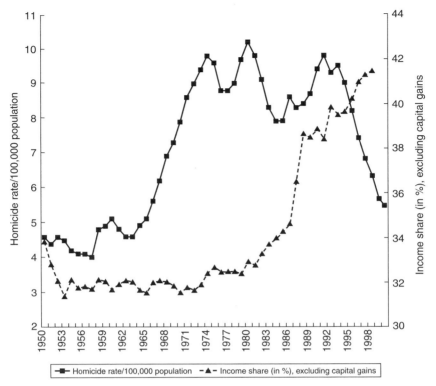

Figure 4-2. Homicide rate in the U.S. and income share of the top decile of the population, 1950–1999. (Income data from T. Picketty & E. Saez, *Income Inequality in the U.S., 1913–1999*. NBER working paper w8467. Cambridge, Mass.: National Bureau of Economic Research, 2001.)

The existence of slavery in the American South largely explains the institutional arrangements that perpetuated income inequality and lack of access to easy credit, to education, and to the franchise.[94] It also explains the low level of membership in voluntary associations that pre-dated the Civil War and persists into the present.[95] Indeed, income inequality is greater in the South than elsewhere in the country and is associated with low levels of spending on education, libraries, and health, with low reading proficiency and low levels of high school graduation, with high unemployment, with a high proportion of people in prison, receiving welfare of various sorts, and without health insurance.[96] It is also the legacy of slavery in the American South that has resulted in weak governments dominated by elites, governments of men, not of laws. In such situations, when justice is not even-handed, the state cannot claim a legitimate monopoly on the use of force, and personal violence is used in its place.[97]

The persistence of weak governments perpetuated the "culture of honor" that had characterized white southern society from its beginning. White southerners had come from both the South of England to the Chesapeake and from the Celtic fringe of the British Isles to the southern highlands. Each had brought an entirely different culture than the Puritans who settled in New England. For the highlanders, it was a culture that was kin-based, and that emphasized the importance of family and personal honor, the spoken over the written word, agrarian over business values, and leisure over enterprise. In this culture, fighting was an accepted means of defending one's honor and of settling disputes both large and small.[98] In Virginia, hierarchical violence of the elite against the poor was common, as it was among the class from which the elite had originated in England.[99]

Recent studies indicate that white southerners are still more likely than people elsewhere in the country to regard certain forms of violence as legitimate, regardless of social class.[100] Violence in defense of one's honor, one's safety, or one's family is more widely acceptable in the South than in other parts of the country, and the type of homicide that accounts for the high rates among white southerners is that resulting from an argument.[101] Indeed, as with age-adjusted and infant mortality rates, the significant association between the Gini coefficient and homicide observed among all 50 states is entirely explained by the pattern in the South (see Appendix 5).

Homicide among African Americans is largely an urban phenomenon, most commonly observed in racially segregated areas of concentrated poverty. In such areas, where the state has abdicated its responsibility to assure its citizens decent housing, education, and health care, and where there is no trusted police presence and little community control over public behavior,[102] one's safety depends upon being willing to retaliate for an offense, whether actual or threatened, and to strike preemptively if one believes oneself threatened or "disrespected." Many homicides, then, are committed in defense of one's self and one's honor, or the honor and safety of one's family and friends. Indeed, a study of the structural and cultural determinants of retaliatory homicides in St. Louis showed that such events are much more common in segregated areas of concentrated poverty, as a consequence of economic deprivation, the absence of a police presence, distrust of the police when they are present, and a culture of honor that requires retaliation for disrespectful behavior.[103] Economic deprivation is important, especially to the degree that it made the drug trade an attractive alternative to unemployment,[104] but by itself is not sufficient to explain the pattern. It is combined with racial segregation and a vacuum where there should be a trusted police presence. The absence of government that can be trusted to exercise justice even-handedly and thus can monopolize force legitimately is similar to what has been described in the South.

It is the weakness of the state and the perceived illegitimacy of the governing authorities that created the context in which individuals feel they have the right—indeed, the obligation—to resort to violence to settle disputes both large and small. Income inequality is part of the context, but inequality *per se* is not enough. For although income inequality is positively correlated with elevated homicide rates among African American men in metropolitan areas, and among whites and African Americans in the southern states, there is no correlation in small nonmetropolitan areas where the rates among African American and white men are equally low regardless of the level of income inequality.[105]

Thus, while inequality is certainly associated with homicide in some settings, the association may not necessarily be causal and is certainly not universal. An explanation that includes as a crucial element the weakness or illegitimacy of the governing authorities is consistent with the long-term decline of homicide in Europe. As states emerged, the high rates found in medieval communities declined to their present levels, the product, as Norbert Elias argued, of the growth of self-control as a concomitant of the growth of the state.[106]

Indigenous Peoples in Liberal Democracies

Another way to approach the question of just how universal is the association between relative inequality and mortality is to consider particularly deprived populations within different countries to see if they differ more or less from the rest of the country, and from one another, with respect to mortality. Table 4-7 displays life expectancy, income, and income inequality data from four advanced industrialized, English-speaking, liberal democracies: Australia, Canada, New Zealand, and the United States. Of the four, Australia and Canada had about the same per capita income, the same life expectancy, and about the same level of income inequality. New Zealand was the poorest but the most egalitarian with respect to income distribution. The United States was the richest and most unequal. They all had life expectancies in the range of 76 to 78 years in the early 1990s.

Table 4-7
Income, Income Inequality, and Life Expectancy at Birth

Country	Life Expectancy (1994)	GNP per capita U.S. $ (1994)	Income per Adult in the Poorest 25% of the Population as a % of the Median Income per Adult (yr)
Australia	77	18,000	46.5 (1985)
Canada	78	19,510	45.8 (1987)
New Zealand	76	13,350	53.6 (1987–1988)
United States	77	25,880	34.7 (1986)

Sources: 1994 data are from World Bank. *From Plan to Market: World Development Report 1996.* New York: Oxford University Press, 1996. Data on income inequality are from A.B. Atkinson, L. Rainwater, and T.M. Smeeding, *Income Distribution in OECD Countries: Evidence from the Luxembourg Income Study.* Organization for Economic Cooperation and Development, Paris, 1995, p. 40.

Table 4-8

Life Expectancy at Birth of Indigenous and Non-Indigenous Peoples

| Country | Years | Life Expectancy at Birth | | Indigenous as a % of Non-Indigenous |
		Indigenous	Non-Indigenous	
Australia	1991–1996	60.4	77.7	77.7
New Zealand	1990–1992	70.5	76.3	92.4
United States	1992–94	71.1	75.5	94.2
Canada	1995	71.9	78.3	91.8

Sources: Australia: W. McLennan and R. Madden, *The Health and Welfare of Australia's Aboriginal and Torres Strait Islander Peoples.* Canberra: Australian Bureau of Statistics, 1997. *New Zealand*: Eru Pomare Maori Health Research Centre, *Hauora: Maori Standards of Health 3: A Study of the Years 1970–1991*. Wellington South, NZ. Wellington School of Medicine, 1995, p. 36. *United States*: Indian Health Service, *Indian Health Trends and Services, 1996*. Rockville, MD: U.S. Public Health Service, Department of Health and Human Services, 1997, p. 134, corrected for misclassification of race. *Canada*: First Nations and Northern Statistics Section, Corporate Information Management Directorate, Information Management Branch, Department of Indian Affairs and Northern Development, *Basic Departmental Data 2001*. Minister of Indian Affairs and Northern Development, Ottawa, Canada.

Table 4-8 displays life expectancy figures for the indigenous and non-indigenous people in each country. Maoris in New Zealand, First Nation peoples in Canada, and Native Americans in the United States all had life expectancies that were similar. Australian Aborigines, however, have remarkably low life expectancy, confirmed in numerous studies, compared to the other three indigenous populations.

A study using 1999 data from the United States and New Zealand reported life expectancies of Maori males and females as 68.0 and 72.3 respectively; non-Maori New Zealand males and females as 76.9 and 81.7; American Indian/Alaska Native males and females, 67.4 and 74.2; and white American males and females, 74.8 and 80.0.[107] Thus, among nonindigenous people, life expectancy in the United States is consistently less than in New Zealand, but among indigenous people the situation is more complicated. Men have similar life expectancy (68.0 and 67.4) but Maori women have life expectancy almost 2 years less than American Indian/Alaska Native women. Moreover, major causes of death such as malignancies, IHD, cerebrovascular disease, chronic obstructive pulmonary disease, and diabetes occur at substantially higher rates among Maoris than among indigenous Americans.

Among Native Americans in 1989, median household income was 66% of the U.S. figure[108] and mean income of Indian men 15 to 64 was 55%, and of women 70%, that of their counterparts in the general population.[109] Among Aborigines in 1991 and 1996, mean per capita income was 61% and 64%, respectively, of the income of the Australian population.[110] Among Maoris in 1996, annual median household income was 79.5% that of non-Maoris, and average weekly income of people 15 years of age and above was 77%.[111]

While the measures are not precisely comparable across countries, they do indicate that the income of indigenous people is substantially less than that of nonindigenous people in their respective countries, and that Maoris are relatively less deprived than either Native Americans or Aborigines. (There are no recent data available for Canadian native peoples.) The results also indicate that Native Americans are relatively more deprived than Maoris, although their per capita income is absolutely the highest because they live in the wealthiest of the four countries. Yet their life expectancy is the same as, or better than, that of Maoris, the least deprived relatively, but certainly more deprived in absolute terms than Native Americans. In addition to higher incomes than the other indigenous peoples, Native Americans have benefited from the equivalent of a universal health care system, the only one in the United States. This system, even with all its flaws, has made an important contribution to the health of Native Americans.[112] Likewise, Australia is far more egalitarian than the United States, and Aborigines have relative incomes somewhat higher than, or the same as, Native Americans. Nonetheless their life expectancy is far lower.

The differences among these populations have been discussed in detail elsewhere.[113] The only point to be made here is that (1) there is no obvious association between the magnitude of income, income inequality, and life expectancy of indigenous people in these countries; (2) if relative inequality were of overwhelming importance, Native Americans would be expected have much lower life expectancy than Maoris and Aboriginal Australians; (3) there are different ways to attain the same end point, in this case, life expectancy; and (4) to argue that inequality *per se* accounts for differences in life expectancy is to decontextualize particular situations. Certainly New Zealand, with a per capita income about half that of the United States, has managed to attain life expectancies for its citizens that are almost the same as those in the United States. Egalitarian policies no doubt play an extremely important part. Looked at another way, however, the United States and New Zealand have achieved similar end points by very different paths. Which of them is socially preferable is not the issue.

Inequality and the Standard of Living Debate

The widespread interest in relative inequality and its association with mortality both among and within nations comes at a time of growing international and national income inequality.[114] And the heightened intensity of interest in inequality also raises in particularly acute ways all the questions that are part of the long-running standard of living debate. Optimists claim that all peoples are experiencing rising incomes, so inequality is nothing to worry about. Pessimists claim that relative disparities are not improving and in many instances are worsening. They use the Standardized Mortality Ratio (SMR) to demonstrate persistent or worsening relative inequality, even in the face of diminishing absolute differences among social classes. They generally call for the reduction in health disparities by redistributing income, limiting the role of the free market, and providing more services to those who are deprived.

Those who take the optimistic side in this current version of the standard-of-living debate believe that interfering in the economy in this way damages the potential for economic growth and is, in the long run, damaging to the very people the pessimists want to help. Richard Epstein writes that public health should not become conflated with social welfare but should stick to what it has traditionally done best: controlling epidemics of infectious diseases.[115] These are conditions the market cannot control. Noninfectious diseases and occupational exposures are best left to individuals and to the free market. He criticizes an essay in which Michael Marmot:[116]

> [E]mphasizes equality first and overall levels of health second. His account of infant mortality in Yorkshire is instructive. In 1901, infant mortality per 1,000 ranged from 247 for the poorest working class groups to 183 for the middle working class, 173 for the richest working class, and 94 for the class fortunate enough to own [sic] servants. One hundred years later, the range of infant mortality from bottom to top was 8.1 to 3.1. In one sense nothing has changed, for the ratio of mortality rates between the least and most fortunate is about 2.6 to 1 in both periods. But to concentrate on income inequalities is to overlook the most mind-blowing feature of the exercise, which is the *overall* decline in infant mortality for all groups, by close to 97 percent! . . . If income inequality has produced these overall savings, then relative deprivation becomes a cause for celebration rather than dismay . . .
>
> The blunt truth is that the ratio from top to bottom is far less important than the massive downshift over time, which tracks the large growth of income and leisure in England during the twentieth century. The question is what drives all of this, and the answer cannot be equality as such, but technical advances in all walks of life whose indirect effects produce massive changes that are hard to track. We should therefore be careful before we slow down the engine, for the price of static equality is a slow-down in dynamic progress.[117]

Epstein argues that the position advocated by Marmot would require so much redistribution of income and wealth, and so much government intrusion into private affairs, that it would destroy the incentives of the free market that have generated the wealth that has made such startling improvements in mortality possible.

> [I]nequalities are allowed to persist because of the benefits that they generate for all people, no matter where they sit in the overall

distribution. The obvious explanation is that the rich are prepared to pay handsomely for new technologies that become available to poorer individuals within the next generation at far lower prices. Leveling incomes through government action, then, will come at some substantial costs of real income available to fund these improvements.[118]

There is no doubt that in historical perspective, the changes in infant mortality in Yorkshire and elsewhere have been truly remarkable. In comparison to the inequalities of a century ago, the contemporary disparities are trivial, and to emphasize the enormity of the relative differences while ignoring the even more dramatic absolute declines experienced by all classes would be to overlook a remarkable social achievement. But to attribute these improvements entirely to the workings of the free market when they occurred concurrently with the improvement and increased accessibility of services made possible by the expansion of the welfare state is a remarkable—even mind-blowing—assertion. Furthermore, to assert that inequality is justified by investments made by the rich in new technologies that ultimately benefit everyone ignores the crucial role played by governments in providing research grants and contracts and funding government laboratories that support, or even do, much of the work on such livesaving technologies.

The data in Table 4-9 show that the percent of Gross Domestic Product spent publicly on health services is significantly correlated with life expectancy in Western Europe and North America, whereas the amount spent privately on health care is not. On the other hand, neither GDP per capita nor government spending as a percent of GDP is correlated with life expectancy.

Table 4-9
Life Expectancy at Birth in 20 Developed Countries,[a] 2000, Correlated With Health Expenditures and GDP Per Capita, 1998 (Pearson's r)

Public health expenditures (% of GDP)	0.47[*]
Private health expenditures (% of GDP)	0.01
Health expenditures per capita	0.18
Total health expenditures (% of GDP)	0.24
GDP per capita	−0.01
Government expenditures as a proportion of GDP	0.14

[*]$p = 0.0365$

[a]Countries: Australia, Austria, Belgium, Canada, Denmark, Finland, France, Germany, Greece, Ireland, Italy, Luxemburg, New Zealand, Norway, Portugal, Spain, Sweden, Switzerland, United Kingdom, United States

Source: World Development Indicators CD-ROM, Washington, D.C.: The World Bank, 2002.

This supports, but does not prove, the claim that neither the magnitude of the government's involvement in the economy, nor the amount private citizens pay for health care, nor the average income of these rich countries is significantly related to life expectancy, but targeted spending on health care by governments is.

Conclusion

Several points are made in this chapter. The first is that inequality of income and wealth has not always been associated with health disparities, even when social differences based upon place and/or culture have been. That economic inequality was not invariably associated with unequal death rates indicates, (1) that culture and behavior made a difference even when infectious diseases were widely prevalent and, (2) that differences in status have not been universally associated with differences in mortality.

Consider as an example the higher death rates of officers than lower ranks in the British army in India in the early twentieth century: 1899–1908, 11.97 per 1000 compared to 11.63; 1909–1913, 6.27 per 1000 vs. 4.74.[119] Philip Curtin writes:

> Medical authorities were greatly concerned, especially about typhoid fever, which was far more serious among officers than among other ranks. They found no good explanation, aside from the obvious fact that enlisted men were under far stricter control outside working hours. In any case, typhoid inoculation soon eliminated the problem.[120]

These observations raise several issues. (1) It appears that officers may have been more susceptible to typhoid than the lower ranks, perhaps because they had been raised in more sheltered environments. (2) They had greater autonomy than the lower ranks, which increased their risk rather than reduced it. (3) The problem was solved by a technological fix, not by changing the social organization of the army.

Of course, typhoid is an infectious disease, but so is tuberculosis, whose differential rates among rich and poor have been invoked by Marmot as a late nineteenth-century example of the importance of, among other things, differences in host susceptibility and resistance.[121] The example is not meant to cast doubt upon the increased susceptibility of the poor to tuberculosis but to state again the point that social context and the prevailing epidemiological regime matter. In the case of the British army in India, every bit as rigidly hierarchical as the civil service in the United Kingdom several generations later, they shaped the association between social stratification and mortality.

The second point is that, on the other hand, in the contemporary world characterized by noninfectious diseases, a gradient of mortality with income, education, or occupational status is widely observed. The fact that there is such a gradient, even among people living well above poverty, has suggested to many that relative rather than absolute deprivation is the explanation. Virtually all observers agree that part of the explanation has to do with access to material resources—decent housing, access to health care and other services, an adequate and balanced diet; part with personal behavior; and part with psychosocial processes. The largest area of disagreement is between those who consider psychosocial explanations most important and those who consider material conditions most important. The former accord much greater weight to the idea of general susceptibility to disease and to the importance of stress as an explanation of the differences in the health of people at different locations in their society. The latter accord much greater weight to exposure than to susceptibility: exposure to poor living conditions, economic deprivation, inadequate diets, hazardous occupations, and the like.

The results of different studies are often in disagreement. (1) Not all diseases follow the same status gradient. (2) The evidence that populations with high income inequality have lower life expectancy than populations with low income inequality is inconsistent and therefore unpersuasive, and the positive associations may be confounded by spatial autocorrelation. (3) Differences in the stress response of nonhuman primates are often said to be associated with differences in status, with high-status animals showing lower levels of stress than their subordinates. This observation is then generalized to human hierarchies. However, in primate populations with stable hierarchies, physiological measures of stress are inversely correlated with rank, whereas in unstable hierarchies no such correlation is observed: that is, higher status animals experience as much, or more, stress as those of lower rank.[122]

The third point is that a similar criticism may be made of those explanations of health disparities that invoke individual decisions about unhealthy "life-styles." No doubt there are occasions when people do make more- or less-well-informed decisions based upon a critical understanding of the relevant scientific findings. Generally, these are assumed to be the well-educated or those living in the south of England. But more often than not decisions about health-related "life-style" issues are made because some self-proclaimed expert has announced a new diet, exercise regimen, stress-reduction program, or child-rearing practice that he or she claims works. The history of Western medicine is littered with such experts. The discussion of fashion was meant to show that what are generally conceived to be individual choices are more often than not choices based upon the culture and values of a particular class. Those of us who write on these topics are members of the bourgeois class whose preferences were described by Bourdieu earlier in this chapter, and the choices he describes no doubt appear to us eminently sensible, what any rational person would choose. It is not obvious that in this we are always correct.

A fourth point is that the optimists' claim to be concerned with the greatest good for the greatest number underpins (1) their objections to redistributive policies, and (2) their criticisms of claims that social class inequalities are widening. The criticism of redistribution is that it will "kill the goose that laid the golden egg" and that, in the not-so-long run, this will harm the poor by increasing unemployment and reducing technological innovations that benefit everyone.[123] In respect of the claim that gaps between the affluent and the poor are widening, the optimists assert that upward mobility has changed the class composition such that many more people benefit now than in the past from improved material conditions. The fact that some are left behind is thus of less concern to them than it otherwise might be because there are relatively few poor, and overall the total population is experiencing improved health.[124] Furthermore, since mortality of all groups is declining, even if relatively the differences are as large as ever, the problem is not nearly as serious as pessimists assert. All of these claims have, of course, been disputed.[125]

The need to disprove the claim that the present system has led to the greatest good for the greatest number also underpins the pessimists' need to show that among rich countries, those that are egalitarian have lower overall mortality than those that are inegalitarian. For, in that case, equality would be associated with the greatest good for the greatest number, not wealth and inequality. Relative differences are thus of the utmost importance.

In the event, international comparisons do not support either position. Among the richest countries, neither inequality nor income per capita is consistently associated with life expectancy. This is not to say, however, that in specific countries the link between income inequality and mortality is not real and significant. Worsening income inequality and high unemployment, coupled with a decline in the real incomes of the poor and weakening of the National Health Service in England in the 1980s and even through the 1990s[126] have almost certainly been important causes of the widening relative and absolute gaps in mortality and the virtual stagnation of life expectancy among working class men of working age. Moreover, there is consistent evidence that the more unequal the income distribution within a country, the higher the infant mortality rate. The mechanism is unclear, but it is fair to assume that infants do not experience much status anxiety and that autonomy—at least for infants, even if not for the elderly—does not extend to, for instance, changing their own diapers. I would hazard the (neomaterialist) explanation that countries with more nearly equal income distributions are also those that provide a broader range of services for the care of infants and support for their families.[127]

A fifth point has to do with the problems that come from seeking universally applicable explanations for patterns of health and disease in populations. Egalitarianism does not in all its forms lead to harmonious and pacific relationships. Relative deprivation is not invariably associated with increased morbidity, anxiety, and mortality. Social status within troops of monkeys and within human populations does not invariably lead to the same gradient of cardiovascular disease. And the workings and failures of the free market cannot explain the international differences and similarities in life expectancy in the rich countries, for some are generous welfare states and others are not, and yet life expectancy is remarkably similar in all of them.

The final point is that the more rapid improvement of mortality among groups of higher than lower status is a widely observed but not inevitable phenomenon. The more rapid decline of mortality among the lower than higher classes in England before 1941, and more rapid declines of tuberculosis and cervical cancer among African Americans than whites in the 1980s and 1990s demonstrate that. It is highly likely, however, without specially targeted programs. For even relatively generous and egalitarian welfare states such as the Scandinavian countries have increasingly unfavorable mortality ratios, although mortality rates for all groups continue to fall.[128] Such special programs have been successful but are difficult to sustain. Thus socially unequal mortality rates and differential rates of decline are likely to persist, for at present there is neither the political will nor power to make a change.

5

Community

I thought: "Well, I've come to the Union—
    The workhouse at last—
After honest hard work all the week, and
    Communion
O' Zundays, these fifty years past.

" 'Tis hard; but," I thought, "never mind it:
    There's gain in the end:
And when I get used to the place I shall find it
    A home, and may find there a friend.

"Life there will be better than t'other,
    For peace is assured.
The men in one wing and their wives in another
    Is strictly the rule of the Board."
—T. Hardy, *The Curate's Kindness: A Workhouse Irony*[1]

Holism and the quest for community during the interwar years were both responses to urbanization and industrialization, and to the atomization and alienation that are believed to be among their most important consequences. The distinctions drawn by nineteenth and early twentieth century writers between *gemeinschaft* (community) and *gesellschaft* (society), between status and contract, and between traditional and legal–rational authority were all attempts to describe the social transformation from a world of small, face-to-face communities in which change was slow, everyone knew everyone else in multiplex roles, and understood their place in the social order to the modern world of rapid change, social and geographic mobility, specialized roles, and disrupted relationships.

The argument of this chapter is that one important contemporary version of the quest for community is to be found in the significant role assigned to social capital. Indeed, the subtitle of an important book on social capital, Robert Putnam's *Bowling Alone*, is *The Collapse and Revival of American Community*.[2] Putnam has been the most visible and voluble advocate of the beneficial effects of social capital on the quality of civic life. "Social capital," he writes, "refers to features of social organization such as networks, norms, and social trust that facilitate coordination and cooperation for mutual benefit."[3] Social capital originates in membership in voluntary associations, and in dense networks of such organizations in any community, because it is in such

settings that people learn to trust, to reciprocate, and to act in concert to de-
mand public services and good government.[4]

Putnam credits James Coleman with having first clearly developed the social capital theoretical framework.[5] Coleman in his turn wrote of social capital that it:

> [I]s defined by its function. It is not a single entity but a variety of
> different entities, with two elements in common: they all consist of
> some aspect of social structures, and they facilitate certain actions
> of actors—*whether persons or corporate actors*—within the structure.
> Like other forms of capital, social capital is productive, making
> possible the achievement of certain ends that in its absence would not
> be possible. Like physical capital and human capital, social capital is
> not completely fungible but may be specific to certain activities. A
> given form of social capital that is valuable in facilitating certain
> actions may be useless or even harmful for others.[6]

He goes on to say that, "Unlike other forms of capital, social capital inheres in
the structure of relations between actors and among actors. It is not lodged either in the actors themselves or in physical implements of production." The
idea of social capital, according to Coleman, is meant to integrate two streams
in social thought, the radical individualism of the economic notion of rational
man, and the "oversocialized" view of man characteristic of much sociology.[7]

Putnam's use of social capital is somewhat different. Social capitalists,
called "the new republican theorists" by Putnam, stand in opposition to "the
defenders of classical liberal individualism."[8] They champion the importance
in public policy of cooperation, community, equality, and inclusiveness as
means of achieving a more just and humane society. Eva Cox has written,
"When Margaret Thatcher said there's no such thing as society, she lost the
plot. Society is the myriad of ways people connect, linked by some common
interests or characteristics." And she goes on to speak of the "often forgotten
but powerful forces that connect us as social beings. These forces—trust, reciprocity and mutuality—survive in our everyday lives but are not reflected in
public policy and therefore are losing ground."[9]

Social capital is often thought of as a societal phenomenon, reflected in
such measures as degree of income equality or membership in secondary groups
such as sports clubs, choirs, Rotary, and so on. As Cox's comment suggests, primary group ties—that is, relationships with kith and kin—are taken for granted.
That is a mistake. Social capital is also produced by primary groups and may or
may not be possessed by individuals. That is a point made by Portes, who writes
that "Social capital stands for the ability of actors to secure benefits by virtue of
membership in social networks or other social structures."[10] Coleman, in the
passage quoted above, and his own study of high school drop-outs, makes a
similar point, for he measures social capital within and outside the family. The
former is measured by the presence of both parents and the strength of relationships among members; the latter by geographic mobility, which attenuates ties

with other families and with the school. Thus, high school students may or may not possess social capital, and its possession diminishes the probability of dropping out of school. That is, social capital is not simply produced by, and reflected in membership in secondary groups, which are regarded as a manifestation of civic culture. It is also reflected in the structure and function of primary groups, or personal communities.[11]

Many of these ideas of social capital have found their way into epidemiology, public health, and health care policy,[12] where they have mingled with and provided a new vocabulary for ideas that have long existed. This chapter examines the way the vocabulary has been used at both the primary and secondary group levels in an effort to explain patterns of morbidity and mortality. The results are mixed, for in some instances there are beneficial effects, and in others, no or harmful, effects.

Social Capital in Secondary Groups

When Alexis de Tocqueville visited the United States in 1831, he observed that the vitality of local governments and of voluntary associations was very different from what he knew in Europe. Both were important, he thought, because the French Revolution had swept away many of the institutions that mediated between individuals and the state. Without such intermediating institutions, the state was in a position to manipulate and coerce its citizens in ways that were not possible when mediating institutions were present. This is perhaps one of the first statements of the dangers of mass society.

Local Government. Tocqueville was only one among many observers to have noticed profound differences among the people who had settled the various American colonies.[13] The men who initially settled the South, he wrote, were adventurers who came without families in search of wealth. They were followed by "a more moral and orderly race of men" who were, however, "nowise above the level of the inferior classes in England." They compared unfavorably with those who settled the North. The people who settled in the North "belonged to the more independent classes of their native country." They were "neither rich nor poor." All were educated and in proportion to their number possessed "a greater mass of intelligence than is to be found in any European nation of our own time." They were sober, moral, family men who were accompanied by their wives and children.[14] They were, he continued, Puritans, and "Puritanism was not merely a religious doctrine, but it corresponded in many points with the most absolute democratic and republican theories."[15]

Other observers noted these same differences. One preacher wrote of the Yankee settlers in the Upper Midwest: "[They] naturally unite themselves into corporate unions, and concentrate their strength for public works and purposes. They have the same desire for keeping up schools, for cultivating psalmody, for settling ministers, and attending upon religious worship; and unfortunately the same disposition to dogmatize, to settle not only their own faith, but that of their neighbour, and to stand resolutely, and dispute fiercely, for the slightest shade of difference of religious opinion." And he contrasted the Yankee settlers in Ohio who, "in the strong exercise of social inclination, expressing itself in habits of neighborhood, [formed] villages, and live[d] in them, . . . to that sequestered and isolated condition, which a Kentuckian, under the name of 'range,' considers as one of the desirable circumstance of existence."[16]

Reflecting the cultural differences between North and South were the political differences observed by Tocqueville. He wrote:

> Townships and a local activity exist in every State; but in no part of
> the confederation is a township to be met with precisely similar to
> those of New England. The more we descend towards the South, the
> less active does the business of the township or parish become;
> the number of magistrates, of functions, and of rights decreases; the
> population exercises a less immediate influence on affairs; town-
> meetings are less frequent, and the subjects of debate less numerous.
> The power of the elected magistrate is augmented, and that of the
> elector diminished, whilst the public spirit of the local communities
> is less awakened and less influential.[17]

That is to say, Tocqueville was describing variations in what is now called "civic culture" every bit as profound as those described by Putnam in northern and southern Italy.[18] He also observed that the introduction of slavery exercised a "prodigious . . . influence on the character, the laws, and all the future prospects of the South."[19]

It is difficult to disentangle the effects of slavery as an institution from the culture of the white settlers who first came to the South. There are, however, places in the South and the border states where slavery never appeared and where there were virtually no African Americans, in which a distinctly southern mountain culture has persisted, for example, in the Appalachian Mountains in eastern Kentucky.[20]

With this brief background in mind, recall some of the studies referred to in the previous chapter of mortality among American states and metropolitan areas. If one inspects the data displayed in those studies, they indicate that southern states have the lowest levels of social capital (measured as a sense of trust and as membership in voluntary associations), the lowest levels of education, the highest levels of income inequality, and the highest levels of homicide and of overall mortality of all the regions of the United States. Indeed, the southern predilection for homicide has been observed for well over a century and is high for both African Americans and whites[21] in places where there was slavery, as well as for whites in places where there was neither slavery nor African Americans, for instance, in the Appalachians.[22]

Clearly, the legacy of the civic cultures implanted in the North and

South in the seventeenth century continues to have profound consequences right down to the present, and at the state and regional level, the advantage seems to be to the North, where social capital is higher and mortality lower than in the South. At the metropolitan level, however, a paradox emerges. In a study of the impact of racial segregation on mortality in metropolitan regions, it was found that segregation was associated with an increase in deaths among African Americans but not among whites.[23] But it was also observed that the most racially segregated metropolitan regions were in the Northeast and upper Midwest, the very areas in which the civic culture that so impressed Tocqueville had taken deepest root. The two are not unrelated.

These cities were America's industrial heartland, and the relatively unskilled jobs available in their factories and mills provided economic opportunities for vast numbers of immigrants. In the nineteenth century, cities in the Northeast grew by annexation. They were able to acquire territory at the fringes and incorporate them within a larger city. This was to everyone's advantage. People in the annexed territory were glad to have city services such as water, sewers, paved roads, and trolley lines, and the city acquired an expanding tax base.[24]

In the late nineteenth and early twentieth centuries, however, as immigrants from Eastern and Southern Europe, and African American from the deep South began flooding these cities, the older inhabitants moved to the suburbs and began erecting barriers that would prohibit annexation without their consent. They drew on the tradition of local community government to protect their economic, ethnic, and racial exclusivity. As a result, these cities became the most racially segregated in the country, as well as the least elastic.[25] That is, they are cities that have failed to expand their geographic boundaries to capture suburban growth. Consequently, the metropolitan areas of which they are a part are divided into many different municipalities, each with their own taxing authorities, school systems, and exclusionary zoning practices. The effect has been to create relatively affluent suburbs and poverty-stricken, unhealthy inner cities.

Thus, the civic culture that impressed so many observers has also worked to strangle solutions to problems that were never anticipated when the colonies were established. And this suggests that local governments may cause as many problems as they solve, for they may introduce rigidity and divisiveness into social structures that require flexibility and integration.

Voluntary Associations. Even more than New England town meetings, voluntary associations have been said to be the seedbed of American democracy.[26] They are, it is claimed, where citizens learn how to work together, to compromise for the sake of realizing a common goal, and to trust one another. Because individuals belong to many associations, it is also claimed that there are cross-cutting ties that bind communities together. Thus they are said to be a cohesive, not a divisive, force in American life.[27]

The state has little role in this version of the story. But there is another version, for both Tocqueville, and later, in the nineteenth century, his country-man Emil Durkheim, saw voluntary associations as not simply the places where individuals learned to work with and trust one another, but as interme-diating institutions between a powerful central government and the unpro-tected and thus easily manipulated citizen. Tocqueville wrote:

> An association for political, commercial, or manufacturing purposes, or even for those of science and literature, is a powerful and enlight-ened member of the community, which cannot be disposed of at pleasure, or oppressed without remonstrance: and which, by defend-ing its own rights against encroachments of the government, saves the common liberties of the country.[28]

Durkheim, whose name and study of suicide are cited and recited like a mantra in virtually every article in the field of social epidemiology,[29] made similar observations. Rates and patterns of suicide were, he argued, just one instance of "the whole of our historical development," the "chief characteris-tic [of which] is to have swept cleanly away all the older forms of social orga-nization." He continued, "The great change brought about by the French Revolution was precisely to carry this leveling to a point hitherto unknown. . . . Only one collective form survived the tempest: the State. . . . [I]ndividuals are no longer subject to any other collective control but the State, so it is the sole organized collectivity."[30] And he used the same metaphor of mass soci-ety used by many of his contemporaries. "Individuals," he said, "tumble over one another like so many liquid molecules."[31] He dismissed the solu-tion proposed by other writers: "the restitution of local groups of some-thing of their old autonomy," and advocated instead a different sort of intermediating institution: corporatism. "The only decentralization which would make possible the multiplication of the centers of communal life without weakening national unity is what might be called *occupational decentralization*."[32]

In 1891, 6 years before Durkheim published *Suicide*, Pope Leo XIII had is-sued the encyclical *Rerum Novarum*,[33] that made a similar point: "[T]he an-cient workingmen's guilds were abolished in the last century, and no other protective organization took their place. Public institutions and the laws set aside the ancient religion. Hence, by degrees it has come to pass that working men have been surrendered, isolated and helpless, to the hardheartedness of employers and the greed of unchecked competition." He supported a wide va-riety of voluntary associations, the most important of which were working-men's unions. "It is [a] natural impulse which binds men together in civil society; and it is likewise this which leads them to join together in associations which are, it is true, lesser and not independent societies, but, nevertheless, real societies." It is an obligation of the state to protect the natural right to join associations, he continued. Or, as the influential Jesuit economist Heinrich Pesch wrote in 1918:

> In the place of egotistical self-interest and atomistic divisiveness
> there must be *a solidarity among members of the same political
> community*. At the same time, political society achieves its natural
> formation by the *solidaristic association of members of the same
> occupation* into vocational organizations which effectively represent
> the interests of their group.[34]

Thus, in the European context, voluntary associations were widely viewed as significant sources of protection for individuals. As Tocqueville observed, they were also important in the United States. Whether as an intermediating institution between individuals and the state, or as a place where individuals learned cooperation, democratic participation, and trust, or both, they had an important place in the United States in the nineteenth and twentieth centuries. Between the Revolution and the Civil War, they proliferated across a growing country, not simply in the Northeast but in other regions as well.[35]

There were many reasons. (1) That there was no official state church meant that many religions and denominations proliferated and competed for members. (2) After the Revolution, "citizenship idealized political participation and initiative."[36] (3) The Second Great Awakening reinforced republican principles of individual volition and noncoercion and made voluntary associations the vehicle for moral crusades, such as antislavery and temperance. (4) Voluntary associations were also practical vehicles for other forms of mutual aid and capitalist enterprise, especially in the absence of strong central authority.[37] Indeed, in the antebellum period, the same laws of incorporation formed the legal basis for civic associations and business enterprises.[38] (5) Voluntary associations were adaptive because the state was weak.[39]

While the antebellum period saw the growth of voluntary associations in cities as diverse as New York, New Orleans, and San Francisco,[40] it was in the period between the Civil War and World War I that voluntary associations enjoyed their greatest growth, both in terms of the number of associations and the proportion of the population that were members. Though it is usually thought that large cities with rapidly growing, diverse populations were especially fertile soil, Gerald Gamm and Robert Putnam have showed, based on a sample of 26 cities, that small cities in the Midwest and West provided even more fertile soil.[41]

Though considered a manifestation of community, much evidence suggests the reverse. On his visit to the United States in 1904, Max Weber observed that the functions of religious sects had changed. He wrote of an American he visited, he "belongs to an 'order' ":

> His credit rating is based largely on this—to which one is elected at
> the suggestion of five members and from which one is expelled for
> bad conduct. It is a health insurance, a burial fund, and a widows'
> pension fund; the members are pledged to mutual aid and obligated
> to grant credit in cases of blameless economic distress; expulsion is
> the punishment for an unmotivated refusal.

Once this was the most important function of American sects. The tremendous increase in the clubs and orders here is a substitute for the crumbling organization of sects.[42]

As Robert V. Hine has observed, "this was the distinction he [Weber] would later make between intuitive, traditional communality with its feelings of belonging, and rational association based on expedient self-interest."[43] Hine shows further that in one Midwestern and Western town after another in the late nineteenth century, voluntary associations were more divisive than integrative.[44] And Page Smith commented that "Such a plethora of organizations is obviously a disease of the body politic in communities which have lost all sense of an integrated community life."[45]

This became evident in studies of Midwestern towns and small cities in the 1920s, 1930s, and early 1940s. All show that voluntary associations worked to reinforce the class structure, not to knit communities more tightly.[46] Memberships were largely limited to one or two classes without much overlap. The higher the social class of a family, the greater was the number of its memberships. Exclusivity was a relatively new phenomenon in the 1920s, according to Robert S. Lynd and Helen Merrell Lynd. In their 1924 study of Middletown, a mid-sized Midwestern city, they found that the early clubs had tended to be relatively inclusive. By the time of their study, however, club life was changing. Upper-class men left the lodges that had been relatively inclusive to join clubs such as Rotary and Kiwanis. These clubs for the business class were said to be civic in nature, but the civic activities in which they engaged were relatively innocuous: driving a crippled student to school, providing a radio for the local orphanage, or, more impressively, making schoolyards available as playgrounds.

> The lack of coherence in the subjects of the speeches to which each of these clubs listens week after week and in the noncontroversial occasional charity which constitutes their civic work suggests that, as in the women's study clubs, the reason for their dominance lies in neither of these activities but in the instrumental and symbolic character of their organization. Not only are they a business asset, but by their use of first names, sending of flowers on birthdays, and similar devices, they tend to re-create in part an informal social intercourse becoming increasingly rare in this wary urban civilization. . . .
>
> Certainly it is true that a wide gap exists between the activities of the civic clubs and the major maladjustments of which Middletown complains . . . [T]he clubs exist primarily as an adjunct to the business interests of their members and as a pleasant way of spending leisure; chiefly as a supplement to these interests and in regions where no enemies will be made or no ructions raised do the clubs become "civic."[47]

What was true of Middletown also seems to have been true of Jonesville, Plainville, and Elmtown. First, associations in the small and medium-sized cities of the American heartland can hardly be seen as a unifying force teaching democratic values, cooperation, and tolerance. Far from it. They functioned to reinforce the class structure and to assure domination of the community by the elite.

Second, the descriptions of the role of associations suggest a reason why associational growth was so much more rapid in places like these than in large cities of the Northeast in the late nineteenth and early twentieth centuries. Clubs and associations were increasingly and largely a way for different classes and ethnic groups to distinguish themselves, and specifically for the well-to-do to separate themselves from those with less income and wealth. Suburbanization served the same purpose, and cities of the Northeast suburbanized earlier than cities elsewhere. Thus, clubs and associations may have been the functional equivalent of suburbanization in places where segregation by residence and school system may have been less easily achieved than it could be in the suburbs of large cities.

Class differences in association membership continued to be important in Middletown into the late 1970s, more than 50 years after the Lynds did their original study. Membership in labor unions was more likely among the working class. There was no difference in the social class membership in veterans' groups, farmers' associations, and political committees. Every other type of organization overwhelmingly involved the business class, as had been the case two or three generations earlier.[48]

Membership in locally based organizations has declined since the 1970s, for reasons that are not obvious.[49] Whatever the reason, the decline in involvement in face-to-face organizations is equated to a loss of social capital, but it is reasonable to wonder (1) whether the club activities described in Middletown, Jonesville, Plainville, and Elmtown really had any impact on improving either the civic good or generalized trust in those communities, and (2) whether declining membership in such organizations is as problematic as is claimed. For the club activities that were described by observers seem more likely to have promoted exclusivity and mistrust than inclusiveness and trust, and mortality declined throughout the twentieth century regardless of the growth or decline of voluntary associations.

Associationalism and Health

Social capitalists assert that membership in face-to-face associations promotes health. There are two closely related components that are said to be important, structural and cognitive.

> The *structural component* of social capital includes the extent and intensity of associational links and activity in society (e.g., density of civic associations, measures of informal sociability, indicators of civic engagement). The *cognitive component* assesses people's

perceptions of the level of interpersonal trust, sharing, and reciprocity.[50]

Although the distinction is often arbitrary, each is considered in turn.

The Cognitive Component. In respect of trust, several studies have shown an association with mortality and self-rated health: the greater the trust, the lower the mortality and the greater the self-rated health.[51] Two measures of social capital—what is also sometimes called social cohesion, membership in voluntary associations and the proportion of people agreeing with the statement "most people can be trusted," are significantly correlated with age-adjusted mortality rates across the 39 states for which data were available. Income inequality is also associated with mortality, and it is argued that social capital—trust and association membership—is the link between them: where income inequality is high, social capital is low, and thus, mortality is high.

The correlations between indicators of social capital (including trust) and mortality are not always as expected, and where they are in the expected direction, social capital may be an epiphenomenon for reasons other than those suggested above. With respect to the unexpected findings, data from Canada indicate that neither trust nor civic participation is associated with self-rated health.[52] It is also significant that in international comparisons among high-income countries, social trust is unassociated with self-reported health,[53] and social trust and organizational membership are weakly, inconsistently, or not at all associated with mortality at different ages and from different causes.[54] For example, the greater the level of distrust, the *lower* the death rate from coronary heart disease among both women and men. The greater the average number of organizations to which people in a country belong, the lower was the death rate from cirrhosis (marginally significant at conventional levels, $p = 0.05$ for both women and men). There was no association between either distrust or organizational membership and life expectancy. Moreover, it was just the period when social capital was said to be declining in the United States, from the 1960s through the 1990s, that saw dramatic decreases in death rates and increases in life expectancy, in the United States as well as in most other developed countries.

With respect to the suggestion that trust is an epiphenomenon in those instances where the association with health is significant, it is noteworthy that all the American states where inequality is high, social capital is low, and mortality is high are in the South.[55] All are states where governments are weak and spending on health, education, and welfare is low. It is perhaps not surprising that in such an environment, trust is low, for lack of trust may be the result of weak political institutions, and those same weak political institutions may be implicated in the high levels of income inequality and low levels of spending on social services that characterize that part of the country.

Conservatives claim that as governments wax, voluntary associations wane.[56] Historically in the United States, this may have been the case, but as a generalization the evidence is not persuasive. Americans are among the most likely to be members of voluntary associations when compared to samples from 14 other developed countries. However, when church membership is excluded, the rank drops very substantially, and it drops even further when only active or working membership is counted.[57] Evidently church membership does not spill over into greater involvement in voluntary community activity in the United States. Why church membership is so high in the United States is a question that goes well beyond the confines of this chapter. It suffices to say that in the absence of a state church, in the presence of great ethnic and cultural heterogeneity, and as a result of aggressive marketing by various denominations, high membership should perhaps not be a surprise.

Furthermore, in Sweden, a generous welfare state, levels of associational participation and trust are high, and people trust both other people (horizontal trust) and institutions of law and order (vertical trust). Bo Rothstein writes, "There seems to be no reason why there should be a causal mechanism between trusting other people and trusting these two particular institutions. One possibility is that the causal link runs the other way around; that is, if you trust the institutions that are supposed to keep law and order, you also trust other people."[58] If the governing institutions treat all who violate the law in a fair and effective fashion, then individuals will trust those institutions, and they will trust others because the chances of their getting away with illegal behavior are small, and they can therefore be counted upon to act within the law. Similarly, Rothstein suggests, precisely because the welfare programs in Sweden are universal, no one benefits unfairly and there is no threat to civil society. Indeed, one may go further and argue that when governing institutions are not trusted, voluntary associations such as militias and racist groups may become prevalent and highly destructive, as happened in Germany between the two world wars.[59]

More generally, Peter Evans has argued on the basis of case studies in several developing countries that the rule of law is "important as a complement to the efforts of less privileged groups to organized themselves . . . [T]he provision and enforcement of universal rules is an invaluable organizational resource for the less privileged."[60] The rule of law and the cooperation of agents of the government with the public in the provision of basic services (e.g., irrigation, health services, law enforcement) generates "relations of trust."

For all these reasons, it seems likely that the association between trust and low mortality, when it exists at all, is best accounted for by the fact that they are both found in places where the governing institutions are viewed as fair and responsive, and such institutions are likely to be perceived as fair when they dispense justice and services evenhandedly and equitably.

The Structural Component. The other component of social capital is structural, including measures of civic engagement. Although some of the data reported immediately above do not support the association between civic en-

gagement and health, it is somewhat more obvious how this component could
be associated with reduced mortality, for voluntary associations may provide
services themselves, and they may lobby some level of government for programs and policies that have a beneficial impact on health.

During the Progressive Era in late nineteenth- and early twentieth-century
America, voluntary associations proliferated and were extraordinarily active in
agitating for reform, particularly at the municipal level but also at the federal
level, and many of the reforms for which they worked were either directly or
indirectly health related, such as garbage collection, street cleaning, milk sta-
tions for the urban poor, and teaching hygiene to immigrants and school children. For example, a partial list of some of the organizations with which John
Collier, a reformer who worked first for the People's Institute and then for Indian rights in the 1910s and 1920s before becoming Commissioner of Indian
Affairs during the New Deal Administration, was associated included the National Playground Association, the National Conference of Community Centers, the Committee on Public Education, the Gramercy Park Community
Clearing House, the National Conference of Social Work, the Greater New York
Community Council, the Child Health Organization, the General Federation of
Women's Clubs, the National League for Constructive Immigration Legislation,
the Boy Scouts of America, the Camp Fire Girls, The California League for
American Indians, the Indian Rights Association, the New Mexico Association
on Indian Affairs, the Eastern Association on Indian Affairs, the National Popular Government League, the League for Political Education, the American Indian Defense Association, and the Wilderness Society.[61] Many of these were
local in orientation, but many were also aimed at shaping federal policy.

Simon Szreter has observed that in Robert Putnam's account of the Gilded
Age and the Progressive Era, government is strangely absent.[62] He makes a point
similar to the one made by Edward Devine in 1913: many of the voluntary associations created in the late nineteenth and early twentieth centuries were
"founded mainly for the purpose of influencing governmental action, either directly, or through the development of public opinion."[63] Much of what reformers did was to work with and mobilize governments to provide better services or
to regulate unscrupulous businessmen and practitioners (e.g., physicians).

Szreter and Michael Woolcock,[64] argue that there are several kinds of
social capital: bonding, bridging, and linking. Bonding "refers to networks
formed from perceived, shared identity relations"—for example, kin groups
and ethnic communities. Bridging refers to networks in which shared identity
relations may not be significant and in which people may come from different
backgrounds and groups.[65] Linking social capital "refers to the relationships of
exchange, which are established between parties who know themselves not
only to be unlike, as in the case of bridging social capital, but furthermore to
be unequal in their power and their access to resources."

> It takes on a democratic and empowering character where those
> involved are endeavoring to achieve a mutually agreed beneficial

goal (or set of goals) on a basis of mutual respect, trust, and equality of status, despite the manifest inequalities in their respective positions. [66]

Much of the work done by social reformers would count as linking social capital. Jane Addams of Hull House, for instance, mobilized immigrants and also worked to improve the quality of the neighborhoods in which they lived through active involvement with the government of Chicago. Clearly, this was meant to promote the well-being of the immigrant community. Another example is the way advocates of compulsory health insurance during this period made cross-class alliances in such organizations as the American Association for Labor Legislation and numerous labor unions.

But bridging and linking social capital could also be used for purposes that many progressives did not support. The National Civic Federation, made up of business and labor leaders strongly and successfully opposed the passage of compulsory health insurance, for instance. Similarly active in opposing compulsory health insurance were the many fraternal lodges that provided health insurance and burial benefits to their members.[67] Thus, bonding, bridging, and linking social capital were present on each side of the issue. Ultimately, such patterns of cooperation and alliances have evolved into the interest-group politics that have been characterized as "iron triangles."[68] More generally, linking social capital may also take the form of nepotism, favoritism, and corruption as exemplified by the urban political machines found in so many American cities in the late nineteenth and early twentieth centuries.

Local governments may involve their citizens in civic life, as Tocqueville suggested, but they may also promote exclusivity and protect citizens from integration into larger regional structures that may be widely beneficial. Associations "for political, commercial, or manufacturing purposes" may protect their own interests, as Tocqueville and Durkheim both suggested, but in the process may be harmful to the health and well-being of the public. This is amply demonstrated by the opposition of the tobacco industry trade association to limitations on cigarette advertising and sales, and by the destruction of President Clinton's plan for health care reform by a coalition of voluntary associations including the National Rifle Association, the Christian Coalition, the National Federation of Independent Businesses, and the Health Insurance Association of America.[69] Churches may be the most integrative institutions in Hispanic and African American communities, but their deep conservatism prevented them from acting early in the AIDS crisis and has contributed to its severity.[70]

The point is twofold. First, social capital of all varieties can be mobilized for very different goals. This means that voluntary associations do not necessarily create "community" and the benefits to health that community is believed to foster. They are every bit as likely to create conflict. Thus, it should not be a surprise that mortality rates from ischemic heart disease declined beginning the 1960s as association membership was also declining nationwide, for there is no necessary connection between associationalism and health, despite Robert Putnam's assertion to the contrary. He has written, "[A]s a rough rule of thumb, if you belong to no groups but decide to join one, you cut your risk of dying over the next year *in half*. If you smoke and belong to no groups, it's a toss-up statistically whether you should stop smoking or start joining."[71] This is clever rhetoric but bad—indeed irresponsible—advice. It confuses relative risk (a measure of causal force) with population-attributable risk (the proportion of a particular disease attributable to a particular cause). Relative risk may be high, or at least statically significant, but the amount of disease actually caused by the risk factor may be quite small. In the case of group membership and smoking, the mixed consequences of the former and the unequivocal ill effects of the latter mean that the decision is not a toss-up, either statistically or for an individual smoker.

Second, voluntary associations as often as not are concerned with trying to get some level of government to do, or not do, something. The remarkable absence of political institutions from consideration in many of the epidemiological studies of the health benefits of social capital results in the idealization of "community" and "trust" without adequately working through how each may be created and destroyed, and work for good or ill, in large and diverse nation states with different histories, cultures, and styles of governance. Social capital may be valuable in facilitating certain actions, as James Coleman wrote, but "may be useless or even harmful for others."[72]

Social Capital and Primary Groups

Just as social capital is fast becoming a paradigm with which to explain inequalities in health at the societal level, so in the form of social support and integration has it become important in studies of the health of individuals.[73] For investigators who write on the association between health and the social support provided by kin and friends have begun to draw on the literature on social capital as well. And as in studies at the societal level, so too at the individual level are there anomalous results that should encourage a more nuanced way of thinking about the processes at work.

The studies of social support and integration on the one hand and subsequent mortality on the other have shown that when support is high, the risk of mortality tends to be reduced, even after controlling for various measures of health status. The effects are particularly strong for white males. They are much weaker or nonexistent for women[74] and for non-whites, including African Americans,[75] Japanese-Americans,[76] and Navajo Indians,[77] all primarily rural populations.[78] One commentator has suggested that such anomalies "have to do with the extent to which women and blacks are deeply integrated into stable, rural communities. . . . Under such circumstances, if these groups routinely obtain large doses of social support, specific measures tapping frequency of contact and size of network may be less differentiating than in less-well-integrated communities.

Furthermore, these sources of support may be so much a part of the normal daily lives of these people that they commonly go unnoticed and, as a result, are underreported in surveys of this sort. In urban areas, where people are more mobile, their awareness of sources of support and frequency of contact may be heightened."[79]

Indeed, it may well be that the differences are simply the result of (1) methodological difficulties; the instruments that have been used to measure integration and support may be too blunt to dissect subtle distinctions among populations where support is generally high, or (2) the fact that the places in which no effects have been observed have so few isolated people that no effect could ever be demonstrated, no matter how good the instruments for measuring isolation.

On the other hand, the notion that these anomalous results may be explained by the pervasiveness of social support rather than by its absence assumes that which must be demonstrated. It may be that there are true differences in the structure, meaning, and functioning of social networks in different populations and settings. For example, in a study in one southern community, it was found that African Americans had lower levels of support than whites,[80] rather than higher levels as suggested in the previous quotation. Moreover, while family networks have been shown to be important sources of support among African Americans, the conflictual and nonsupportive side of such networks has also been noted.[81]

Furthermore, in a variety of studies, women are found to report higher use of support than men, but they are also more likely than men to provide support. "Thus, women may be more likely to be exposed to negative social outcomes regarding both themselves and others than is true for men. Women with larger networks may be more involved in dealing with the stresses of others and thus experience more stress than women with smaller networks or than men."[82] Indeed, the study of "caretaker stress" has become something of a cottage industry, and the results consistently show that people who care for disabled kin are more susceptible to a variety of illnesses than people who do not.[83]

Finally, living in poverty, living in a rural area, or living in a poor country means that informal social networks and primary groups are called upon to provide a broader range of services than they are in settings where the availability of, and access to, formal services are greater.[84] Without an infrastructure of public health services, widely accessible health care, public schools, a legal justice system, and other formal institutions, the establishment and maintenance of personal networks—what has been called "bonding" social capital—are a matter of survival.[85] But social networks may also impose heavy burdens, for example when reciprocity is required by other members, when gossip and other forms of coercion are used to control behavior, or when no social services are available to ease the burdens of family caregivers. That, of course, is one of the reasons people have fled small towns for large cities. Kinship and friendship networks are not unambiguously supportive and may exact very high costs.[86] This is especially true where poverty and the absence of formal institutions force people to depend upon informal networks for all forms of assistance both large and small.

Not only are different contexts associated with differences in the services provided by personal networks, but the structure of networks is different as well. In general, "studies in several Western countries show that close relatives, especially parents, continue to be of central importance in personal networks. There are, however, differences between rural and urban populations and between social strata in the importance of extended kin as compared to friends and acquaintances. In larger cities as well as in middle classes, relations with extended kin become looser, while those with friends and acquaintances gain in importance."[87]

And network structure has profound consequences, even among different social strata in the same society. For example, in secure settings such as those in which the middle and upper classes in developed countries live, loose networks based upon friendship—perhaps meeting the criteria of "bridging" social capital—are particularly well suited to obtaining jobs as well as needed services from a broad array of formal organizations.[88] In contrast, dense networks in urban ghettos in the United States—perhaps an example of "bonding" social capital—isolate people from information about the availability of jobs and services elsewhere in the city.[89]

Some of the complexities of the associations between social context and the structure, function, and effectiveness of social networks are suggested by the results of several studies among Navajo Indians in the American Southwest. Indian reservations such as the Navajo's are generally rural and characterized by high rates of poverty and unemployment. Traditionally, extended families have been both a common as well as the ideal form of social organization and, in many instances, still are because they are adaptive to the prevailing unstable economic conditions.[90] This pattern is changing substantially, however, as people move to towns on and off the reservation.

In a study of social integration and subsequent mortality among Navajo men and women 65 years of age and above, only marital status was significantly associated with an increased risk of death, and only among men over the age of 75. No other measures of isolation or integration were significant.[91] This was because in the Navajo context social integration meant that the family had to carry a heavy burden. For instance, a significant number of the elderly lived with adult children with physical or psychological disabilities for whom no institutional or day care services were available, and for whom the elderly parent was a major source of financial and other support. Rates of depression were significantly higher among these respondents than among people without such burdensome responsibilities.

Among women of childbearing age, use of contraception was more likely by those who were not living with their kin than among those who were, even adjusting for parity and education. This was because in a generally pronatalist setting, women of childbearing age who lived in extended family arrangements were subjected to intense social pressure, and sometimes physical coercion, from their mothers and husbands not to use contraception, whereas those living in independent households were more autonomous and able to exercise choice.[92]

But the freedom associated with independent households is a mixed blessing. Young people who grew up in extended families learned to use alcohol in settings that emphasized responsibilities to kin and therefore shaped their careers as drinkers. While heavy drinking often led to serious difficulties, it was generally outgrown before catastrophe occurred.[93] However, as the livestock economy has declined, people have left rural areas and residence within extended families and moved to reservation towns where they live in independent households, near unrelated neighbors, and attend school with nonrelatives. In these new settings, the cross-generational fabric has been torn and a youth culture has emerged which, at the extremes, is characterized by gangs, violence, drug use, and high-risk drinking.[94] As a result, the homicide rate has tripled on the Reservation since the 1960s. Thus, the same freedom from kin which has increased the likelihood of contraceptive use has also resulted in the creation of social networks that encourage destructive and self-destructive behavior.

These brief examples have been meant to suggest some of the ways in which the larger context may influence the structure, functions, and effectiveness of social networks, and how these may, in turn, influence various dimensions of peoples' health and use of services. That is to say, social relations are not always supportive and may be damaging. This is particularly so when poverty, unemployment, insecurity, and inadequate infrastructure of formal institutions are prevalent. Under such conditions, people have little choice in those upon whom they must depend, and the consequences of enforced dependence on kinsmen may be quite mixed, for they may be oppressive as well as supportive. This is unlike the situation of the well-to-do in developed countries, where a good deal of freedom may be exercised in the choice of network members, where networks are looser, and where in any event the need for support from informal sources is less than in many other parts of the world. It is this sort of complexity that explains why social relations that are often assumed to be a form of social capital and of positive value may be of little value or actually harmful.

The Roseto Effect

The community studies of Middletown, Elmtown, Jonesville, and Plaineville, not to mention all the urban sociological studies in Chicago and other major cities, have not had an impact on the methodological individualism of epidemiological studies of Framingham, Evans County, Alameda County, Tecumseh and Whitehall. Virtually all the data from the latter studies are ego-centered and nothing much is ever said of the historical and sociocultural context of each setting. One would never know, for instance, that the study in Evans County, Georgia was done during the years of the civil rights movement. Did that make a difference in the results? We don't know. Certainly the reader is never given an adequate understanding of how the social organization and culture of each place may have shaped the results. We know there are "neighborhood" effects on mortality and self-perceived health in addition to those reported for individual level risk factors,[95] but "neighborhood" remains a black box and we are left with the impression that the results from the individual level analyses are generalizable to other populations.

An important exception to this observation is the study of Roseto, a town in Pennsylvania that had been established in the late nineteenth century by immigrants from a town of the same name in southern Italy. It was of interest to medical investigators because a local physician had observed that people in the community had an unusually low incidence of heart attacks, unlike those from neighboring towns,[96] and the resulting study is widely cited as an important example of the health-promoting effects of equality and social capital.

After several rounds of medical examinations, interviews, and reviews of historical records and vital statistics, Stewart Wolf and John Bruhn concluded that the low incidence of heart attacks in Roseto was attributable to the egalitarianism and cohesiveness of the community and to the commitment of family members to one another. On the basis of changes in local values and ways of living, they predicted in the 1960s, as the third generation was reaching maturity, that the incidence of heart attacks would increase, as indeed it did. The third generation was said to aspire to independence, comforts, and even luxuries that were unknown to their parents and grandparents, and it was this growth of inequality and individualism that the investigators believed would cause the increase. "While Rosetans were becoming better educated and more prosperous as their contacts with the outside world broadened, they were also becoming less family-centered and less cohesive, less willing to sacrifice for family, friends, and neighbors. As a community, they were also becoming less self contained."[97] "It is intriguing," they wrote elsewhere, "to try to relate the striking shifts in the social environment of Roseto to the equally impressive change in the death rate from coronary disease and in the prevalence of coronary disease among the living. The timing of the two events fits quite well our original hypothesis that social cohesion and cooperative attitudes were protective against coronary disease in Roseto and that contrary attitudes are destructive."[98] In their conclusion they wrote:

> There are elements of the Roseto story that, during the short interval of a hundred years, parallel in miniature the history of great powers in ancient Western civilization, Greece and Rome. In each case there was a coming together under early influence of inspirational leaders, followed by a period of comfortable prosperity. Ultimately, there

developed signs of self-indulgence with a weakening of commitment to traditional values and a lack of responsibility for the community.[99]

Roseto in the first half of the twentieth century was a cohesive community, more so even than the village from which the original immigrants had come, and more than many other villages in southern Italy as well.[100] This was the result of hostility on the part of non-Italians in neighboring communities, as well as other hardships. Even among the first generation of settlers, however, the seeds of subsequent changes were evident in the envy, lack of trust of those outside the family, and competition—what has been called amoral familism—that have been described by Clement Valletta, an anthropologist who studied the community.[101] It appears that external pressure made the first generation "much less concern[ed] with appearing different or a 'little better' in having . . . material objects" than the second generation.[102] Nonetheless, their decision not to remain peasants, their ambition, and their early involvement in industry (slate quarrying and blouse manufacturing) set the stage for the differentiation that developed in the second generation. "[W]anting to progress, Carnetans [the name used by Valletta instead of Roseto] opened their own small plants with the money they saved. Once this happened, the spiral of . . . imitative competition was begun. This experience was also followed by padrones [family heads], in the construction business, who competed as a family business for contracts . . . [C]ooperation among the mills was so difficult that owners were 'cutting each other's throats' for work. One padrone wanted the town council to control the number of new entrants into the business," but this proved impossible.[103]

In addition to the competition created within the community by the establishment of several mills and construction businesses, another major force for change internally was the number of second-generation women who worked in the blouse factories and who earned income they used to purchase better material goods. This too led to competition among families. For example, a second-generation mother objected when her son and his wife decided to place their television set in their bedroom, fearing that "others might think that the couple could not afford a television."[104] Externally, growing acceptance by neighboring communities and the larger society made the internal cohesiveness less of a necessity as well.

The impression from Valletta's study is that consumerism did indeed increase over the three generations, but envy and competition had always been present. Thus, even though at midcentury homes and cars looked similar, there were important status differences and competition for business opportunities and income that make one wonder whether the harmony and community spirit that also existed in the town were sufficient to keep the first two generations protected from heart attacks.

These two ways of seeing community life in Roseto, as characterized by conflict or cooperation, mirror a long-standing debate in the social sciences about the nature of peasant communities in general. On one hand is the romantic view of preindustrial communities as just that, *communities*, characterized by face-to-face, supportive relationships. On the other hand is the view of peasant villages divided by family loyalties, feuds, and jealousy. In a frequently cited and contentious article in this latter tradition, George Foster wrote:

> By "Image of Limited Good" I mean that broad areas of peasant behavior are patterned in such fashion as to suggest that peasants view their social, economic, and natural universes—their total environment—as one in which all of the desired things in life such as land, wealth, health, friendship and love, manliness and honor, respect and status, power and influence, security and safety, *exist in finite quantity* and *are always in short supply*, as far as the peasant is concerned. Not only do all these "good things" exist in finite and limited quantities, but in addition *there is no way within peasant power to increase the available quantities.*[105]

Foster argued that much peasant behavior could be understood as shaped by this image of limited good. "People who see themselves in 'threatened' circumstances, which the Image of Limited Good implies, react normally in one of two ways: maximum cooperation and sometimes communism, burying individual differences and placing sanctions against individuals, or extreme individualism. Peasant societies seem always to choose the second alternative."[106] Cooperation, Foster wrote, was neither necessary nor common in peasant villages, but since goods are finite, success of any individual or family could only be achieved at the expense of others. Thus, to avoid jealousy or worse, it was common not to "reveal evidence of material or other improvements in [one's] relative position, lest [one] invite sanctions."[107] According to this view, the egalitarianism in Roseto was a manifestation of the fear of sanctions characteristic of peasant communities.

Foster's conception of the nature of peasant life is not without its critics. There is substantial evidence from both Europe and America that cooperation was a significant—indeed necessary—fact of peasant life. Peasant villages could not have survived without it. For example, in Europe, communal governments managed the use of resources such as common land, and communal cooperation and unity were reinforced by the necessity to jointly meet obligations to the seigneur and the sovereign.[108] In northern New Mexico, to take but one North American example, Hispanic villages could not have survived without irrigation that was managed by the community, and many scholars believe that cooperation rather than atomism and competition characterized these villages.[109]

What seems most likely is that both aspects of peasant village life were present. Cooperation was necessary for survival, but factions, feuds, and individual and family ambition were not infrequent either. As external forces requiring cohesion lessened—the decline of seigneurial obligations in Europe, the decline of hostility toward Italian immigrants in America, the loss of common land to the U.S. government and to Anglo-Americans by Hispanic villages in northern New Mexico—village cohesion became less necessary for survival and individualism and factionalism could be expressed more openly. Thus, in Roseto, the egalitarianism and cooperation invoked by Wolf and Bruhn were no doubt real and the result of external forces excluding Italians from participation in the wider life of the area, but equally real and always present were the amoral familism, conflict, and competition described by Valletta that became more obvious as external pressure for solidarity lessened. Because conflict, competition, and status distinctions were always present, one must wonder how much of the increase in heart disease can be explained by their increasingly visible display.

In addition, there have been a number of questions raised about the validity of the reported results with respect to death rates from heart disease.[110] The population is very small and the number of events even smaller. Even assuming that the rates are accurate and do differ significantly from those of neighboring non-Italian towns,[111] however, there is an alternative explanation to the one usually offered. John Lynch and George Davey Smith[112] have proposed that the original settlers, who came from Italy, had different diets from their neighbors, who were of German, English, Welsh, and Scots-Irish origin. Indeed, we know that the first generation in Roseto raised and prepared all their own food,[113] that most of the men engaged in hard physical labor, and that, in general, Italian immigrants and their first-generation descendants typically had lower rates of coronary heart disease than immigrants from northern Europe.[114] Their resistance to heart disease was lost within one or two generations, however, as diets and exercise patterns changed, suggesting that such changes were very likely an important cause of the increase in coronary artery disease and deaths from myocardial infarctions.

Thus, there are two reasons to be wary of citing the Roseto Effect as evidence for the importance of social capital as a protection against heart disease. One has to do with the fact that the community may not have been as cohesive and cooperative as has usually been presented. The other is that a plausible alternative explanation is ready at hand. Nonetheless, despite these serious reservations, this is an important and all-too-rare kind of study, for it is one of a very few that actually attempts to grapple seriously with the nature of the community being studied and the way changes over a long period have affected the health of its people. For that alone we should be grateful.

Conclusion

Social capital is but the most recent manifestation of the quest for community that has run through much of Western thought for the past two centuries.[115] Many of the most powerful social thinkers of the nineteenth and twentieth centuries have feared that the destruction of communities and the alienation and anomie that followed would leave only the omnipotent state confronting unprotected individuals. Tocqueville and Durkheim were too realistic to think that an idealized world of small, local communities could ever be reconstituted after the great transformations brought about by industrialization and the French revolution. They thought, however, that intermediating institutions such as voluntary associations might protect individual citizens from the worst excesses of the state.

But voluntary associations can be anti- as well as pro-civic. They may be most "civic" when the institutions of the state are most effective. Sheri Berman has observed that the answer to the question of "when civil society activity produces social or unsocial capital?" is that "It depends heavily on the political context."

> If a country's political institutions are capable of channeling and redressing grievances, then associationism will probably buttress political stability and democracy by placing its resources and beneficial effects in the service of the status quo. This is the pattern Tocqueville described.
>
> If, on the other hand, political institutions are weak and/or the existing political regime is perceived to be ineffectual and illegitimate, then civil activity may become an alternative to politics for dissatisfied citizens, increasingly absorbing their energies and satisfying their basic needs. In such situations, associationism will probably undermine political stability and have negative consequences for democracy by deepening cleavages, furthering dissatisfaction, and providing rich soil for oppositional movements.[116]

Dissident activity is not always a bad thing, of course, depending upon the government and issues involved. Nonetheless, the point is that civil society activity is not always pro-social. Berman points out that in the United States, charter schools, gated communities, private police and guard services, and right-wing militias all meet Tocqueville's criteria of classic American voluntary associations, and yet they may be regarded in some senses as deeply antisocial.[117] The same may be said of the privatization of a wide variety of public services. They represent a failure—or perhaps more accurately, the destruction—of political institutions, not simply the vitality of civil society.[118]

The illegitimacy of political institutions has an impact not only upon secondary associations but upon (1) the level of trust in institutions and other citizens expressed by respondents to surveys, and (2) the structure and functioning of primary groups. Where political institutions are distant, inequitable, and illegitimate, trust is likely to be low, and primary groups are likely to be relied upon heavily.

In the United States, the federal government was created according to a model brought by the earliest settlers who came from England before the parliamentary revolution. As a result, American political institutions are not as centralized as they were becoming in England and on the Continent in the seventeenth century, and the federal government has been relatively weak, for political authority has been dispersed through many institutions and levels of government. In many respects, this is no bad thing. On the other hand, with much power devolved to states and lower levels of government, in such a highly diverse country with such different regional histories, economies, and cultures, the potential for inequity in some places is very real. This has been the case especially in cities of the Northeast and in the American South.

In the South, the legacy of slavery as well as the culture of settlers from the Southeast of England and from the Celtic fringe of the British Isles have left a lasting imprint.[119] Political institutions were dominated by and run for the benefit of a white elite; poor whites and African Americans were set against one another; and there continue to be (1) low levels of support for education and health care, (2) high levels of income inequality, (3) high levels of distrust, and (4) worse mortality rates than in other regions of the country. That is to say, social capital is lower in the South than elsewhere because the political institutions are perceived by many to be inequitable. Low levels of expenditure on services and inequity have led to continuing high rates of mortality. The result is an association between low social capital and high mortality, but this is because both are the result of a common cause, the failure of local and state governments to deal equitably with all their citizens and to provide the services that are the *raison d'etre* of governments at this level.

The quest for community represented by the recent great outpouring of interest in social capital is also associated with the pessimistic position in the standard-of-living debate. The destruction of traditional communities and the freeing—indeed, the creation—of individuals is precisely what the pessimists regard as the excessively high costs of economic expansion. This is clear from the assertions of the strong association in rich countries between income inequality and the decline of both civic participation and generalized trust. It is also clear in the statement quoted previously by the investigators who studied heart disease in Roseto: "Ultimately, there developed signs of self-indulgence with a weakening of commitment to traditional values and a lack of responsibility for the community."[120]

The generalizability of the beneficial health consequences of social capital, whether of the bonding, bridging, or linking type, is questionable, as other writers on the topic have mentioned in passing.[121] But more is needed than a passing reference. What is needed is a better understanding than we now have of the conditions under which different forms of social capital emerge and how they exert their effects, for good and ill, on the health of populations. Case studies are one way, perhaps the best way, to accomplish this. Without them, more ecological correlations and multilevel regression analyses will simply be sterile exercises.

6

Globalization

You mean that you keep clear of your father because he differs
from you about Free Trade, and you don't want to quarrel with
him. Well, think of me and my father! He's a Nationalist and a
Separatist. I'm a metallurgical chemist turned civil engineer. Now
whatever else metallurgical chemistry may be, it's not national. It's
international. And my business and yours as civil engineers is to
join countries, not to separate them. The one real political conviction that our business has rubbed into us is that frontiers are hin-
drances and flags confounded nuisances.
—G.B. Shaw, *John Bull's Other Island*[1]

Globalization, generally understood as increasing liberalization of international
trade, has entered public debate only in the past 20 years or so, although as the
epigram from Shaw demonstrates, it was a very live issue at the beginning of
the twentieth century as well. This chapter focuses on the association between
openness to international trade—measured as imports plus exports as a percent of gross domestic product (GDP)—and its consequences for the health of
populations, as well as on the debates about its beneficial and harmful effects.[2]

There are, of course, other measures of globalization: the growth of international organizations and the increasing volume of international mail, telephone, television, radio, and internet communication, to list only a few.[3] Many
of them no doubt have an impact on health. However, international trade and
financial flows are widely acknowledged to be among the most significant aspects of globalization. They have important health consequences, they can be
measured more reliably than many other features of globalization, and debates about their significance bear an important relationship to many of the
themes that have run through this book. Those debates recapitulate debates
about the standard of living and the loss of community that have been described in previous chapters. For example, one critic of trade liberalization has
written of the advocates of globalization:

> The visions they offer us are unfailingly positive, even utopian:
> Globalization will be a panacea for our ills.
>   Shockingly enough, the euphoria they express is based on their
> freedom to deploy, at a global level—through the new global free

trade rules, and through deregulation and economic restructuring regimes—large-scale versions of the economic theories, strategies, and policies that have proven spectacularly unsuccessful over the past several decades wherever they've been applied. In fact, these are the very ideas that have brought us to the grim situation of the moment: the spreading disintegration of the social order and the increase of poverty, landlessness, homelessness, violence, alienation, and, deep within the hearts of many people, extreme anxiety about the future. Equally important, these are the practices that have led us to the near breakdown of the natural world, as evidenced by such symptoms as global climate change, ozone depletion, massive species loss, and near maximum levels of air, soil, and water pollution . . .

[T]he deep ideological principles underlying the global economy are not so new. . . . They include the primacy of economic growth; the need for free trade to stimulate the growth, the unrestricted "free market"; the absence of government regulation; and voracious consumerism combined with an aggressive advocacy of a uniform worldwide development model that faithfully reflects the Western corporate vision and serves corporate interests.[4]

This critique is from the left of the political spectrum, where the belief is that globalization will eviscerate hard-won regulations regarding occupational health and safety and environmental quality and will destroy the benefits of the welfare state. In addition, it will lead to inequality both within and among nations, to environmental degradation both at home and in poor countries to which corporations flee, to the destruction of democratic participation in policy-making, to the homogenization of cultures,[5] and to massive unemployment,[6] resulting in what Ross Perot described as "a great sucking sound" caused by the movement of jobs from the United States to low-wage countries.[7]

The fact that Perot and the political left agreed was itself remarkable and exemplified the fact that antiglobalists are a heterogeneous lot from all points along the political spectrum. Though they disagree about much, they share a concern that globalization will destroy national sovereignty, will lead to loss of American jobs as industries move overseas to low-wage countries, and will make "the nation subservient to multinational corporations."[8] Patrick Buchanan, speaking as a defender of capitalism and as a conservative, has called globalization "The Great Betrayal." For example,

- "In the 'knowledge industry'—authors, economists, lawyers, journalists, bankers, brokers, entertainers, whose labor foreign workers cannot easily replicate—wages continue to rise. It is Americans who make things with their hands, tools, and machines who are paying the price of free trade."
- "As expanding trade creates new bonds with foreign countries, it dissolves old bonds of patriotism."
- "If one's allegiance is to one world, who cares if America is the dominant power. To a citizen of the world, a hollowing out of America's industrial

power is an inconsequential, even a positive, development. It matters deeply only to American patriots."[9]

Those who favor globalization are also found along most points on the political spectrum. They all agree, however, that international trade raises living standards in all those countries that participate;[10] that it is not a cause of increased inequality within or among countries;[11] that even when inequality is increasing, it leads to greater philanthropic giving;[12] that openness to trade does not require the weakening of governments; and that the benefits of openness are translated into improved health and well being more generally. The editors of *The Economist* write:

> All kinds of qualifications and elaborations are needed, obviously, to fill out the argument properly. . . . But it is essential to understand one point from the outset. The liberal case for globalisation is emphatically not the case for domestic or international laisser faire. Liberalism lays down no certainties about the requirements of social justice in terms of income redistribution or the extent of the welfare state. It recognises that markets have their limits, for instance in tending to the supply of public goods (such as a clean environment). A liberal outlook is consistent with support for a wide range of government interventions; indeed a liberal outlook demands many such interventions.
>
> But the starting point for all liberals is a presumption that, under ordinary circumstances, the individual knows best what serves his interests and that the blending of these individual choices will produce socially good results. Two other things follow. The first is an initial skepticism, at least, about collective decision-making that overrides the individual kind. The other is a high regard for markets—not as a place where profits are made, it must be stressed, but as a place where society advances in the common good.[13]

This is a widely shared view among advocates of openness to trade. For instance, Jagdish Bhagwati writes: "The beneficial outcomes are only what economists call a "central tendency," which is to say that they hold for the most part but not always. They leave room for downsides, and we must have institutional mechanisms to cope with such adverse outcomes if and when they materialize."[14] David Dollar has written, "[I]t has to be a concern that some poor households are hurt in the short run by trade liberalization. Thus, it is important to complement open trade policies with effective social protection measures, such as unemployment insurance and food-for-work schemes."[15]

At a minimum, however, and for many writers, these institutional protections refer to the rule of law and to the sanctity of private property. Francis Fukuyama writes that, "Milton Friedman, dean of free-market economists, said a couple of years ago that his advice to former socialist countries 10 years earlier had been to "privatize, privatize, privatize." "But I was wrong," he added. "It turns out that the rule of law is probably more basic than privatization." The cost of learning this lesson was high."[16] And Martin Wolf answers the question, "So what role does the state have to play to make a market economy work?" as follows:

> At the broadest level, it has three functions: first, to provide things—known as public goods—that the market cannot provide for itself; second, to internalize externalities or remedy market failures; and, third, to help people who, for a number of reasons, do worse from a market or are more vulnerable to what happens within it than society finds tolerable.[17]

Thus, advocates of globalization generally regard government as having an important, though limited, role to play with respect to the untoward consequences of globalization. But they also consider many of the occupational, health, safety, and environmental regulations so valued by trade unionists, environmentalists, and nationalists as nothing more than nontariff barriers (NTBs) to trade—legislation passed as protectionist measures rather than as a way to guard the health of workers or the public—that in the long run do more harm than good.[18]

The Quest for Community. Globalizers are cosmopolitans whereas antiglobalizers are nationalists. Nationalism, moreover, is often understood as the quest for community writ large. This is captured in a useful though admittedly incomplete typology, first developed by Dudley Seers and subsequently adapted by Herman Daly and John Cobb, Jr., that suggests that the distinction between right and left is only one dimension and that another equally important one is nationalist/antinationalist, communitarian/anticommunitarian.[19] That is, the nation is understood to be a great community, a community of communities.[20] The distinction between egalitarian and antiegalitarian is inaccurate in one sense, for neoclassical liberals would argue that they are not antiegalitarian but believe in equality of opportunity and a meritocracy. The results may be indirectly antiegalitarian.[21]

	Egalitarian	Anti-egalitarian
Anti-Nationalist/ Anti-Communitarian	Marxist socialists	Neoclassical liberals
Nationalist/Communitarian	Dependency theorists, Populists, Neo-Marxists	Traditional conservatives

Samuel Huntington has observed "The central distinction between the public and elites is not isolationism versus internationalism but nationalism versus cosmopolitanism."[22] Despite disagreement on many key issues, members of the globalizing American elite share certain basic assumptions, whether they work for transnational corporations, international nongovernmental organizations, or evangelical missionary groups.[23] Most do not have "ongoing face-to-face involvement with local cultures and people they serve."[24] They use a similar vocabulary, "global speak," "derived from social sciences, human rights, the market, and multiculturalism."[25] "If epistemological authority for these elites is grounded in the language of social science, moral authority is grounded in the *language of universal individual rights and needs*,"[26] rights to soft drinks, fast foods, running shoes, abortions, health care, free speech, Christianity, and information. For these elites, national boundaries have become porous. They think of themselves as citizens of the world who happen to carry an American passport.[27] The president of National Cash Register is quoted as saying, "I was asked the other day about U.S. competitiveness, and I replied that I don't think about it at all. We at NCR think of ourselves as a globally competitive company that happens to be headquartered in the United States."[28]

Antiglobalists of the political right and of the political left instead identify the nation and nationalism with community and communitarianism. Pope Pius XI wrote in his encyclical *Quadragesimo Anno*, "[A]s to international relations, two different streams have issued from the one fountain-head: On the one hand, economic nationalism or even economic imperialism; on the other, a no less deadly and accursed internationalism of finance or international imperialism whose country is where profit is."[29]

Echoing the papal encyclical, Patrick Buchanan, writes, "The winners in a world of free trade and floating exchange rates are regimes whose central bankers manipulate currency values for national benefit, and a global corporate elite that can shift production from one country to another and calls no country home. Losers are the rooted people, the conservative people tied by the bonds of family, memory, and neighborhood to one community and one country."[30]

From a different point on the ideological spectrum, Wendell Barry has written, "A new political scheme of opposed parties . . . is beginning to take form."

> This is essentially a two-party system, and it divides over the fundamental issue of community. One of these parties holds that community has no value; the other holds that it does. One is the party of the global economy; the other I would call simply the party of local community. The global party is large, though not populous, immensely powerful and wealthy, self-aware, purposeful, and tightly organized. The community party is only now coming aware of itself; it is widely scattered, highly diverse, small though potentially numerous, weak though latently powerful, and poor though by no means without resources.[31]

Globalization and the Welfare State

The social compacts characteristic of Western Europe, the United States, Canada, Australia, and New Zealand in the post–World War II era had their genesis in the late nineteenth century and were further expanded during the Great Depression, when "governments tried to take control of their economies at the same time as they tried to resuscitate them. Having seen the chaos generated by orthodox finance and relatively unfettered markets, they opted for more planning and control."[32] Peter Temin continues that although there were great differences among them, this amounted to a socialist response to the crisis of the Depression, socialism characterized as, "(1) public ownership *or regulation* of 'the commanding heights' of the economy; (2) heavy government involvement in wage determination; and (3) a welfare state providing everyone with . . . 'a social dividend constituting the individual's share in the income derived from the capital and the natural resources owned by the society.' "[33] It surfaced again after World War II as what was called a mixed economy,[34] the result of an historical compromise. "International liberalization was coupled with a domestic social compact: Governments asked their publics to embrace the change and dislocation that comes with liberalization in return for the promise of help in containing and socializing the adjustment costs."[35]

John Gerard Ruggie has shown what has often been forgotten, that this compromise was fundamental to the liberalized trading rules negotiated after World War II. He shows further that liberalized trade is not under threat from the "new protectionism" as is frequently argued but rather that the social safety net that was integral to the social compact, what he has termed "embedded liberalism," of the pre- and postwar years has been jeopardized in large measure by increasingly liberalized rules of international trade.[36] This threat has arisen for several reasons.

1. As point of entry tariff barriers have been reduced, domestic economic structures have become increasingly salient as barriers to fair trade. Such barriers had little to do with protectionism, although they could be captured by interest groups with a protectionist agenda.[37]
2. Originally, trade meant trade in tangible things. In the 1970s, however, it was first suggested that services were also trade items. Because the United States was a major exporter of services (financial, professional, information, etc.), the U.S. government actively promoted this expanded definition. Services have typically been more highly regulated than manufacturing, and as services were increasingly considered trade items, regulations that impeded their flow were viewed as nontariff barriers to be dismantled.[38]
3. Multinational corporations have become transnational. It has thus become increasingly difficult to determine what products are manufactured by American firms and which are not. A study of what the balance-of-trade would be if the net global sales of American-owned and foreign-owned firms were taken into account, showed that the U.S. trade surplus would have been $24 billion in 1991. Using standard measures of sales, that is, by place of production, the United States has a large deficit. "The strategies of

US-owned multinationals, as well as the assessment of these firms by stock markets, reflect this broad US position in world markets. US labour, in contrast, lives in the world of the standard balance-of-trade figures. The growing gap between the two expresses a fundamental source of dislocation in the American political economy."[39] A large deficit, of course, contributes to the perception that the social safety net, so fundamental to the implicit bargain between governments and their publics with respect to globalization of trade, has now become too expensive to sustain.

There are other factors that have also led to the fraying of the safety net: the oil shocks of the 1970s, the decline of fertility and the associated aging of populations of developed countries, increasing costs of services, especially to people above the age of 80,[40] taxpayer revolts, and, of course, profound ideological assaults on the ability of governments to adequately provide services and on the desirability of their doing so, especially by the Reagan and Thatcher governments.

The 1970s was also the time when Thomas McKeown's arguments about the ineffectiveness of health care became widely popular among policy makers, and when health care, like other services, began to be considered a commodity. McKeown's work was widely understood to have discredited the achievements of medicine and public health, and thus to have legitimated cost containment. In such a climate, what has been called the "economizing model" of health care became widely popular.[41] This model emphasizes, in addition to cost containment, improved efficiency, minimizing risks to third-party payers, improved functioning of markets, and income-graduated cost sharing. It has replaced older models in which health care was considered a special service and a matter of distributive justice.

Not surprisingly, the social and economic changes and accompanying ideological debates in rich countries have had strong parallels in disputes about policies in poor countries, including the provision of public and personal health services. The so-called golden age in the rich countries, from the 1940s to the 1970s, was reflected in their policy of economic development for poor countries. And just as the oil shocks profoundly affected the rich countries in the 1970s, so they had an equal, indeed greater, impact in poor countries. Beginning in the late 1970s and accelerating since then, retrenchment of the welfare state and increasing liberalization of trade have affected poor countries as they have rich.

In 1984 Richard Feinberg described the shocks to which developing countries were then being subjected, and some of the consequences.

First, they have had to accept lower living standards to offset the higher costs of oil and capital, the global recession, and, most recently, the retrenchment in international financial markets. Second, they have had to alter investment priorities and relative prices to adjust to the changing costs of energy, food, and other internationally traded goods. Third, their productive structures have been battered by the accelerating pace of technological innovation and by the changing international division of labor as comparative advantage in many industries has shifted dynamically from one country to another. Fourth, countries are under increasing pressure to expose themselves more fully to the international phenomena—that is, to liberalize their economies. These pressures have come from the Bretton Woods institutions, which are advising policies of austerity and liberalization; from the commercial banks, which refuse to fund programs that merely postpone adjustment; and from the market itself, the most relentless foe of illusions.[42]

The high level of debt incurred in the 1970s did not just happen. The petrodollars acquired by the oil-exporting countries as a result of increased prices were deposited in western banks, and much of it was loaned to poor countries for projects that were not scrutinized carefully with an eye to whether they would ever be successful enough to repay the loans.[43] When the day of reckoning came, the result of rising interest rates in the early 1980s as the United States Federal Reserve Board dealt with the savings and loan crisis,[44] the effect abroad led to what in Latin America has been called the "lost decade." But the consequences were also felt in Africa and in the Balkans, contributing to the break-up of Yugoslavia.[45] It was in this context that adjustment policies were developed and implemented by the International Monetary Fund and the World Bank.

Adjustment policies include both stabilization and structural adjustment.[46] The former refers to "reducing imbalances in the external accounts and the domestic budget by cutting down on expenditure . . . , and reducing credit creation and the budget deficit." The latter refers to changing the structure of the economy by expanding trade and the supply of exports. Currency devaluation is often part of the package, as is reduction of the government sector and increased privatization. Adjustment policies and practices have changed over the years in response to criticisms and to the experience of some of its deleterious consequences. Thus, social safety nets have increasingly been included in newer programs.[47] Nonetheless, the overall policy remains the same: to shrink the role of government in the economies of developing countries, to increase privatization, and to open them to trade in both goods and services.

Rich Countries' Health Policies with Respect to Poor Countries[48]

In the immediate post–World War II period, there were strong continuities with public health policies that had been pursued earlier in the United States as well as internationally. The belief in the idea of causal necessity held by administrators and investigators working for the Rockefeller Foundation's hookworm eradication campaign justified the narrow focus on the eradication of hookworm, leaving economic and social institutions untouched. The idea of multiple weakly sufficient causes of pellagra was used to justify changes in those same institutions. Similar differences emerged in international health after the war, where they were institutionalized in what came be called horizontal and vertical programs.

The idea of causal necessity supported vertical programs narrowly focused on the eradication or control of a particular disease. Among the most articulate spokesmen for this position was Fred Soper, who had begun his career working for the Rockefeller Foundation's Sanitary Commission on the eradication of hookworm and then went on to work on similar projects until the early 1960s. Soper hailed Charles Chapin, the influential health officer of Providence, Rhode Island at the turn of the twentieth century, with "having the vision and the voice of a prophet; he recognized instinctively that the rejection of spontaneous generation and the acceptance of the germ theory of disease implied the concept of contagious disease eradication. Were Chapin alive today . . . he would be championing the cause of world eradication programs."[49]

Soper pointed out that in the 1920s and 1930s the idea of eradication had been discredited as a result of the resilience of jungle yellow fever. By the end of World War II, however, much had changed.

> However justifiable the complacent acceptance of the persistence of preventable diseases may have appeared 30 years ago, it is no longer defensible. The success of local and national eradication efforts during the past three decades, the discovery of new methods of disease prevention, and the increasing participation of all nations in coordinated international health programs have led to a rehabilitation of the eradication concept. Today the nations of the Americas are committed to the eradication of the *Aedes Aegypti* mosquito, malaria, smallpox, and yaws; the nations of the world have joined in the global eradication of malaria, and the demand for the eradication of other preventable diseases is inevitable.[50]

This extreme view of eradication was not widely accepted, certainly not for tuberculosis, one of the diseases for which it was advocated in the 1950s. Most experts accepted the more modest goal of "eradication as a public health problem," rather than total eradication.[51] Malaria, too, had been a target for eradication, and the failure to do so had helped discourage further attempts at disease eradication more generally, despite the success of the campaign against smallpox, the one disease to have been successfully eradicated.[52]

The eradication ideal was most popular during the 1950s, at a time when development theory seemed to imply that money spent on health programs was being misapplied because it would only lead to increased population, which would vitiate the effects of economic development.[53] It was believed that funds should be invested productively, and that in the long run the resulting economic development would lead to improved health for the entire population as benefits trickled down from the top to the bottom of the social hierarchy.[54] The appeal of eradication programs in this context was that they were economical as well as humane, that they did not require the expansion and restructuring of the health services of less-developed countries or income redistribution and long-term commitments of aid, that they were visible and very broad based, and, therefore, that they were an effective propaganda tool in the contest with Communism.[55]

By the 1960s, the ecological approach to epidemiology was becoming more popular. As early as 1952 in his historical account of American epidemiology, John Gordon had written:

> If communicable disease is a pure ecologic process, its aim is that of all biologic processes, namely, to permit survival of both living elements. Nature is as much concerned with the welfare of the parasite as with that of the host. This has an important bearing on principles designed to guide prevention and control. The practical objective is not so much to eradicate disease, as to modify it to innocuousness.[56]

In his now-classic studies with Scrimshaw and Taylor of the interaction of nutritional status and infection, this ecological approach was used to great effect.[57] In these studies, it was shown that the nutritional status of the host had a significant bearing upon the severity of infectious diseases, and likewise that an episode of disease—most importantly diarrhea—could cause significant deterioration in the nutritional status of the host. Thus, the relationship between host and parasite was determined not simply by the virulence of the parasite but by the condition of the host. Disease, then, was multicausal.

This position became increasingly popular in the 1960s for several reasons. First, the studies were well conceived and well executed. Second, by the 1960s, the significant causes of morbidity and mortality in many developing countries were less often the "named" diseases than the "pneumonia-diarrhea complex," which was the result of any number of infectious agents and which was sensitive to the nutritional status of the host.[58] Third, as noted above, the failure to eradicate malaria had encouraged a rethinking of the eradicationist philosophy.

And fourth, development philosophy had begun to change. One important variant was the "human capital" approach, in which population itself was considered a valuable resource. Thus, investment in health and education was investment in the improvement of human capital, which would ultimately lead to economic development through increased productivity.[59] This meant that broadly based (horizontal) health programs were increasingly favored by development specialists rather than vertical, disease-oriented programs. Gordon and his colleagues wrote:

> It should not be forgotten that a high prevalence of debilitating infectious disease may also affect the nutritional status of a population by reducing the ability of many of its members to produce or earn

their food supply. Populations with a great deal of endemic malaria, severe hookworm disease, schistosomiasis, and other infections common to tropical, underdeveloped areas are likely to lack the physical stamina to be efficient in agricultural and industrial labor. Heavily parasitized farm animals give a poor return for the food they consume and for the effort in caring for them. These direct effects on economic development provide major justifications for expanded health programs.[60]

In its programmatic implications, the multicausal, ecological conception of disease was compatible with the human capital approach, for it advocated the expansion of health systems horizontally to cover a wide assortment of major causes of morbidity and mortality. The approach was adopted by the World Health Organization and the United Nations Children's Fund and ultimately came to be called primary health care. It was considered an alternative to the sophisticated health care available to the upper classes of most developing nations, as well as to the disease-eradication programs that had characterized the 1950s.[61] Djukanovic and Mach wrote:

> The relative emphasis on programmes to control specific diseases may also have hindered the development of basic health services over the past 25 years. As early as 1951, when the efforts of many developing countries were centred on specialized mass campaigns for the eradication of diseases, the Director-General of WHO pointed out in his annual report that these efforts would have only temporary results if they were not followed by the establishment of permanent health services in rural areas to deal with the day-to-day work in the control and prevention of disease and the promotion of health.[62]

The WHO-UNICEF conference at Alma Ata in 1978 formally endorsed primary health care, which addresses the main health problems in the community and provides promotive, preventive, curative, and rehabilitative services as one of the ways to deal with the disparities between the people of the developed and the developing countries.[63] The goal was health for all by the year 2000. The conference report was as much a political as a public health document, based upon the assumption that declines in mortality and improvements in health could only be accomplished by broad changes in social and political organization, as well as massive expenditures on health and social services. Indeed, the report was placed within the context of economic and social development based upon a New International Economic Order requiring the transfer and redistribution of wealth from the developed to the developing countries.

> The Conference considered the close interrelationship and interdependence of health and social and economic development, with health leading to and at the same time depending on a progressive

improvement in conditions and quality of life. The Conference stressed that primary health care is an integral part of the socioeconomic development process. Hence, activities of the health sector must be coordinated at the national, intermediate, and community or local levels with those of other social and economic sectors, including education, agriculture, animal husbandry, household water, housing, public works, communications, and industry. Health activities should be undertaken concurrently with measures such as those for the improvement of nutrition, particularly of children and mothers, increase in production and employment, and a more equitable distribution of personal income; anti-poverty measures; and protection and improvement of the environment.[64]

This policy was in sharp contrast to those that had been pursued in both the colonial and postcolonial periods when the concern was first for the health of Europeans working in tropical areas, and then for the health of workers in European-owned enterprises, to help assure their productivity. Such narrow and technologically-based health interventions had historically been seen as one way to achieve economic development.[65] Alma Ata represented a reversal. Development was one of the ways to achieve better health.

Such a reversal and the necessary transfer of resources from the rich to the poor nations to support it were unlikely even in the best of times, and the late 1970s was scarcely the best of times. The oil shocks of the 1970s had had significant effects on the world economy, and conservative administrations were soon to take control of the governments of both the United States and Great Britain. Alma Ata was the end of an era, a very short era, in fact, not the beginning of a new one.

Criticism of the broad-gauged approach of primary health care was almost immediate. Judith Walsh and Kenneth Warren from the Rockefeller Foundation considered the Declaration of Alma Ata well meaning, even noble, but hopelessly unrealistic. They remarked: "The goal set at Alma Ata is above reproach, yet its very scope makes it unattainable because of the cost and numbers of trained personnel required. Indeed, the World Bank has estimated that it would cost billions of dollars to provide minimal (not comprehensive) health services by the year 2000 to all the poor in developing countries."[66] The alternative they proposed, known as selective primary health care, was characterized as follows.

On the basis of high morbidity and mortality and of feasibility of control, a circumscribed number of diseases are selected for prevention in a clearly defined population. Since few programs based on this selective model of prevention and treatment have been attempted, the following approach is proposed. The principal recipients of care would be children up to three years old and women in the childbearing years. The care provided would be measles and diphtheria-pertussis-tetanus (DPT) vaccination for children over six months old, tetanus toxoid to all women of childbearing age, encouragement of long-term breast feeding, provision of chloroquine for episodes of fever in children under three years old in areas where malaria is prevalent and, finally, oral rehydration packets and instructions.[67]

A subsequent elaboration of this approach was based upon consideration of the ways in which a number of low-income countries had managed to reduce mortality rates without substantial foreign support.[68] It was generally agreed that vertically organized categorical disease programs were an essential ingredient, but beyond that were a number of other important factors. Warren wrote, "One just can't wait for affluence."

> For the last decade at least there has been a model for health in the developing world which I shall call the Northern paradigm. The evolution of good health in the developed world or the North, in the terminology of the Brandt report, has been related particularly by McKeown to the process of development, i.e., the growth of a literate population living in spacious housing provided with piped water and sanitary facilities and supplied with the fruits of industry and agriculture via good roads and communication facilities. The allopathic medical system which gained ascendancy in the North had little to offer prior to the late 1930s or early 40s. Therefore, the governments of the developing world, aided and abetted by multilateral, bilateral and non-governmental aid agencies have been attempting to institute the Northern model of health. The cost of this approach is staggering . . .
>
> In the meanwhile, it appears that certain countries of the South have quietly evolved a different model, which I shall call the Southern paradigm, resulting in a remarkable reduction in infant and child mortality rates and increases in life expectancy. The basic elements of this approach as described by China, Kerala State, and Costa Rica appear to be only four:
>
> 1. Political and social will.
> 2. Education for all with emphasis on primary and secondary schooling.
> 3. Equitable distribution throughout the urban and rural populations of public health measures and primary health care.
> 4. Assurance of adequate caloric intake for all.[69]

The model of economic development that is said to have been responsible for mortality decline in developed countries was judged inappropriate for developing countries, but high-technology medicine was also inappropriate, for it too is expensive and does not address the needs of the population. The necessary ingredient is "political and social will," the functional equivalent at the national level of responsibility for one's own lifestyle and health at the individual level, the exercise of which will allow poor countries to improve their mortality patterns independent of economic development and without having to depend upon large amounts of money from the industrialized countries.

Critics called selective primary health care a repackaging of vertical disease-control programs.[70] W. Henry Mosley has observed that such modifications of the original vision of primary health care (PHC) represent an implicit acknowledgement of the difficulties of implementing the fundamental political commitments that are necessary to bring it to fruition. "As a result, PHC, rather than being a revolutionary force for change, is more often simply added as another appendage to the assortment of vertical programs directed to the masses."[71] "There remains [a] rather truncated definition of PHC which is essentially a top-down strategy to reach the community with some simple but theoretically effective preventive and curative technologies along with health motivation using various types of village level workers."[72]

Despite these and other criticisms, selective primary health care has become a large part of the package of reforms that have been advocated by influential westerner institutions since the 1980s. For example, the 1993 edition of the World Bank's *World Development Report* was concerned entirely with health, and made the linkage between selective primary health care and structural adjustment programs explicit.[73] Early adjustment programs, the authors wrote, had had an adverse impact on health and had slowed the rate of improvement. "As a result of this experience, most countries' adjustment programs today try to rationalize overall government spending while maintaining cost-effective expenditures in health and education."[74]

Cost-effectiveness was to be assessed by the use of Disability-Adjusted Life Years (DALYs). Those interventions that had the largest impact would be part of a basic package of services, both public health and essential clinical services that were similar in concept to selective primary health care. Public health activities included "immunizations, school-based health services, information and selected services for family planning and nutrition, programs to reduce tobacco and alcohol consumption, regulatory action, information, and limited public investments to improve the household environment, AIDS prevention."[75] Essential clinical services include pregnancy-related care, family-planning services, tuberculosis and STD control, and "care for the common serious illnesses of young children."[76]

Unsurprisingly, the question of payment was crucial. In poor countries, targeting free services to the poor was considered by the World Bank to be a necessity, for without targeting there would not be sufficient resources to provide the essential package of services to the poor.

> Public financing of a national essential clinical package can be justified because the package creates positive externalities and reduces poverty.

The case for government financing of discretionary clinical health care—services outside the essential package—is far less compelling. In fact, governments can promote both efficiency and equity by reducing—or, when possible, eliminating—public funding for these services. Doing so requires recovering the cost of discretionary services provided in government health facility and cutting subsidies to private and public insurance schemes that finance discretionary care. By reducing spending on these services, governments can concentrate public expenditure where it will do the most good—in public health and cost effective clinical services.[77]

By providing free only the essential services as defined by the World Bank, the maximum number of disability-free years of productive life would be saved while at the same time countries could meet the adjustment goals set for them as conditions for the receipt of loans to pay off their debts, finance further development, and open their economies to increased trade. This is an entirely different vision of the role of health in development than that promulgated at Alma Ata. It is consistent with the goal of health care as it has been most frequently defined since the colonial period, goals that have been made even more explicit in the World Health Organization's Report of the Commission on Macroeconomics and Health, *Macroeconomics and Health: Investing in Health for Economic Development*.[78] Good health is seen not primarily as a human right but as a commodity and as one of the means for promoting economic development.

Privatization of services, the diminution of the role of governments in the provision of health and other services, and the imposition of the economizing model of health care have all been the subject of numerous analyses and critiques.[79] Among the criticisms have been that the use of DALYs implicitly devalues people who are disabled and/or not in the most productive or potentially productive years of life; that shrinkage of governments' regulatory powers has lead to more, not less, corruption and inefficiency; that private insurers and HMOs have been allowed to pillage public social security funds for their own profit in poor and middle-income countries; that selective primary health care, now called the essential package of services, depends upon technical interventions implemented by vertically organized programs to improve health rather than treating public and personal health services as one element in the development process; and that the definition of public health has been narrowed and is essentially the same whatever the particular needs of different populations. In a book of essays by Indian scholars critical of the 1993 World Development Report, *Investing in Health*,[80] Mohan Rao wrote:

> Thomas McKeown, a medical doctor less well known than he ought to be both among health professionals and policy-makers, offered us startling new insights into the remarkable advance in human longevity and health made over the last two centuries. His revelatory findings

in the 1970s as a historian of health have profound implications for
health policy and planning.[81]

Rao went on to argue that in the West the decline of mortality had been the
result primarily of improvements in the standard of living, not medical technology, and that World Bank policies devised for India and other poor countries flew in the face of the very conditions needed to improve life expectancy.
"As the prospects of 'Health for All through Primary Health Care' recede, we
see again the dominance of the magic bullet approach to public health technology accompanying what Renaud describes as eliminating society from disease
where disease occurrence is ascribed to individual proclivities and failures."[82]
This is not an entirely fair criticism because the evidence is very persuasive that even poor countries can raise the life expectancy of their populations
without becoming rich. But it is accurate to say that vertically organized programs targeted to specific conditions and based upon an assumption of necessary causes of disease have generally been seen to be a more economical
way to improve the health of the poor than horizontally organized programs
that require the mobilization of many resources and that are usually based
upon the assumption of multiple weakly sufficient causes of disease. It is
also an entirely fair political criticism if equity is the major concern. For the
position of the World Bank and other international organizations is that
there are inexpensive interventions that can improve life expectancy and
health more generally, and that improved health will generate greater
wealth. Health, then, is a means to an end, not an end in itself to be achieved
by the kind of social transformation envisioned by the signatories of the declaration of Alma Ata.
If the World Bank and the International Monetary Fund have been the
targets of severe and extensive criticisms, they have not been targeted in quite
as dramatic a fashion, at least in recent years, as the third and newest of the
Bretton Woods institutions, the World Trade Organization (WTO).[83] Quite
apart from street demonstrations, however, there have also been severe criticisms of the WTO insofar as trade includes, in addition to manufactured and
agricultural products, financial, educational, medical, and other services. National laws and regulations related to occupational and environmental health
and safety, as well as to public and personal health services, have increasingly
been considered nontariff barriers to trade. The fear of critics, and the hope of
advocates, is that they will be dismantled as a means of increasing openness.
Furthermore, trade in services is understood to mean that foreign firms must
be allowed access to domestic markets on the same terms as local providers of
health care. The result in both rich and poor countries, it is widely believed,
will be diminution of the welfare state, privatization of services, and growing
inequality of access to care.[84] In addition, intellectual property rights as applied to pharmaceuticals has meant that poor countries cannot obtain the
drugs they need to treat such conditions as HIV-AIDS and sleeping sickness.[85]
Thus, trade liberalization and the increasing involvement of countries in the

international economy potentially have profound consequences for the health of populations.

The Health Consequences of Globalization

Policy debates have not occurred in an atmosphere devoid of evidence. The studies reviewed in this section suggest, however, that the evidence regarding the health consequences is mixed. The optimistic side of the globalization debate is based upon the frequently observed positive association between per capita income and life expectancy. Average life expectancy in rich countries is higher than in poor ones, and the association is linear, except at the highest incomes where more money is not associated with substantially longer life. Thus, to the degree that openness is associated with high income, optimists argue that openness of a nation's economy will promote the health of its population. This is the argument made by Richard Feachem, who argues further that globalization has social and political benefits as well as economic ones. For example, he writes,

> Many very poor people in the world do not have governments that are concerned for their welfare and their interests. Such poor people are given hope by an interconnected world in which information and ideas flow rapidly and protest and action can be mobilised in the face of oppression, corruption, and genocide.[86]

He goes on to say, "[W]ithout a trend towards global moral and ethical standards, more Chinese women would still be crippled by foot binding, more African women would still be genitally mutilated, and more Indian women would be killed or beaten in disputes over dowries."[87]

David Dollar and Aart Kraay have analyzed data from a group of developing countries that have increased openness to trade more than other developing countries in the period since 1980.[88] They show that the economies of these countries grew more rapidly than those of other developing countries. In another study, they have shown that income growth is not associated with increasing income inequality.[89] These findings have been contested. For example, Branko Milanovic has shown that globalization (openness to trade) is associated with increased income inequality in poor countries and decreased inequality in rich countries.[90] Nonetheless, Dollar and Kray argue that on average everyone's income improves with increasing openness. And additional analyses, to which I return below, demonstrate that increasing incomes are associated with declining mortality, especially among infants and children under 5 years of age. The more rapidly income increases, the more rapidly does mortality decline.[91]

Advocates of openness generally support their position with macro-level studies rather than case studies of particular segments of populations, presumably because they are concerned with the greatest good for the greatest number. An exception is a case study of young women textile workers in Bangladesh (of whom there were about a million at the time of the study) that found, contrary to what has often been claimed, [92] that for most of them employment was a welcome alternative to heavy agricultural labor. While they continued to share their earnings with their families, they also accumulated dowries, which gave them more control over the choice of a husband; they became less timid and developed self-confidence in dealing with employers and strangers; and, because virtually all were unmarried, they postponed marriage and childbearing, which benefited their health[93] and did not create the added burdens of child care which are such a problem for working mothers.

This is not to say that factory work was ideal. Exploitation was real, unwelcome encounters with men were not uncommon, and young women who worked in factories were regarded as lower status than those who did not do factory work. Nonetheless, most of them believed it to be a better alternative than they would have had otherwise.

> All of these beneficial outcomes of garment-industry jobs have been experienced largely by women who started working as teenagers, many of them at ages that would put them into an illegal category in terms of existing Bangladeshi child-labor laws. However, where choices are extremely limited, and where education is rarely a realistic option, factory work in the garment industry may be regarded as a positive opportunity enabling girls to delay marriage and motherhood and to reduce their reliance on alternative and more risky forms of employment.[94]

Openness to trade is not the only measure of economic globalization. The 1980s was a decade of slow growth, massive indebtedness of many poor nations, and the emergence of structural adjustment programs requiring that, in exchange for loans from the Bretton Woods institutions (The World Bank and the International Monetary Fund), borrower countries reduce government expenditures, devalue their currencies, and engage in export-led growth.[95] These arrangements were a means of shrinking the size of government, privatizing services, and creating a surplus with which to repay the loans. Many observers have argued, however, that these policies worsened the health of people in the affected populations. The evidence is mixed.

Studies of Latin American countries indicate that there were some deleterious effects but that the reversals of the decline of mortality, when they occurred at all, were minor and did not reach statistical significance.[96] There was, however, a consistent pattern that emerged among particularly vulnerable groups, children and the aged, who were somewhat more likely to die of infectious diseases during the economic shocks of the 1980s than they had been previously.[97] Likewise, in Argentina in the 1980s and early 1990s, mortality due to motor vehicle accidents and violence increased among young men in association with deteriorating socioeconomic conditions.[98] The same pattern of worsening mortality among particularly vulnerable groups was found in a World Bank study of the health consequences of Structural Adjustment Programs in several African nations in the 1980s.[99]

A study of international indebtedness and life expectancy into the early 1980s (before the AIDS crisis had truly erupted) found that there was a significant inverse association between the level of debt and the rapidity with which life expectancy improved: the greater the debt, the less the improvement. In no case, however, did the improvements cease or reverse.[100] Analyses of infant mortality in Yugoslavia in the 1980s before the break-up of the country showed that the rate of decline slowed as the economy deteriorated, the result of a high level of international indebtedness, economic restructuring, and massive inflation.[101] Indeed, worldwide, the rate of decline of the infant mortality rate slowed during the period of globalization beginning in the 1980s.[102]

The break-up of the Soviet Union and the increasing integration of its former republics and of the former Eastern bloc countries into the international economy has also had mixed effects. Among all of them there was a decline of male life expectancy immediately following 1989, but in the Czech Republic, Slovakia, Poland, and the former German Democratic Republic, life expectancy improved dramatically thereafter. The situation was different in the former republics of the Soviet Union and other Eastern bloc countries, where the decline persisted for at least several more years. Of those remaining countries, only in Hungary had male life expectancy improved by 1996 compared to 1989. The patterns were essentially the same for women, with a few exceptions.[103]

Likewise, in the former republics of Yugoslavia there have been mixed results. Before the collapse of the country, there had been continuing improvement of mortality in all the republics, even though there had been a slowing of the decline in the 1980s. After the break-up, existing inequalities widened and in some cases deterioration occurred (Figure 6-1). The former republics, now nations, that did best, Slovenia and Croatia (especially the former), were the ones that had been richest before the break-up and were best prepared to enter the international economy and benefit from it.

The late 1990s saw the collapse of some of the Asian tiger economies and the spread to other countries, including Russia, of the financial crisis that had engulfed them; the result of massive borrowing by businesses and banks "on short term in foreign currency and invested long term in dubious domestic assets . . . facilitated by a premature opening up of their capital markets to free entry of short-term, speculative funds."[104] A study of child labor, school attendance, and health in Indonesia, based upon surveys before and after the financial crisis found little if any impact.[105] On the other hand, a study of child and maternal health found a reduction in high-quality foods that resulted in anemia.[106] Furthermore, Cornia cites "World Bank studies of the impact of the Mexican and Thai financial crises [that] show that, even after the economies of these two countries recovered, health status was still affected. During the transitory but acute recessions, children were taken away from their schools, entered hazardous jobs or prostitution rings, or sustained permanent brain damage if they suffered from acute malnutrition."[107]

Using data from the World Development Report, I have compared infant mortality rates in the 2 years prior to the 1997 crisis to the 3 years following

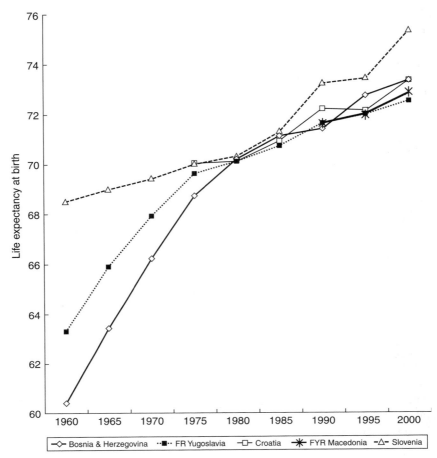

Figure 6-1. Life expectancy at birth in countries that comprised the former Yugoslavia, 1960–2000. (*Source*: World Bank, *World Development Indicators*, CD-ROM. Washington, D.C., 2002.)

for the five Asian countries most affected: Indonesia, Thailand, Malaysia, South Korea, and the Philippines. Recognizing that these data are often of questionable validity, it is nonetheless worth noting that there was no significant slackening in the rate of decline from before to after the crisis.[108] On the other hand, "In the Russian Federation the standardized death rate rose by almost 20% in the wake of the financial crisis of August 1998."[109]

Several qualifications must be offered. (1) The validity of much of the mortality data is often questionable, and most questionable in the poorest countries. For example, infant mortality and other vital rates often differ widely for the same year and country when reported by the United Nations and by the World Bank. (2) What have been observed are often short sharp shocks to which families and public institutions have been able to adapt. Longer crises, such as those in the former Soviet Union and in some of the former Yugoslav republics, tax the resources of both and are associated with worse health outcomes. (3) Long-term consequences of even short sharp shocks have generally not been determined and are obviously difficult to assess. (4) Mortality is only the most visible outcome. Morbidity and micronutrient deficits are less easily and less frequently measured but, as many observers note, are extremely significant outcomes as well, having implications, for instance, for the development of cognitive abilities.

Despite these qualifications, the mixed results of the studies cited above suggest that globalization, measured as openness to trade, structural adjustment, and/or financial crises are the consequence of great differences among nations, which have been summarized by Giovanni Andrea Cornia as follows:

> If properly managed, globalization can lead to important health gains. Global market forces work efficiently in settings where domestic markets are competitive and non-exclusionary, regulatory institutions are strong, asset concentration is moderate, access to public health services is widespread, social safety nets are in place, and rules of access to global markets are non-exclusionary. Under these conditions, globalization reduces opportunistic behaviour, rewards effort and entrepreneurship, captures economies of scale in production, increases employment opportunities, and improves welfare by raising earnings, and reducing the prices of consumer goods . . .
>
> However, the domestic and international conditions for successful globalization have been met in relatively few countries. In several countries, growth has been hindered and improvements in health have been slowed down by premature, unselective, and poorly sequenced globalization.[110]

That is, nations fortunate enough to have governments that can manage globalization in the ways described by Cornia have done reasonably well. Those that are not competent, whatever the reason, have done poorly. Of course, conditions imposed by the International Monetary Fund and the World Bank with respect to shrinking the role of government are not conducive to the development of a competent civil service able to administer and regulate either public or private programs, thus opening the door even wider to the very corruption that is said to be endemic in many poor countries, not to mention among the foreign firms that seek to do business in them.

Openness and Health

In this section, data from the World Bank's *World Development Report*[111] are used to consider in more detail the association between openness and health. The first point is that small countries are generally much more open to international trade than large countries. This has been widely observed and is a consequence of the need for small countries to buy and sell in larger markets than exist within their own borders. This is the case, for instance, for the Scandinavian countries, the Low Countries, and Austria and Switzerland.[112] It is also true of Singapore, Hong Kong, and Malaysia. Indeed, there is a strong inverse correlation between openness (exports + imports as a percent of GDP) and population size.[113] In 1980, the correlation was -0.59 (p < 0.0001), and in 2000 it was -0.41 (p < 0.0001): the larger the population of a country, the less open the economy. The weakening of the association over the 2 decades is because large countries increased in openness more rapidly than small countries.[114]

Changes in openness are significantly and positively correlated with changes in GDP per capita from 1980 to 2000, just as advocates of openness argue.[115] Moreover, the greater the change in GDP per capita, the greater the percentage decline in the infant mortality rate. There was, however, no association with changes in life expectancy at birth. These results should be regarded with some skepticism because the quality of the mortality data in many countries is highly suspect. Nonetheless, they are consistent with more sophisticated analyses using only data from countries in which the validity is considered to be good.[116] These data suggest that at the national level the greater the increase in openness to trade, the greater is the increase in incomes, and the greater the increase in incomes, the greater is the decrease in infant mortality (but not life expectancy at birth).

However, the relationships are somewhat more complex than reported above. GDP per capita in 1980 (in constant 1995 U.S.$) is not associated with subsequent changes in openness or GDP per capita, but it is strongly and inversely associated with changes in infant mortality rates. The higher the income, the greater the subsequent decline in infant mortality.[117] (There is no association with changes in life expectancy at birth.) When change in infant mortality is regressed onto GDP per capita in 1980 and subsequent changes in income and openness, only income per capita is significant.[118] That is to say, changes in openness and in GDP per capita over a 20-year period are not associated with declining infant mortality when GDP per capita at the beginning of the period is also included in the analysis.

Because rich and poor countries are so different in their economies and institutions, it is common to analyze them separately. Thus countries with per capita GDP (in 1995 U.S. $) of $5000 and above and less than $5000 in 1980 are next considered separately. Among the wealthy countries, there was no association between the percent change in openness and the percent change in GDP per capita on the one hand, and changes in either life expectancy or infant mortality on the other. In poor countries (N = 92), there was a significant inverse correlation between the percent increase in GDP per capita and the percent decline in infant mortality rate,[119] as well as a significant association between increasing openness and increasing GDP per capita.[120] However, in a multiple regression analysis similar to the one described above, when GDP per capita in 1980 was included, neither change in openness nor change in GDP

Table 6-1
Infant Mortality and Life Expectancy at Birth of Post-1980 Globalizers and Non-Globalizers; Countries with 1980 GDP per capita <$8,000 (1995 U.S. $)

Mortality	Globalizers	Non-Globalizers	p-value
Life expectancy 1980 (N)	58.5 (34)	58.0 (65)	0.7990
Life expectancy 2000 (N)	62.4 (35)	62.1 (71)	0.9111
Infant mortality rate 1980 (N)	80.1 (35)	77.4 (65)	0.7684
Infant mortality rate 2000 (N)	50.2 (35)	47.7 (71)	0.7470
Mortality rate children <5 yr 2000 (N)	75.7 (35)	75.6 (64)	0.9956

per capita was associated with change in infant mortality. (Again, there was no association with change in life expectancy.)

Recall the findings of Dollar and Kray that hyperglobalizers increased their incomes faster than countries that were globalizing laggards. In 1980, the highest income (GDP per capita) among the hyperglobalizers was in Argentina: $7785 in 1995 U.S. dollars. The hyperglobalizers are next compared with all the other countries with 1980 incomes per capita of less than $8000 (in 1995 U.S. $). There were no differences in infant mortality or life expectancy in 1980 or 2000 or in the percentage change in infant mortality or life expectancy between 1980 and 2000 (Table 6-1). Thus, whatever the differing benefits that may have accrued with respect to improved incomes were not reflected in changes in mortality.[121] Others have recently questioned the seemingly strong association between improvements in income and declining infant mortality rates as well.[122]

These data suggest that the higher the per capita income, the greater the life expectancy and the lower the infant mortality. They also indicate that openness is associated with improvements in income. The most open countries do not necessarily have more favorable mortality rates than other countries, however. To explore further why this is so, the next analyses use data from developed countries. The first analysis involves the same set of 18 countries discussed in Chapter 4 (see Table 4-6). Comparable to what was observed in the world sample, there is a significant inverse correlation between population size and openness in 2000.[123] Openness, however, is unrelated to infant mortality, life expectancy at birth, per capita income, and income inequality.

When the countries are compared by the type of political regime that has been dominant since World War II (as in Table 4-6), the results are as shown in Table 6-2. There is no difference in respect of openness, but the Social Democratic countries are the most equal with respect to income and have the lowest infant mortality rates. Life expectancy at birth does not differ, and income per capita is highest in the Liberal countries and lowest in the Ex-Fascist countries.

These results suggest that political institutions mediate between openness to trade and the health of populations.[124] We see something similar when an

Table 6-2
Type of Government, Trade Openness, and Mortality, 2000

Type of Government	Openness	Gini	GDP/cap ppp	Life Expectancy	IMR/1000
Christian Democrat (6)	91.0	30.8	$25,759	78.4	4.6
Ex-fascist (3)	61.9	34.0	$17,754	77.2	4.9
Liberal (4)	81.8	36.6[a]	$28,839	77.4	5.9
Social Democrat (5)	82.3	26.6	$26,716	78.0	4.1
p-value	0.7772	0.0017	0.0007	0.3514	0.0118

[a]Gini coefficient for Ireland is not available.

overlapping set of countries is examined using measures of economic openness gathered from different sources than the World Bank data used thus far.[125] The analyses in Table 6-3 show that infant mortality rates in 1995 are unassociated with GDP per capita, capital controls, trade openness, and outward investment but are significantly inversely correlated with international borrowing, government revenues, civilian government employment, and the public share of health expenditures. None of these variables is associated with life expectancy at birth.

Table 6-3
Correlations of Infant Mortality Rates and Life Expectancies With Measures of Trade Openness and Government Spending, 17 Welfare States, Early 1990s

Variable	Infant Mortality Rate		Life Expectancy	
	r	p-value	r	p-value
GDP/capita	0.12	0.6228	0.04	0.8500
Capital controls	0.03	0.8871	−0.01	0.9508
Trade openness	−0.12	0.6439	−0.07	0.7853
Outward investment	−0.04	0.8532	0.28	0.2683
International borrowing	−0.59	0.0121	0.10	0.6931
Government revenue*	−0.65	0.0064	0.08	0.7550
Government expenditure	−0.39	0.1176	0.08	0.7523
Social Security expenditure	−0.47	0.0513	0.20	0.4245
Public pension	−0.31	0.2186	0.17	0.5067
Civilian government employment[a]	−0.55	0.0262	0.16	0.5423
Public share of health expenditure	−0.55	0.0212	0.25	0.3149

[a]Data for New Zealand not available.

Sources: E. Huber and J.D. Stephens, *Development and Crisis of the Welfare State.* Chicago: University of Chicago Press, 2001, pp. 228–229. Infant Mortality Rates and Life Expectancy in 1995 are from the *World Development Indicators 2002.*

Table 6-4
Types of Welfare States and Measures of Trade Openness, Government
Involvement in the Economy, and Mortality

Measure	Christian Democrat	Liberal	Social Democrat	Wage Earner	p-value
Capital controls	3.8	3.8	3.8	3.8	0.1039
Trade openness	75	62	62	47	0.6917
Outward investment	2.6	1.8	2.7	3.7	0.8282
International borrowing	2.8	4.6	7.2	3.9	0.0266
Government revenues	45.5	38.5	55.7	34.0	0.0022
Government expenditures	50.2	43.7	58.7	47.5	0.0617
Social Security expenditures	20.0	13.7	20.2	13.0	0.0099
Public pensions	66.4	37.2	63.7	55.5	0.0621
Civilian government employment	9.4	11.2	20.0	11.0	0.0027
Public share of health expenditures	74.2	69.0	86.5	73.5	0.1614
IMR 1995	5.5	6.3	4.3	6.2	0.0030
Life expectancy	77.3	76.5	77.0	77.2	0.7014
GDP per capita 1995	$22,460	$22,439	$22,228	$19,705	0.6915

Sources: See Table 6-3.

Table 6-4 displays the mean values of these various measures according to the classification of type of welfare state. The groups of countries do not differ in respect of capital controls, trade openness, outward investment, government expenditure, public pension, public share of health expenditures, and GDP per capita. They differ significantly in respect of international borrowing, government revenues, social security expenditures, civilian government employment, and infant mortality rates. In general, governments of Social Democratic and Christian Democratic welfare states are larger, spend more on services and transfer payments, and the infant mortality rates of these countries are on average lower than those in the other types of welfare states.

Like the results described above, these results suggest that while trade openness does not differ among these different kinds of welfare states, the policies pursued by their governments do differ, and those differences are reflected in differences in infant mortality. [126] The countries with the more activist governments have the lowest infant mortality rates, although once again life expectancy at birth does not differ.

One sees something similar in three small Asian states: Singapore, Hong Kong, and Malaysia. According to the World Bank, all three are more open to trade than the most open European nations,[127] and M. Ramesh and Ian Holliday have shown that they have achieved remarkably low mortality at relatively low cost.[128] Health care expenditures per capita in 1996 were U.S. $1214 in

Hong Kong, $140 in Malaysia, and $979 in Singapore, respectively 4.6%, 2.9%, and 3.3% of GDP. Life expectancy was 78.7 in Hong Kong, 71.6 in Malaysia, and 77.1 in Singapore. Hong Kong and Singapore would count as high-income countries; Malaysia as a middle-income country, and as Ramesh and Holliday show, their life expectancies are as good as, or better than, the averages of countries in each of those income groups.[129]

Part of the reason for the superior performance of these small countries is that they have much younger populations than those of their European equivalents. This would not explain the life expectancy patterns, but it is associated with the caregiving function of families. A tradition of family support for the sick exists in each country, and the young age structure means that there are people available to provide care for the elderly. Furthermore, densely settled populations with centralized administrations also contribute to bureaucratic efficiency in the management of government programs.

Ramesh and Holliday argue that these factors cannot be a complete explanation because many countries have similar features and do not perform as well. Neither can health care financing mechanisms explain the results, which differ substantially among them. However, "State dominance of secondary care provision is," they claim, "a common feature of these three countries and marks them out as a distinctive cluster. It is also a feature of the British NHS, after which the three health care systems are loosely modeled."[130] And, they continue, "In each of these countries the large state presence in the provision of secondary care has played a significant role in keeping down costs in this notably expensive part of the health care service."[131]

Lance Taylor has summarized the results of studies of the impact of trade liberalization in nine poor and middle-income countries. He shows that liberalization had different consequences among them, though in none could it be considered a brilliant success.[132] Figure 6-2 displays GDP per capita in each of the countries but Cuba, for which the World Bank provides no data,[133] and Figure 6-3 displays a measure of trade openness (Imports + Exports as a percent of GDP). Table 6-5 displays correlations between GDP per capita (in 1995 U.S. $) and openness from 1980 through 2000. Income did not increase uniformly in all of them, and trade openness was also highly variable, as were the correlations between openness and GDP per capita. They were significant and positive in five of the countries and unassociated in the other three, Russia, Zimbabwe, and Korea (Cuba is not included due to absence of data). Income rose most impressively in Korea, despite the fact that openness actually declined into the early 1980s, and despite a major financial crisis in 1997. Income declined in Russia and stagnated and declined slightly in Zimbabwe despite increasing openness.

The details of the policies pursued in each country are too complex to be described here. Taylor describes some of the social policies very broadly as follows. "Colombia, Cuba, and Korea introduced social policy programs to offset some of the negative consequences of liberalization." "Russia, Turkey and Zimbabwe faced fiscal resource constraints during external liberalization and were

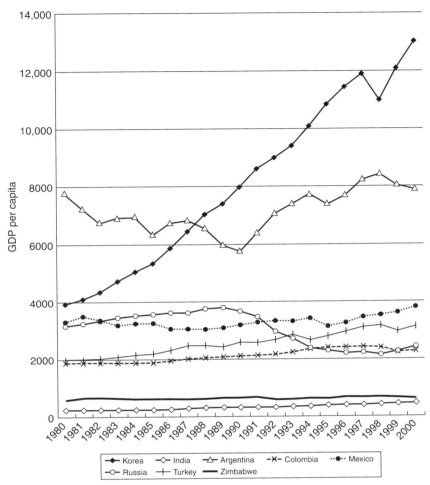

Figure 6-2. GDP per capita in eight countries. (*Source*: World Bank, *World Development Indicators*, CD-ROM. Washington, D.C., 2002.)

forced to cut back on social programs." "In Argentina, India, and Mexico, external liberalization has not been accompanied with increased social spending."[134] Russia and Zimbabwe are described as "disasters,"[135] and it is significant that in these two countries there has been a substantial decline of life expectancy from the late 1980s, as displayed in Figure 6-4,[136] even as openness has increased. That the decline in life expectancy in each of these countries is measurable at the national level suggests just how profound the crises are in each of them, for the impact of economic turmoil is often observed in particularly vulnerable segments of the population and may not be discernible in national figures.

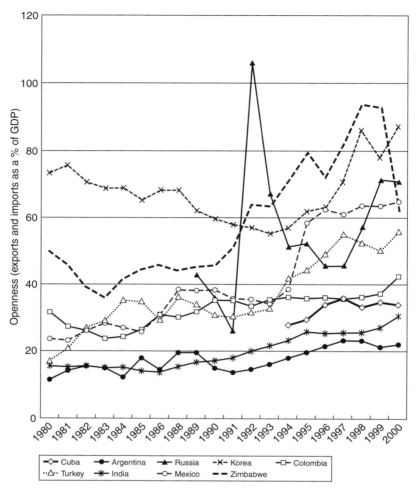

Figure 6-3. Openness in nine countries. (*Source*: World Bank, *World Development Indicators*, CD-ROM. Washington, D.C., 2002.)

Table 6-6 displays correlations between life expectancy on the one hand and GDP per capita (in 1995 U.S. $) and openness on the other. In all countries but Argentina there is a significant association between life expectancy and GDP per capita, although in Zimbabwe it is negative. Life expectancy there has declined despite essentially stagnant or slightly declining income, presumably largely a reflection of the impact of HIV/AIDS and the inability to obtain the necessary drugs at an affordable price. In Russia, Korea, Mexico, and Zimbabwe, there is no association between life expectancy and openness.

Cuba is one of the countries included in the comparative analyses summarized by Taylor, but aside from data on mortality, there is not much data in

Table 6-5
Correlations Between Trade Openness and GDP per Capita
(in 1995 U.S. $), 1980–2000

Country	Correlation Coefficient	p-value
Argentina	0.53	0.0140
Russia (1988–2000)	0.29	0.3575
Korea	0.10	0.6495
Colombia	0.85	<0.0001
Turkey	0.88	<0.0001
India	0.94	<0.0001
Mexico	0.47	0.0365
Zimbabwe	0.35	0.1289

the World Development Report on income and openness until the mid-1990s. This is a pity, for as Figure 6-4 demonstrates, life expectancy of the Cuban population was higher than of any other population included in the comparative analyses. Much has been written about Cuba's remarkable achievements with respect to health status and low mortality rates,[137] especially in light of the economic problems it has had stemming from its unpopularity with the government of the United States.[138] Those difficulties became even more formidable after the collapse of the Soviet Union, which had been Cuba's major trading partner, and a tightening of the U.S. embargo. Cuba has been forced to engage in trade with new partners, and the result has been growing inequality and the emergence of a small, highly controlled, market economy.[139] What has not changed is the government's commitment to maintaining the high level of health services and education.

Figure 6-5 displays GDP per capita in Cuba and Costa Rica from 1980 through 2000 from the United Nations *Statistical Yearbook*[140] and openness for the available years from the World Bank's *World Development Report*. Costa Rica is included because it too is a Caribbean nation that is often cited as an example of a small, democratic, open, poor country with remarkably high life expectancy.[141] Costa Rica suffered a severe financial crisis at the end of the 1970s, which is reflected in the steep drop in GDP per capita from 1980 to 1981. Since then, income has increased relatively smoothly. GDP per capita remained more or less constant in Cuba over the same period, with a drop beginning in 1990, the start of the so-called "special period" after the collapse of the Soviet Union.

In addition to having substantially higher GDP per capita, Costa Rica has a far more open economy than Cuba's, even after the latter's cautious trade liberalization starting in the early 1990s. And although Costa Rica has among the most egalitarian income distributions in Latin America, a region with the least egalitarian income distribution in the world, it is nonetheless a highly unequal society, with a Gini coefficient of 0.46 in the late 1990s.[142] Comparable

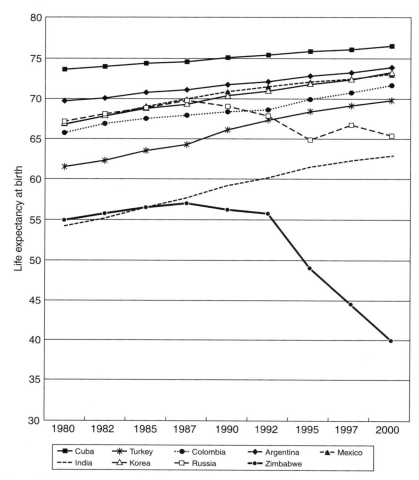

Figure 6-4. Life expectancy in nine countries, 1980–2000. (*Source*: World Bank, *World Development Indicators*, CD-ROM. Washington, D.C., 2002.)

data are not available for Cuba, but it is certainly the case that the Cuban commitment to equality has resulted in a far lower Gini coefficient than that. (By way of comparison, the Gini coefficient for the United States was 0.41 [in 1997] and for Sweden 0.25 [in 1992].[143])

Keeping in mind the substantially lower GDP per capita of Cubans than Costa Ricans, the consistently lower infant mortality rate in Cuba than Costa Rica (Figure 6-6) is remarkable. On the other hand, life expectancy at birth has improved somewhat more rapidly among Costa Rican than Cuban men. The reverse is true for women, among whom the improvement for Cubans was more rapid than for Costa Ricans. By 2000, life expectancy was the same for men in each country as well as for women. This comparison, like those

Table 6-6
Correlations of Life Expectancy at Birth With GDP Per Capita and Trade
Openness for Various Years, 1980–2000

Country	No. Observed	GDP per capita		Openness	
		r	p	r	p
Argentina	8	0.41	0.3057	0.82	0.0118
Cuba			Insufficient data		
Russia	12	0.85	<0.0001	0.26	0.3991
Korea	8	0.99	<0.0001	0.14	0.7144
Colombia	8	0.63	0.0186	0.93	0.0027
Turkey	8	0.88	0.0039	0.98	<0.0001
India	8	0.88	0.0034	0.94	<0.0001
Mexico	8	0.90	0.0023	0.34	0.3848
Zimbabwe	9	−0.75	0.0181	−0.12	0.3572

reported previously, again suggests that while openness may be associated with increased average income per capita, it is not the case that good health necessarily follows the same path.

Of course, it is not even necessarily the case that high income is invariably associated with openness, or with better mortality. Figure 6-7 displays the openness of the Canadian and American economies from 1965 through 1995. Because of its relatively small population and the size of its neighbor to the south, Canada has been far more open than the United States, and the difference has only increased with the passage of NAFTA. On the other hand, Canadian per capita income is lower than in the United States. Nonetheless, as demonstrated in Chapter 3, the Canadian health care system has done a far better job of reducing mortality among Canadians than the U.S. system has among Americans, both black and white, and at about half the cost per capita.

Globalization and Local Culture and Institutions

To drive home the point that globalization does not have the same effects everywhere and that the impact is refracted through the lens of local institutions and economies, I describe briefly the collapse of Yugoslavia and the different institutional arrangements in the United States and Canada that underlie the differences in mortality described previously in this chapter and in Chapter 3.

The Collapse of Yugoslavia.[144] The Kingdom of Serbs, Croats, and Slovenes (what became Yugoslavia after World War II) was largely an undeveloped country in the interwar years. High taxes, declining agricultural prices

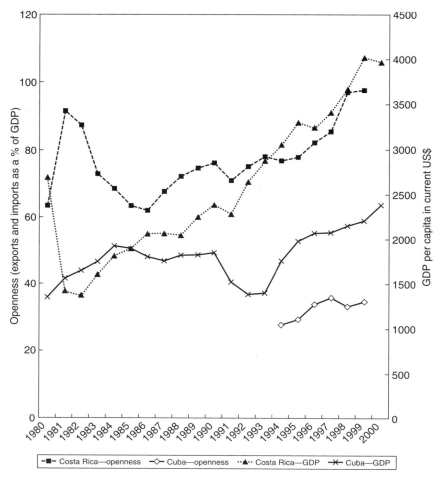

Figure 6-5. Cuba and Costa Rica, GDP per capita and openness, 1980–2001. (*Sources*: GDP from *UN Statistical Yearbook*, 47th issue, CD-ROM. New York: United Nations, 2003. Openness from World Bank, *World Development Indicators*, CD-ROM. Washington, D.C., 2002.)

during the depression years of the 1930s, and poverty contributed to the peasants' hostility to the government and to their support for the Partisans during World War II, which was as much a civil war as a war against the German invaders.

That they had fought their own war of liberation and had had their own communist revolution gave the Yugoslavs a certain degree of independence in their dealings with the Soviet Union and other Communist nations. In particular, the Yugoslav leadership wished to develop their own industry rather than be dependent entirely upon the Soviet Union for manufactured goods. Conflict

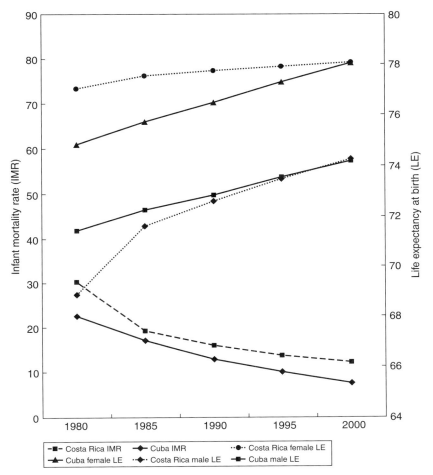

Figure 6-6. Infant mortality rate (IMR) and life expectancy (LE), Cuba and Costa Rica, 1980–2000. (*Source*: World Bank, *World Development Indicators*, CD-ROM. Washington, D.C., 2002.)

with the Soviet Union over this and other issues resulted in expulsion from the Comintern in 1947 and increasing economic and political isolation.[145]

As a result, Yugoslavs became increasingly critical first of Soviet foreign policy and then of domestic policy, what they called *etatism*; that is, centralized, bureaucratized government planning and control. In response to the threat of invasion by the Soviet Union, and to maintain the allegiance of the people, most of whom were non-Communists, a new form of socialism, called self-management, was developed, which involved both decentralization and inclusion of workers in decision-making in the enterprises in which they worked.[146] There was growing openness toward, and dependence upon, the

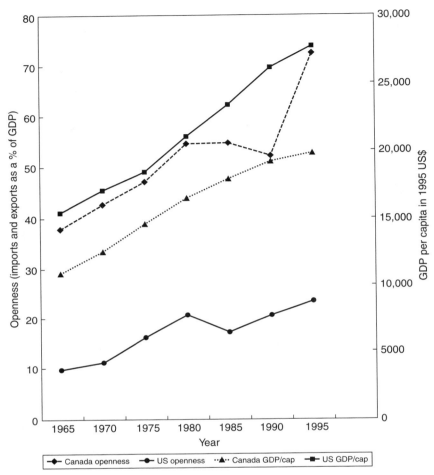

Figure 6-7. Openness and GDP per capita, USA and Canada, 1965–1995. (*Source:* World Bank, *World Development Indicators*, CD-ROM. Washington, D.C., 2002.)

West as trade with the Eastern bloc declined. This took several forms including foreign aid, foreign investment in Yugoslav enterprises, an increasingly market-oriented economy, and, increasingly through the 1970s, loans from commercial lenders.

The benefits of international integration were real but also dangerous. Incomes increased substantially from the early 1950s to the late 1970s but then began a precipitous fall as inflation destroyed the economy.[147] The economic decline was due to severe deficits in the balance of payments, the result of increases in the price of oil and other imported goods beginning in the early 1970s; declining competitiveness of Yugoslav exports in the world market; and increasing resort to short-term commercial loans at high and rising interest rates caused by the savings and loan crisis in the United States.[148] Despite the establishment of an IMF-supported economic stabilization program in 1979, inflation accelerated through the 1980s.[149] From 1970 to 1980 inflation had averaged 18.4% per year. It was between 85% and 105% annually in the early 1980s, reached 800% to 900% by the end of the 1980s, and averaged 123% annually from 1979 to 1989.[150]

Complicating and exacerbating the economic crisis was the policy toward nationalities pursued by the Yugoslav government, similar to that pursued by the Soviet government.[151] Nationalities were recognized as having cultural rights (to be educated in their own language, for instance). This was seen as a necessary but transitional phase; necessary to gain the loyalty of the many different nationalities; transitional because it was believed they would ultimately become one people. In both the Soviet Union and Yugoslavia, nationalities were territorially based in the different republics of the federation, but significant minorities were found in other republics, for instance, Serbs in Bosnia, Croatia, and the autonomous province of Kosovo (part of Serbia and the poorest region of Yugoslavia); Croatians in Bosnia; Albanians in Macedonia; and Hungarians in Vojvodina (also an autonomous province and part of Serbia and among the richest regions in the country). The notion that nationalities were ethnocultural communities (an idea with too long and complex a history to recount here[152]) was thus encouraged by government policy. Among other things, it meant that Serbia had an interest in the treatment of Serbs outside of Serbia, and that Croatia had an interest in the treatment of Croats in other republics. The policy with respect to the equality of nationalities also required equalization across the republics; that is, a transfer of wealth from the rich to the poor republics, which had been a continuous source of resentment.

It was in this context of hyperinflation that first Slovenia and then Croatia seceded from Yugoslavia in 1991, for these were the two wealthiest republics. Their citizens had supported decentralization and liberalization and had long resented what they perceived to be the confiscatory taxes levied by the central government to pay for equalization, including development projects and services in the poor republics and in the Autonomous Province of Kosovo. While the taxes and redistributive policies they supported may have been tolerable when real incomes were rising, they became intolerable when the economy had fallen apart.

In addition to inter-republic tension, however, there was the additional problem that Yugoslavia, like the Soviet Union, was a single-party state. There was no organized opposition party that crossed republic lines and that could unite people once the dominant party had been discredited. Indeed, the policy with regard to nationalities had created local elites in each republic ready to assert their claims to independent nationhood, and in both Serbia and Croatia demagogic leaders arose whose appeal to their constituents was based on religious and ethnic loyalties that, once unleashed, could not be controlled.[153]

In a very real sense, the route to the collapse of the Yugoslav federation, like the collapse of the Soviet federation, was paved by the policy toward nationalities that each had pursued, but it was precipitated by involvement in the global economy, to which the domestic political culture and institutions were unable to adapt. As described earlier in this chapter, the consequences for the health of people in the poor (now former) republics has been profound, and the lack of foreign aid to replace the income transfers they had received when the country was still intact suggests that recovery in future will be slow and uncertain.

Political Institutions and Health in the United States and Canada[154] Globalization in peripheral and semiperipheral countries has more obvious effects than in the core countries of northwestern Europe and the Americas north of Mexico. As described above, Canada has a far more open economy than the United States and substantially lower income per capita. If income were the determinant of health, the United States should have higher life expectancy and lower cause-specific mortality than Canada. That would also be the case if trade liberalization were so catastrophic. As demonstrated in Chapter 3, however, the expectations of neither optimists nor pessimists have been realized. Despite a more open and less opulent economy, Canadian life expectancy and cause-specific mortality are more favorable than those of Americans, both white and black. To understand why, it is necessary to consider the political culture and institutions of each country.

An important feature of the American presidential system is that "individual members of the legislature owed their primary loyalty to their constituencies," powers are divided among the branches of the government, and party discipline is weak. This system, according to Samuel Huntington, an inheritance of the Tudor model of government, was made obsolete by the parliamentary revolution in England even as it was being implanted in America.[155]

In contrast to the presidential system, the parliamentary system centralized authority in Parliament. MPs were no longer responsible primarily to their constituencies but to the nation as a whole;[156] executive and legislative powers were merged; policy making was "concentrated in a relatively small and cohesive Cabinet, and the crucial debate on issues comes before they are presented in the legislature for consideration."[157] Party discipline is strong, which means that dissidents within a political party may be forced to look elsewhere "rather than try to influence major parties from within."[158] Third parties are thus more likely to emerge and persist in this sort of system than in the presidential system, in which party discipline is much weaker and parties far more diverse.

The pervasive importance of the presidential system goes a considerable way toward explaining both the differences between African American and white life expectancy, and the difference between American and Canadian life expectancy. The persistent disenfranchisement of African American citizens after the Civil War meant that southern politics was dominated by whites, and because the Republican Party was the party of Lincoln, the Democratic Party dominated the South. Long-serving white Democrats thus came to represent the South in both the House of Representatives and the Senate where, because of the seniority system, they ultimately controlled the chairmanships of many important committees.[159] Thus, by the time of the Great Depression of the 1930s when the Democratic Party came to power under Franklin Roosevelt, it comprised an unwieldy coalition of conservative southern whites jealously guarding the rights of states and the status quo with respect to race relations, and largely independent of the control of the party, and northern representatives of industrial workers and urban political machines. The urban reform movement and what would have been a socialist or social democratic party were submerged within this coalition, and it was this coalition that was largely responsible for the shape of the historic welfare legislation passed during the New Deal.

Details are available elsewhere. Suffice it to say that all the titles of the Social Security Act contained mechanisms that discriminated against African Americans.[160] Similarly, the National Labor Relations (Wagner) Act of 1935 did not bar discrimination on the part of unions,[161] and the National Housing Act of 1934, which created the Federal Housing Administration (FHA), did not provide loans for homes in African American or mixed neighborhoods and encouraged restrictive covenants prohibiting sale of homes to African Americans. Housing policy went further, however, for the Housing Act of 1937 allowed local authorities to use tax-free bonds to build public housing projects, with federal funds being used to subsidize rents for the poor. In practice, housing projects were built in racially segregated neighborhoods.[162] Thus, home ownership was for whites, rentals were for African Americans, and working class neighborhoods remained racially segregated, with important long-term consequences for residential patterns as well as the intergenerational accumulation of wealth.[163]

One important piece of legislation that failed in the face of resistance from the conservative congressional coalition of Republicans and southern Democrats during the New Deal was the inclusion of compulsory health insurance in the Social Security Act. This is a story that has often been told and does not require retelling. The only point to make here is that as southern Democrats became less influential in the party during World War II[164] and began shifting their allegiance to the Republican Party, a universal entitlement to health care became ever less likely to being made the law of the land.

Many observers have commented upon the impact of historic patterns of inequality on health care and health status in the South right down to the present.[165] As noted in Chapter 4, mortality in the southern states has consistently been higher than elsewhere. But, as southerners have been among the first to point out, racial segregation is not a uniquely southern phenomenon. Racial segregation in cities of the Northeast and Midwest has been described in Chapter 5. It suffices to say here that the federal government's housing legislation reinforced existing racial prejudices and helped to create what David Rusk has called "inelastic" cities, cities that have not been able to expand to embrace their spreading regional populations.[166] There are several important consequences. The first is that racial segregation is greater in metropolitan areas with inelastic cities, as a result of exclusionary practices in the towns surrounding these cities, than in metropolitan regions characterized by elastic cities.[167]

Second, the tax base of inelastic cities is relatively small, and diminishes even more as the relatively well-to-do flee to the suburbs. As the tax base shrinks, local services, including schools, health care providers, mass transit, and local shops, all decline in number and quality as well. The number of physicians practicing in central cities has declined just as other services have, and inadequate Medicaid reimbursement rates and the great need for health services by poor populations conspire to lead to high rates of closure of urban hospitals. Indeed, the proportion of a hospital's patients and the proportion of the population in a hospital's neighborhood who are African American are among the best predictors of hospital closure.[168]

Third, inelastic cities are the very ones in which old industries have declined, throwing many out of work. These were the industries in which workers, including those living in segregated urban neighborhoods, had health insurance. With the loss of those jobs, health benefits have been lost as well, more by African Americans than whites, and with measurable negative consequences.[169] New employment opportunities requiring literacy and numeracy are not locally available but tend to be located in suburban office parks. Because of the deterioration of urban school systems, many young people do not possess the necessary skills for such jobs, and inadequate mass transit makes them relatively inaccessible anyway.[170] Many of the jobs that are available are in the nonunionized service sector and do not carry with them health care benefits.

All these factors contribute to the disparities between white and African American life expectancy, and among their sources is the presidential system that, while possessing many advantages, has also perpetuated racial segregation and diminished access to employment, education, and health services, injustices that have only slowly and imperfectly been addressed.

If the legacy of slavery and racism has shaped the health disparities between African Americans and whites, it is political institutions that have largely shaped the way that legacy has found expression. And it is those same institutions that contribute so substantially to the differences between the United States and Canada. For just as the presidential system in the United States is part of the reason there is no universal entitlement to health care, so the parliamentary system that was adopted in Canada is an important part of the explanation of the creation of national health insurance there.[171] But as the American example demonstrates, the larger political culture and economy also have a profound effect. The absence of a social democratic party in the United States is an important reason there is no compulsory health insurance, and the fact that there is not a parliamentary system in the United States may be a partial explanation of why there is no social democratic third party.[172] It does not explain, however, either why one of the two major American parties is not social democratic,[173] or why the most important third party in Canada is.

In both Quebec and English Canada, a certain degree of conservative collectivism has been prominent, that is, the belief that the state had the duty to intervene in economic affairs, that the collectivity takes precedence over individuals, and that society is necessarily hierarchical.[174] According to this explanation, socialism in Canada resulted from Tory collectivism and could only develop where collectivist traditions already existed.[175]

Another important part of the story is federalism. If race and the unjust treatment of African Americans is still one of the great unresolved moral and political dilemmas in the United States, regionalism is the unresolved issue in Canada.[176] Morton Weinfeld has noted that "The binational origin of the Canadian state paved the way for full acceptance of the plural nature of Canadian society and acknowledgement of the contributions, value, and rights of all Canadian minority groups." Moreover, the binational origin of the state, and "the fact that Canada's largest minority, French Canadians, control a province, Quebec" means that Canadian federalism is more fissiparous than the American version has been since the Civil War.[177] And, Seymour Martin Lipset continues, "smaller provinces seeking to extend their autonomy have been able to do so because Quebec has always been in the forefront of the struggle."[178] The nature of Canadian federalism, the presence of a social democratic party at both provincial and federal levels,[179] and the role of the welfare state in tying together the country all go a long way toward explaining the passage of national health insurance in Canada.[180]

Social democracy was not crucial for the development of the welfare state in Canada,[181] but with respect to national health insurance, it is significant that the socialist government of Saskatchewan was the first in North America to attempt social insurance, starting with universal, publicly administered hospital coverage in 1947, and followed by more complete protection in the late 1950s and early 1960s.[182] These policies had a national impact.[183] Despite business opposition, as well as Conservative opposition at the provincial level, at the federal level, Conservatives were virtually unanimous in their support of both hospital insurance in the 1950s and physician reimbursement plans in 1972, a unanimity made possible by the party discipline that can be enforced in parliamentary systems such as Canada's.[184]

Thus, just as American attitudes towards race as expressed through political institutions contribute much to the differences in health between African Americans and whites, so have the differences between American and Canadian political cultures and institutions had a profound impact on the differences in health care and mortality between the two countries, even in the presence of great differences in per capita income and trade liberalization. The fact that Canada has a more open economy and lower income per capita than the United States and yet has better life expectancy demonstrates again that neither income nor trade liberalization is necessarily associated with good or bad health. Everything depends upon whether governments have the will and the capacity to protect their publics.

Conclusion

All these examples suggest that openness to trade is not incompatible with good health of the population affected, but neither is it a guarantee. Much of the difference in mortality among countries depends upon the strength and policies of their governments and the degree to which they can protect their populations and communities from the vicissitudes that openness involves, while still benefiting from its positive effects.

However, the social compact that characterized welfare states in the several decades after World War II had been based upon a bargain governments made with their publics: in exchange for the turmoil of trade liberalization, governments would provide help to those who experienced the dislocation that followed. In the past generation, that agreement has been jeopardized by a variety of forces, not the least of which is trade liberalization itself.[185] For one of the paradoxes, perhaps contradiction would be a more accurate term, of liberalization has been that the very protections that were put in place to buffer people from its damaging effects have been weakened as those protections have increasingly been defined as nontariff barriers to trade in services as well as goods. Economically advanced countries may be able to withstand some of these pressures. Poor, heavily indebted countries with already weak or ineffective governments will not be able to do the same. It is probable that many countries in this situation will be unable to benefit from liberalization.

There is another paradox of globalization, however, that also threatens the generous benefits provided by welfare states. The aging of their populations, the consequence of severely diminished fertility, is a major impediment to their continued generosity. One of the ways in which this problem has been addressed is by allowing increasing immigration to respond to demands for labor, an aspect of globalization that has not been dealt with in this chapter. The paradox is that the generosity of welfare states is inversely correlated with the ethno-linguistic heterogeneity of their populations: the more diverse the population, the less generous the benefits.[186] To the degree that immigration increases heterogeneity, social solidarity and the willingness to be generous to fellow citizens may well decline.[187] Thus, internal developments may conspire with forces of globalization to threaten the social compact that was meant to buffer the disruptive effects of liberalization. But for the moment, it is still accurate to say that while openness has not resulted in the benefits promised by the optimists, neither has it had the deleterious consequences for the health of many populations that the pessimists predict.

7

Masterful Images

Players and painted stage took all my love,
And not those things they were emblems of.
—W.B. Yeats, *The Circus Animals' Desertion*[1]

Three related themes have run through this book. The first is the role that inherited ideas about the consequences of social and economic change and of causes of disease have had on explanations of the social determinants of the health of populations. The second is the way these inherited ideas have been assimilated into different political ideologies that influence the choices we all make of the evidence we accept and ignore. The third is the importance of particular contexts—including, but not limited to, political institutions—for understanding the health of populations. In this concluding chapter, I should like to draw together some of these themes, first by using debates about HIV-AIDS for illustrative purposes, and then by returning to the issues raised in the Preface, (1) the significance of the distinction between the cognitive styles of hedgehogs and foxes, and (2) the importance of anomalies and what they can tell us about the generalizability of theories about the social determinants of death and disease.

AIDS, Exemplary Disease

All of the ambiguities considered so far are manifested in the debates surrounding AIDS. It is in this sense that AIDS is an exemplary disease.

Necessary and Sufficient Cause. It is now widely agreed that HIV is a necessary cause of AIDS. Without it, there would be no such disease, no matter how poor, how malnourished, how wretchedly unhappy, how isolated, how sexually active, or how drug dependent one is. The debate is between those who believe HIV is *the* cause to which everything else is subordinate and those who believe that it is the social environment that accounts for the patterns observed worldwide. On the one hand are those who believe AIDS is "a single disease with a single cause."[2] The implications of this position are important. Recall the doctor satirized in the epigraph of Chapter 1 who said, "What is the remedy? A very simple one. Find the germ and kill it." Compare that to what Lewis Thomas wrote of HIV/AIDS:

> [I]t seems to me self-evident that the only sure way out of the dilemma must be by research. This is not to say that education and behavioral change will not be valuable in the short run as ways to limit the spread for the time being, to slow down the pandemic for a while. Obviously we should be instructing all young people in what the virus is and what we already know about how its contagion works, and surely we should be trying whatever we can, including more methadone clinics and the free distribution of sterile needles within the heroin-addicted community. But these are not the answers for the long run. If we are to avert what otherwise lies somewhere ahead, we will have to find out how to kill this virus without killing the cells in which it is lodged, or how to immunize the entire population against the virus, or both.[3]

This view of social interventions—what to do until the doctor arrives—is an example of the kind of "biomedical discourse"[4] that drives mad those who, on the other hand, believe that what is uppermost in importance is vulnerability, the conditions that put individuals and communities in situations in which they are likely to contract the virus and develop the disease.[5] Increasingly, those conditions are defined as poverty and powerlessness, particularly the powerlessness of women.[6]

These are not trivial differences, as the debate about South Africa's President Mbeki questioning the centrality of HIV as the cause of AIDS makes clear.[7] For the president was not simply questioning the significance of the virus as the necessary cause of AIDS, but also asserting that the poverty of black South Africans was the cause, and he assembled an advisory committee of scientists who shared his skepticism about the importance of the virus.[8]

The difference between these ways of understanding causality reflects differences in what is to be explained, the disease or the epidemic.[9] The disease is caused by the virus. The epidemic is best explained by characteristics of populations. This was the argument Thomas McKeown made when he claimed that it was not necessary to know the underlying mechanisms of diseases in order to prevent them.[10] That the mechanism by which smoking caused lung cancer, and contamination from autopsies causes childbed fever were unknown did not mean that each could not be prevented, the first by not smoking, the second by thoroughly washing one's hands after an autopsy. What counts as a cause is thus a pragmatic issue, although for the past century it has been common to define as most fundamental deep biological explanations.

This does not exhaust the matter, however, for as Lewis Thomas argued, the notion of necessary cause also implies a particular kind of intervention in the epidemic, ideally an immunization that will make other social interventions unnecessary in the long run. Indeed, he was right: an effective vaccine made widely accessible would make other kinds of interventions unnecessary. That seems unlikely, at least in the near future, and perhaps in the distant future as well. For the most promising vaccines may not prevent absolutely the spread of the virus but only contain it and slow the progression of the disease in infected individuals.[11] In the meantime, and for a very long time, as many observers have noted, there are several different AIDS epidemics that may respond to different kinds of interventions.

For instance, Shirley Lindenbaum has suggested that, as described in Chapter 1, pellagra offers one model and hookworm another. "Among gay men and hemophiliacs in developed countries a simple intervention—a change in blood bank procedures and new ways to express love and affection (adopted voluntarily by many gay men)—can interrupt transmission of the virus. To understand and prevent continuation of the epidemic among intravenous drug users and their sexual partners, however, hookworm provides the better model. Here, the behaviors to be modified require vast social and economic change."[12] The latter is also true of AIDS in poor countries.

Individual and Social Responsibility. Nowhere are issues of blame and responsibility more evident than in debates about homosexuality and intravenous drug use and their association with HIV and AIDS. Those who in Chapter 1 I called voluntarists argue that since these are volitional acts under the control of those who engage in them, the individual himself or herself is responsible for the consequences, not society or insurance companies.[13] Moreover, voluntarists of a conservative persuasion have used the AIDS epidemic as a reason to urge abstinence even among heterosexuals who are at very low risk.[14] Determinists believe that little, if any, free choice is involved in these behaviors, that the weight of social circumstances determines them, and that the approach must be not abstinence but harm reduction and changes in the social and economic circumstances of the victims.

The same issue is played out on a much larger scale in discussions of AIDS in poor countries, particularly in Africa. Sanjay Basu writes that "Sex is not as much the issue as the context under which sex occurs, yet public health workers studying AIDS are guilty of trying to define an African 'system of sexuality' and render sexual behavior the problem rather than examining why sex among the poor seems to lead to HIV transmission so much more often than sex among the wealthy."[15] Similarly, Wende Elizabeth Marshall has written:

> In the United States, scientific and biomedical discourses on AIDS
> are often tangled with older narratives about the sociocultural (read
> "racial") pathology of black women's reproduction and the welfare
> state. In African nations, the discourse on HIV and AIDS maps onto

narratives about the degraded and dysfunctional nature/culture of African people and politics. In the US and African nations, as well as elsewhere in the [African] diaspora, a "blame the victim" ideology is a persistent subtext of health development discourse.[16]

Contrast this anthropological reductionism to Philip Setel's account of AIDS in Tanzania.

Communities in which risk behavior takes place ought not to be conceptualized as traditional versus modern, promiscuous versus monogamous, or urban versus rural. Rather, sexual risk can be understood to vary for individuals according to context, and to require a model that accounts for the character of risky contact among infected and noninfected persons in the early stages of a lengthy epidemic, a political economy of itinerancy, interaction with cash economies, and social dislocation.[17]

That the spread of HIV and AIDS is associated with recent vast economic and social changes is beyond dispute. But it is also embedded in different cultural and economic contexts that shape the epidemic, some of which may have very deep historical roots,[18] others of which are more recent. To reduce it to either individual irresponsibility or to poverty and powerlessness does violence to the reality of lived experience in which people, even in some very poor places, think of themselves as moral agents and not simply as victims of social forces beyond their control.[19]

Inequality. There can be no doubt that inequality and differences in social power have had a profound impact upon the course of the AIDS epidemics. Examples abound of women with no economic alternatives for whom sexual partners provide an important source of income, and a source of infection as well.[20] Moreover, in developed countries, the epidemics are largely found among the poor and socially marginal. The same does not seem to be as clear in Africa, where evidence suggests that male political leaders, teachers, and government bureaucrats are contracting the disease and dying at very high rates.[21] For example, data from Tanzania, Rwanda, and Uganda reveal that HIV-positive individuals have disproportionately high educational and income levels and that the largest single group is comprised of civil servants.[22] In a series of case studies of women in Zaire, Brooke Grundfest Schoepf writes of a woman married to a man "from the ruling party's inner circle":

For such men, the company of stylish young women is a prerequisite of the job, a routine part of the socializing integral to politics. Mistresses are also part of the intelligence-gathering networks that no man in high politics can do without. The government's ideology of "authenticity," promulgated partly to undermine the influence of the Catholic church, has made polygyny respectable. As in the slaving period prior to this century, access to numerous women is a symbol of power and wealth.[23]

That high-status men exploit women, often very young women,[24] clearly reflects a difference in power, but it does not diminish the fact that the high-status men who infect their sexual partners are themselves HIV positive and likely to develop AIDS. There is some suggestive evidence that the prevalence of HIV is declining more rapidly in wealthy than in poor segments of the population, at least in Uganda,[25] and presumably when the wealthy fall ill, they have greater access to treatment. Nonetheless, across the continent mortality among the political and other elites remains high, so much so that it is further jeopardizing already unstable political regimes and the possibilities of future economic growth.[26] Thus, while poverty may be a fundamental cause of AIDS in wealthy countries, it is not so obvious that it is equally fundamental as an explanation of differences in vulnerability within Africa. Victimizers may themselves be victims.

But inequality is relative as well as absolute, and evidence from 72 developing countries from the mid-1990s indicates that income (GNP per capita in 1994 U.S. $) is inversely, and income inequality (the Gini coefficient) is positively, correlated with the percent of urban adults positive for HIV. That is, the lower the income and the greater the inequality, the higher is the prevalence of HIV.[27] Inequality may well be reflected in lower levels of support for prevention and treatment programs, and is also likely to be associated with predatory behavior of the powerful and dependence of women upon the selling of sexual favors as a means of economic survival.

Community and Social Cohesion. It is useful to think of community and social cohesion in respect of, firstly, exposure to HIV and, secondly, responses to AIDS. The evidence suggests, for example, that for gay men in the United States, integration into a network of other gay men substantially increases the risk of exposure to HIV.[28] On the other hand, when the gay "community" was mobilized,[29] prevention of unsafe sex and an impressive reduction in transmission of HIV occurred. And when people are HIV-positive and develop AIDS, the support they and their caregivers receive is also significantly enhanced by integration into a social network, though even then support from family members may result in additional stress for caregivers.[30] Thus, social networks among gay men have had mixed effects, both supporting increasing risk of exposure and providing support when sick. Similarly, integration of intravenous drug users into a network of other drug users also substantially increases risk of exposure to HIV. Unfortunately, the social networks of drug addicts do not support either safe sex or safe drug use. A change of networks is generally required. [31] The consequences of integration into personal communities of various sorts are thus ambiguous.

The same ambiguity is observable when social cohesion at the national level is considered. For example, Tony Barnett and Alan Whiteside argue that social cohesion is a preferable measure to income inequality. They present a typology of countries based upon wealth and social cohesion and argue that the prevalence of HIV and AIDS will be low where social cohesion is high, and high where social cohesion is low, regardless of the wealth of the country.[32] They define countries as having high social cohesion if they have "strong religious cultures or good governance or integrating ideologies." Countries have low social cohesion if they were "experiencing civil war or economic collapse."[33] Their example of a country with high social cohesion and high wealth was the United Kingdom. Countries with high social cohesion and low wealth were the Philippines, India, and Senegal. Those with low social cohesion and low wealth were Uganda and the Ukraine. And those with low social cohesion and high wealth were South Africa and Botswana.

The ambiguity of these concepts of high and low social cohesion is to be found in the breadth of their defining characteristics. Can the United Kingdom really be considered a cohesive society, despite its "good government," when the magnitude of inequality and social stratification are taken into account. Nor is it clear why India with its caste system, great diversity of populations, different religious faiths, and growing income inequality, is considered cohesive. And indeed, as Barnett and Whiteside observe, the incidence and prevalence of HIV positivity and of AIDS are unknown in India. The low prevalence of HIV and AIDS in the Philippines is attributed to the "moral authority of the [Catholic] Church, the vibrancy of the NGO community and the strength of family discipline . . . in the face of large-scale public corruption and political uncertainty."[34] And Uganda, which has both low income and low social cohesion, is one of the few examples of an African nation in which seroprevalence of HIV is declining. None of which is to deny that the disruption of established relationships and obligations is implicated in the spread of HIV. Rather, it is to suggest that measuring social cohesion at the national level in the way suggested above raises far more questions than it answers. Income inequality, often considered a proxy for social cohesion, at least has the virtue of being a more readily defined—though difficult to measure—concept, and as already noted is associated with the percent of HIV positive adults in urban areas of poor countries.

Globalization. That AIDS is a global epidemic does not distinguish it from many other epidemics that have devastated human populations. The Black Death swept from Central Asia to Western Europe in the fourteenth century. Syphilis was widespread across Europe during and after the Renaissance and spread to newly conquered lands, along with smallpox, measles, hookworm, malaria, and yellow fever, all brought to the Western Hemisphere from Africa and Europe as a result of exploration and trade. And the influenza pandemic circled the globe in the early twentieth century. Nor is the globalization of the "hegemonic western discourse" on AIDS unique.[35] Hegemonic western discourse has been around for a long time.

AIDS is a product of contemporary globalization because it erupted simultaneously with, and was exacerbated by, the economic crisis that engulfed many poor countries, especially in Africa, in the 1980s. That crisis had measurable demographic effects beyond those attributable to HIV and AIDS,[36] and though they were not AIDS-related, they prepared fertile ground in which the disease could take root. For reasons described in the previous chapter, living standards as well as government services and programs all declined. One result has been that many government workers have become unemployed. Another "result of the crisis at the macro level is to render the already crowded informal economic sector increasingly less profitable for many small operators."

> [M]any women who formerly could rely upon steady contributions from partners or from their extended families report that both sources are dwindling because they too are hard-pressed to make ends meet. Women often seek occasional partners, *pneus de rechange* (or "spare tires"), to meet immediate cash needs. As economic conditions continue to worsen, the social fabric is tearing apart, and sexual strategies that maximize returns become increasingly important.[37]

Furthermore, with jobs scarce, more people migrate in search of work, or return to their rural villages, and this too increases the spread of HIV, even as structural adjustment programs and worsening terms of trade diminish the capacity of governments to provide needed drugs and services. Compounding the difficulty of obtaining antiretroviral drugs has been the increasingly strenuous enforcement by the World Trade Organization of intellectual property rights that makes the production of inexpensive generic versions extremely difficult.

All of this is well known and appropriately lamented. What is less obvious is another, emerging, aspect of globalization. The behavior of the pharmaceutical industry during the AIDS crisis is an example, for it has provoked a reaction on the part of many nongovernmental organizations as well as governments and the press, that has forced the industry to lower prices to make antiretrovirals more available. For many, this is a case of too little too late, and it may indeed be nothing more than a sop to public opinion. However, John Gerard Rugie argues that it is illustrative of another side of globalization, the emergence of what he calls a global public domain in which NGOs (also called Civil Society Organizations) have sprung up to challenge the dominance of transnational corporations.[38]

Globalization has contributed to the weakening of the so-called Westphalian system in which nation-states dealt with each other but in which intranational issues, such as human rights, were not matters for international intervention. That system has changed significantly since World War II, and the emergence of transnational corporations is one of the most important reasons. But, Ruggie argues, "[T]he interplay between civil society organizations and transnational corporations . . . is engendering and instituting new expectations concerning the global responsibility of firms."[39] This is so because as borders have become more open to transnational corporations, demands for accountability have grown. The way transnational corporations deal with HIV/AIDS in their workforces and the communities in which they operate in poor countries has been a concern around which civil society organizations have mobilized, as is the pricing of antiretroviral agents. The results, while as yet not overwhelming, have not been negligible either and may well become greater in future. Thus, many of the same actors responsible for the opening of markets and the commodification of services are now increasingly being pressured to assume responsibility for the consequences. It is still early in the process, though too late for millions of people who have suffered and died needlessly, and the outcome is by no means a forgone conclusion. Indeed, there is good reason for skepticism.[40] Nonetheless, it is not Pollyannaish to suggest that globalization carries within itself the seeds of its own reform—if not destruction, as the Gilded Age was followed by the Progressive Era, and the roaring '20s by the New Deal.

Historical and Predictive Sciences

I began this book by invoking Isaiah Berlin's famous distinction between hedgehogs and foxes and by declaring myself an advocate for foxes. For foxes do not hew to a single-overarching theory that explains how social conditions affect the health of populations. The evidence presented throughout the preceding chapters reveals far too many anomalies for any general theory to be as broadly valid as we might wish. This position will no doubt be distasteful to many readers for, they will say, science is predictive and if there are no broadly true theories, then those of us who wish to understand the social determinants of disease cannot claim to be doing science.

There are two points to make. One has to do with whether predictive power is a necessary criterion to qualify a field of intellectual endeavor as a science. The other is what kind of cognitive style results in the most accurate predictions of social phenomena?

In respect of the first point, it is useful to distinguish between historical and predictive sciences.[41] Predictive sciences, whose model is Newtonian physics, deal with reversible phenomena. Historical sciences deal with irreversible phenomena. Fields like cosmology, geology, evolutionary biology, and genetic linguistics, are concerned with reconstructions of the past, both distant and recent, as are the social sciences upon which social epidemiology is based. They are sciences because they have methods that allow for the testing of hypotheses, even if they cannot enunciate laws that allow for the prediction of the emergence of new species, or the precise time and place of an earthquake.

This does not mean we should not try to predict the impact of social change and public policies on health, but it does mean we need to think about the bases upon which predictions are made. Here the distinction between hedgehogs and foxes is useful. For there is persuasive evidence that foxes are more consistently accurate in predicting the consequences of social phenomena than are hedgehogs, precisely because foxes are not committed to an overarching theory but are able to learn from their mistakes and remain open to new information. In a study of the forecasting accuracy of political experts, Philip Tetlock[42] found that those who were least accurate looked very much like hedgehogs: "[T]hinkers who 'know one big thing,' aggressively extend the explanatory reach of that one big thing into new domains, display bristly impatience with those who 'do not get it,' and express considerable confidence that they are already pretty proficient forecasters, at least in the long term."[43] They are people who are likely to "trivialize evidence that undercuts their preconceptions and to embrace evidence that reinforces their preconceptions."[44]

Those who were more accurate "look like foxes":

[T]hinkers who know many small things (tricks of their trade), are skeptical of grand schemes, see explanation and prediction not as deductive exercises but rather as exercises in flexible "ad hocery" that require stitching together diverse sources of information, and are rather diffident about their own forecasting prowess, and . . . rather dubious that the cloudlike subject of politics can be the object of a clocklike science.[45]

Foxes have a "more balanced style of thinking about the world—a style of thought that elevates no thought above criticism."[46]

Both styles of thought among political forecasters are spread across the ideological spectrum, though there is a significant tendency for foxes to be centrists.[47] The same appears to be true of writers on the social determinants of disease, as material on voluntarists and determinists in Chapter 1 should have made clear. And as with political forecasting, overarching theories of the social determinants of disease are also likely to result in misleading predictions. Accurate prediction is unlikely to rest upon deductive science, whether ideologically driven or not, and much more likely to result from stitching together all that one can know about the context—institutional, cultural, political, epidemiological—in which particular populations live and work. This may be disquieting for those who equate doing science with having a theory that makes possible accurate predictions, but we have seen that there are so many anomalous findings that a general theory of everything, or even of most things, is unlikely to emerge any time soon, if ever. Thus, social epidemiology is scientific as it reconstructs the past and explains the present, but it is not likely to be powerfully predictive. When it is successfully predictive, it is not likely to be because it is based upon deductions from scientifically valid generalizations that are true across time and place, but because analysts understand more or less intimately the people and places with which they are concerned.

The Fallacy of Misplaced Concreteness

In literary criticism, art history, and the philosophy of science, debates often erupt between internalists and externalists. The former seek to understand works of literature, art, or science as emerging from within a tradition or school. The latter look to the larger context to understand a particular work and how it came to be produced. This book has been written from an externalist perspective. For the argument has been that the ways in which social determinants of the health of populations are understood derive from the experience of the West, where industrialization, urbanization and the rise of nation-states over the past two centuries have shaped our culture, including the way we understand the association between social phenomena and the health of individuals and peoples. Ideas about the importance of individual and social responsibility, community and alienation, living standards and governing institutions, equality and inequality have thus become part of social scientific discourse, and inevitably they have influenced the ways in which the scientific revolution in medicine in the late nineteenth century has been interpreted and used to explain diseases in populations.

But while inevitable, such deeply embedded ideas may also lead us astray, especially when they reinforce the need scientists feel to infer abstract principles from concrete cases. Induction is, after all, the essence of what we consider science, and these inherited ideas give added force to, perhaps even determine, the way data are interpreted and abstractions are drawn. This has further encouraged what Alfred North Whitehead labeled the fallacy of misplaced concreteness, inferring abstractions from empirical evidence that is inevitably limited.[48]

> The disadvantage of exclusive attention to a group of abstractions, however well-founded, is that, by the nature of the case, you have abstracted from the remainder of things. In so far as the excluded things are important in your experience, your modes of thought are not fitted to deal with them. You cannot think without abstractions; accordingly, it is of the utmost importance to be vigilant in critically revising your *modes* of abstraction . . . A civilization which cannot burst through its current abstractions is doomed to sterility after a very limited period of progress.[49]

What is true of a civilization is also true of scientific disciplines, which is why it is so important to attend to anomalies, to the things excluded. For doing so may help us burst through current abstractions. Thomas Kuhn,[50] writing as an internalist, observed that scientists ignore anomalies for as long as they are able, sweeping them under the rug until the pile under the rug becomes so large they fall over it. When ideologies whose sources are to be found in the larger, external culture reinforce and help to shape the paradigms in a field, there may be an even greater temptation than usual to infer abstract principles from what are inevitably a small number of selected cases, and to ignore anomalies. For in such a case one is often criticizing the status quo and/or making claims about the way society ought to be. This is not simply about one's professional status but reflects as well deeply held values and moral commitments.

Over and over in the preceding chapters discrepant findings from different studies of the same phenomena have been reported. The same measure of living standards (whether height or income) is associated with different life expectancies, no matter how important living standards are believed to be; inequality has not always been associated with differences in mortality, no matter how offensive inequality may be to one's moral sensibilities; social support and membership in voluntary associations have no inevitably beneficial impact on health, no matter how much we may value our family and friends; and trade liberalization does not have the inevitably harmful or beneficial effects on health that are claimed by its critics and advocates.

Different results may of course result from methodological differences and errors. But, for the most part, that does not explain away discrepant findings. More significant is the fact that the settings in which studies were done are substantially different. England and Germany in the nineteenth century were very different; the social organization of work in the British civil service and an American corporation differs; the American South and North have had very different economies, cultures, and social structures; the demands made of informal social support systems differ depending upon the network of formal organizations that are also available; and globalization has different effects depending upon the wealth and political regime of particular nations. That is to say, context matters, because the influences on the health of populations are so numerous that only by attending to the context may otherwise incomprehensibly discrepant findings be resolved. The observations may be valid; their generalizability often is not. Since we cannot do without abstractions, as Whitehead wrote, it is of "utmost importance to be vigilantly critical in revising [our] modes of abstraction."

This requires that we be attentive to the potential uniqueness of the concrete situations from which our abstractions are drawn. Yeats ended the poem from which the epigraph at the head of this chapter comes with this final stanza.

> Those masterful images because complete
> Grew in pure mind, but out of what began?
> A mound of refuse or the sweepings of a street,
> Old kettles, old bottles, and a broken can,
> Old iron, old bones, old rags, that raving slut
> Who keeps the till. Now that my ladder's gone,
> I must lie down where all the ladders start,
> In the foul rag-and-bone shop of the heart.

All generalizations about the social determinants of health and disease begin in the lived reality of particular people and places. It is to that reality that our masterful images must be compared, and against which they must be judged.

Appendix 1
Period and Cohort Life Expectancies

Cohort analyses follow people born in the same year or 5-year period over a particular length of time. In this case, average heights are displayed for men ages 25 to 29 born in successive quinquennia. The life expectancy figures are based upon the probability of death of people of different ages within that same 5-year period. Cohort life expectancy data are available for the English population from 1841,[1] however, and I have compared those to the period life expectancy figures in Figure A-1 of this Appendix. The period life expectancies are lower than the cohort life expectancies because the period figures include individuals from older ages who carried the risk of dying incurred at an earlier and less healthy time. Nonetheless, the correlations are strong between the period data I have used and the cohort data, which is as expected since they come from the same source. The correlation between the period life expectancy of the entire population and the cohort life expectancy of men at birth is 0.96 ($p < 0.0001$). The correlation between the period data and male cohort life expectancy at 1 year of age is 0.94 ($p < 0.0001$). On the other hand, there is no significant correlation between the average height of a cohort and life expectancy at age 0 or at age 1 for the same cohort ($r = 0.42$ for each, $p = 0.2592$), although there are only nine periods when the cohort life expectancy and height data overlap (Figure A-2 of this Appendix). Thus, using period life expectancies does not appear to have distorted the results.

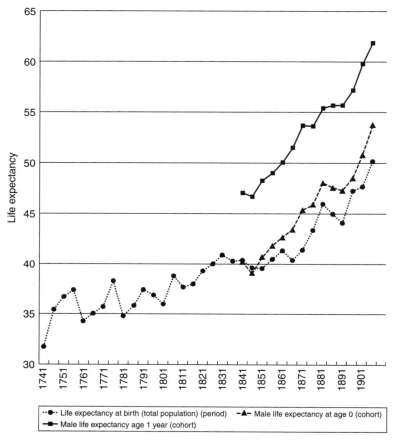

Figure A-1. Period and cohort life expectancy, total population and males in England. (*Sources*: E.A. Wrigley, et al., *English Population*; *Human Mortality Database*; refer to Notes, Chapter 4, note 14.)

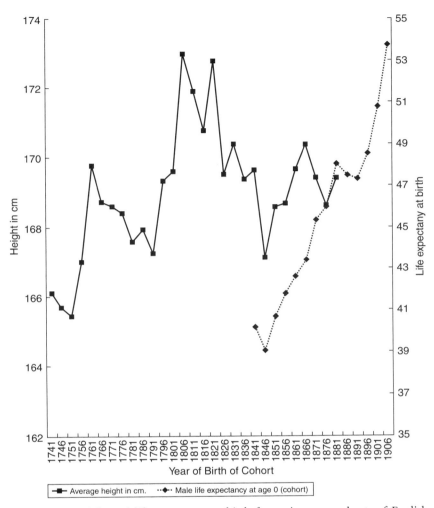

Figure A-2. Height and life expectancy at birth for various age cohorts of English males. (*Sources*: E.A. Wrigley, et. al., *English Population*; Floud, et al., *Height, Health, and History*; and *Human Mortality Database*; refer to Notes, Chapter 4, note 14.)

Appendix 2

The Conundrum of Tuberculosis

Tuberculosis was the single leading cause of death in the second half of the nineteenth century, and its decline was as momentous as it has been mysterious. Because of its overwhelming importance and the role it played in the general decline of mortality, it deserves more attention than I have given it so far. Several types of explanations have been offered for its decline: (1) reduced exposure to the bacillus; (2) increasing resistance on the part of the human population, either from improved nutritional status, biological selection, or reduced exposure to predisposing causes; and (3) reduced virulence of the tubercle bacillus. I consider each in turn.

Arthur Newsholme's book, *The Prevention of Tuberculosis*,[1] is perhaps the clearest and most impressively documented argument for the importance of the reduction of exposure as the single most important reason for the decline of tuberculosis. Newsholme showed that in England, in the nineteenth century, tuberculosis had declined more rapidly than all other causes of mortality combined. He argued that it could not be attributed to declining virulence or to selection of the population for increasing resistance. And he showed that in cross-national comparisons, the decline was not associated with urbanization, crowding, the price of wheat, the amount of food consumed, average wages, or the cost of living. He continued:

> In Norway, Ireland, France, and Austria, the same influences of improved general health, well-being, and sanitary education have operated as in Great Britain, Germany, Belgium, and the United States, side by side with widely different variations in the respective death-

rates in these countries from tuberculosis. Similar discrepancies have been seen when other elements of sanitary environment have been compared with the variations of the disease.

It will next be seen that the only constant correspondence between the variations in the prevalence of tuberculosis and in any element of sanitary environment consists in the relation to tuberculosis of the institutional segregation of patients.[2]

He went on to show that the proportion of the population dying in institutions had approximately doubled between 1866 and 1903, and the death rate from phthisis had declined by about half.[3] Among the institutions in which people died, workhouse infirmaries were the most important. This was due to a change in the Poor Law with regard to indoor and outdoor relief. It was not specifically aimed at the segregation of tuberculous patients, although that was the effect, according to Newholme.

[O]f the total pauper population, who, as we have seen, are the most subject to disease of all kinds and notably to tuberculosis, the segregation in workhouses in 1848–49 amounted to about one-eighth, and was increased by 1902–03 to over one third. The fact expressed in these figures is explained by Mr. Fleming, who speaks of "the great change in the character of workhouse inmates during recent years. . . . The able-bodied inmates are gone and the sick inmates have come." When the frequency of tuberculosis is remembered, these figures and this fact become equivalent to the statement that, as has been seen already for the total institutions of England and Wales, there has been during a period of vast reduction in tuberculosis also a vast increase in the extent of segregation of tuberculous patients in workhouse infirmaries.[4]

Moreover, he argued, the pattern of institutional segregation in other countries paralleled the changes in tuberculosis mortality as well, explaining both the decreases and the increases.

At the time Newsholme was writing in the first decade of the twentieth century, the tuberculin test was not widely used for diagnosis or for epidemiological screening of the population for exposure to tuberculosis. He himself was opposed to its use for diagnostic purposes, believing that it would activate existing infection.[5] Subsequently, however, studies using tuberculin tests in England and elsewhere showed that exposure to tuberculosis was well nigh universal as late as the early twentieth century, with 97% of adults reacting positively to tuberculin tests.[6] Thus, even with segregation of a large number of paupers with active tuberculosis, exposure was still common.

Evidence from the United States regarding the effect of isolation of patients with active tuberculosis is mixed. Barbara Bates has shown that institutionalization could not have had any significant impact on tuberculosis in Philadelphia until the 1920s, although the decline began 40 to 50 years previously.[7] An analysis of data from Massachusetts suggests a similar conclusion. Mortality due to tuberculosis had been declining since the mid-nineteenth century, but institutionalization only became frequent in the early twentieth century, at which time the decline accelerated.[8] On the other hand, Leonard Wilson has argued that in New York, Massachusetts, and Minnesota, the prevention of tuberculosis by isolation had a profound impact on its spread and on the rate at which deaths declined.[9]

Newsholme had rejected the explanation that human populations had become more resistant to the disease either as a result of improved well-being, or as a result of Darwinian selection. But the idea remains attractive. Indeed, there is evidence that there are biological differences in susceptibility. Moreover, the same evidence used by Newsholme has been used more recently to argue the case for selection. Because there was no association between improvements in crowding and average real earnings on the one hand and decreasing mortality from tuberculosis on the other from 1850 to 1910, selection of the human population for resistance has been proposed as a reasonable "residual" explanation. This is supported by a "hypothetical model" that assumes the disease reached its zenith in the first half of the nineteenth century and then as a result of selection declined rapidly thereafter.[10]

Tuberculosis was, however, almost certainly highly prevalent in the British Isles, and no doubt elsewhere in Europe, well before the early nineteenth century.[11] Exposure to the tubercle bacillus was probably universal well before the nineteenth century. It is possible, however, that active disease became more common in the early nineteenth century as people moved into crowded urban quarters and the intensity of exposure, frequency of re-infection, and magnitude of the infecting dose all increased. The rapid decline of tuberculosis mortality during the second half of the nineteenth century, however, is very unlikely to have been due to selection of people who were genetically resistant for several reasons: (1) 60 years is too short a time for such a profound change to have come about; (2) the annual loss from the nineteenth-century population due to tuberculosis was far too small to affect the genetic susceptibility of those who remained;[12] and (3) most of the deaths occurred beginning in young adulthood, after many of the victims would have already had children.

The explanation that has received most attention in the past several decades has been the nutritional hypothesis described previously. Better nutrition, measured as increased stature, is said to be responsible for the decline of tuberculosis mortality. Hans Waaler, whose study of height and mortality in Norway has been the basis for much of this work, wrote: "When it comes to the causes of death, it is relatively clear that the rates for tuberculosis, obstructive lung diseases and cardiovascular diseases are negatively correlated with the body height. For all cancer there is no correlation."[13] There is, however, no evidence in the publication that tuberculosis deaths were related to height. There is striking evidence that in both men and women 50 to 64 years of age, the risk of death from tuberculosis was elevated among those with a body mass index (BMI) below 21 or 22 (BMI is weight in kg/height in m^2).

Evidence from studies done among American servicemen in World Wars I and II as well as subsequently indicates that height is positively correlated with risk of developing active tuberculosis: taller men were at increased risk of developing tuberculosis. The greatest risk was among tall men whose weight was low for their height. The lowest risk was in short men with a high BMI.[14] Thus, the evidence is consistent in showing that BMI is negatively, and height positively, correlated with the risk of developing tuberculosis.

James Riley[15] and Roderick Floud[16] have both shown that the BMI of the British male population in the second half of the nineteenth century was on the order of 21 to 23, above the level shown by Waaler to be a risk factor for death from tuberculosis. These data therefore suggest that (1) improved nutritional status in childhood, as it is reflected in adult height, is not an adequate explanation of the decline in mortality from tuberculosis, and (2) improved nutritional status as reflected in BMI was also unlikely to be an adequate explanation for the decline.

Moreover, although there is disagreement on the course of tuberculosis mortality in France, at the very least, its failure to decline as significantly as it did in England and Sweden during the second half of the nineteenth century is surely important. For this was a time when meat consumption was expanding, heights were increasing, and mortality in general was declining. [17] This too indicates that nutritional status of the population was not an important influence, which is not to deny that during periods of acute starvation, as in concentration camps during World War II, or in populations with a high prevalence of rickets due to vitamin D deficiency, or among individuals who lose weight suddenly as a result of a gastrectomy,[18] active cases are highly likely to develop among people who harbor the bacillus.

One of the important acquired factors affecting resistance to tuberculosis is "acute viral infections especially measles in children."[19] Measles did not decline in the nineteenth century, but smallpox, an even more severe viral disease of childhood, did. A.J. Mercer has made the point that the dramatic decline of smallpox as a result of vaccination in the nineteenth century may well have influenced the subsequent decline of tuberculosis.[20] Indeed, after the smallpox epidemic of 1870 to 1872, efforts at vaccination were redoubled. In the subsequent 2 decades, more than 90% of children were vaccinated. The proportion declined in the 1890s as smallpox largely disappeared and an anti-vaccination lobby gained increasing influence.[21] The decline of mortality from tuberculosis that began at about that time occurred in a cohort-specific fashion, with successive age groups dying at lower and lower rates all through the life course. This is what would be expected if somehow smallpox increased the risk of tuberculosis. As children were increasingly effectively vaccinated against smallpox, and as smallpox virtually disappeared during the second half of the century, each successive cohort would therefore be more resistant to tuberculosis than the one before it. Other countries also encouraged or required vaccination, with France an important exception.[22] There compulsory vaccination only began in 1902, which may help account for the failure of tuberculosis to decline as it had among France's neighbors.

Unfortunately, the evidence that smallpox reduces the resistance to tuberculosis, for either short or long periods, is nonexistent. There is some evidence that measles and scarlet fever suppress resistance to tuberculosis during the active phase of each disease,[23] but there is no evidence of a lasting effect. More significantly, there is no clinical or experimental evidence of any association of tuberculosis with smallpox. It is known, however, that lower respiratory tract diseases in childhood are a risk factor for bronchiectasis (a chronic lung infection) in adulthood, and death due to bronchitis (which has been mistaken for bronchiectasis) did decline in the second half of the nineteenth century among adults above the age of 45.[24] This condition, in turn, predisposes to active tuberculosis in adulthood among those who harbor the tubercle bacillus. The mechanism is not known but may be related to compromised immune response and/or mechanical injury to the lungs. Thus, a decline of lower respiratory tract diseases in childhood could be associated with the decline of tuberculosis. Unfortunately, it is difficult to determine from the very different disease categories used in 1861 to 1870 and 1901 to 1910 whether there was a diminution of nonfatal lower respiratory tract infections among children 1 to 4 and 5 to 9 during these years.[25]

More generally, it has been shown in studies in the late twentieth century that adults who reported a history of serious sickness in childhood were at increased risk of a variety of serious diseases in adulthood. Specifically, "[T]he occurrence of an infectious disease during childhood results in a four-fold increase in lung conditions in middle age, even when controls for later-life comorbid conditions are included."[26] This means that any number of serious infectious childhood diseases (perhaps including smallpox) may be associated with increased risk of pulmonary problems in later life, and that in turn may increase the risk of developing active tuberculosis among people who have been infected with the tubercle bacillus.[27]

As already noted, age-specific, all-cause mortality rates declined in successive age cohorts from the mid-nineteenth century onward, indicating that serious illness did decline in successive birth cohorts.[28] Not surprisingly, the same was true for tuberculosis, as the data displayed in Figure A-3 indicate.[29] These curves show that mortality declined by about 50% (from 116/100,000 to 55/100,000) among boys 5 to 14 from 1851–1860 to 1901–1910. Almost equally large declines were recorded in most of the older age groups during the same period. Each cohort had lower death rates from tuberculosis at every age than the one before, perhaps reflecting improvements in the lives of children starting around the mid-nineteenth century.[30]

Because the rate of tuberculin test positivity was very high in the early twentieth century, indicating widespread exposure to the tubercle bacillus even after half a century of declining tuberculosis mortality, there is good reason to think that the conversion rates from infection to active disease had declined very substantially.[31] This probably resulted from a decline in both the magnitude of infecting doses during primary exposures in childhood and in

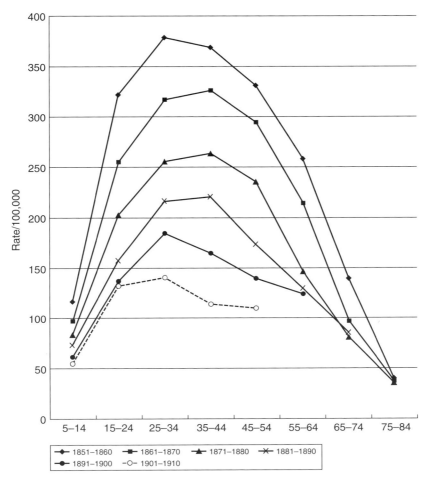

Figure A-3. Mortality rates from tuberculosis for male cohorts who were ages 5–14 in successive decades, England and Wales, 1851–1860 to 1901–1910. (*Source*: Derived from V.H. Springett, "An interpretation of statistical trends in tuberculosis." *The Lancet*, March 15, 1952, pp. 521–552.)

the rate of re-infection of adults who had been previously exposed. Both primary exposure and re-infection are risk factors for the development of active disease, and both could have declined in the late nineteenth century as they did in the twentieth century.[32] In Philadelphia in the late nineteenth century, for instance, reduced crowding was associated with reduced mortality from tuberculosis. Studies in the twentieth century have shown that housing quality is inversely correlated with rates of tuberculin skin test positivity.[33] And Newsholme claimed that there had been a reduction in spitting, at least in homes, if not publicly.[34] He wrote in 1908:

When we remember the immense change which has taken place in our national habits as to spitting, it will be realised what progress has already been made in preventing the spread of infection by sputum. Not many decades since nearly every home was supplied with spittoons, and spitting into the fire or fireplace was common. Now spittoons are almost unknown except in public-houses and barbers' shops, and domestic spitting seldom occurs. If it does, the person finding it necessary to spit retires to a lavatory or water-closet.[35]

The diminution in exposure to large infecting doses of tubercle bacillus in childhood, as well as to re-infection of already infected adults, could have occurred as the degree of crowding within homes decreased and as personal behavior changed. Such changes could also have led to a reduction in the rate and severity of lower respiratory tract infections in childhood. Thus, skin test positivity could have remained high, as we know it did, but the probability of conversion to active disease could well have declined. In the pre-antibiotic era, the case-fatality rate (the proportion of people with active disease who died of it) was said to be about 50%. We do not know if this rate was the same in the nineteenth century.[36] The average duration of active disease was about 2 years. The cumulative lifetime risk of developing active disease after infection (that is, the conversion rate to active disease of people with a positive skin test) has been said to be 10%, although this is age- and time-dependent.[37] It is unknown whether the risk was similar in the nineteenth century, but it appears likely that with almost universal skin test positivity in the early twentieth century, even in the presence of declining death rates, conversion to active disease was declining. And as active cases declined in number, the number of exposed contacts in the population would have declined, even if the case-fatality rate had remained high among those with active disease.

It is also conceivable, though admittedly highly speculative, that virulence decreased as a result of diminished exposure. Paul Ewald has suggested that diseases such as smallpox and tuberculosis are highly virulent, although they are transmitted from person to person, because the causal organisms are stable outside the body for long periods.[38] Just as vector-borne diseases are not dependent on the mobility of the host to spread, and thus virulent causal microorganisms are not at a selective disadvantage, so is the same true for microorganisms that can remain viable until another host happens by. Virulence could have declined, however, if the effect of changed personal behavior and of segregating patients with highly virulent active disease had been to generate selective pressure towards reduced virulence.

I am inclined to believe that mortality from tuberculosis in the nineteenth century declined as a result of improvements in child health that occurred in the second half of the nineteenth century, and as a result of reduced re-infection at later ages. Since both total and tuberculosis-related mortality declined, it seems likely that: (1) the disease experience of successive cohorts was less severe than it was for preceding cohorts; (2) exposure to tuberculosis remained widespread but less intense among children in each successive cohort; (3) the diminution during childhood of disease severity in general and of tuberculosis severity in particular reduced the likelihood of active disease and of severity of active tuberculosis at older ages in successive cohorts; and (4) diminished severity in adulthood along with changes in behavior (e.g., reduced spitting) would have reduced the risk of re-infection of older adults as well as children. Thus, skin test positivity could have remained high while conversion to active disease declined. While it is by no means certain that this was the causal sequence, at the very least, it does not appear that improved nutrition played the major role McKeown had assigned to it.

Appendix 3
Body Mass Index and Mortality

Body mass index (BMI) is weight in kg/height in m^2, a measure of weight for height. It is generally agreed that presently in rich countries increasing BMI is associated with an increased risk of premature death from a variety of conditions, most notably cardiovascular diseases. However, there are discrepant results reported from a variety of studies, which have to do with whether the association is a straight line, U-shaped, or J-shaped: that is, whether the risk of mortality increases at very low levels of BMI. With a variety of other risk factors controlled, it appears that the risk of death from cardiovascular diseases increases in a straight line with increases in BMI.[1] This appears to be especially true among nonsmokers.[2]

On the other hand, when considering all-cause mortality, and not controlling for other risk factors, a large study of the Norwegian population found that the association is J-shaped, with the risk of death increasing slightly at the lowest levels of BMI, and substantially at increasing levels of BMI. The optimal BMI for men ranged from 21.6 at ages 20 to 29 to 24.0 at ages 70 to 74; for women the figures were 22.2 and 25.7, respectively. However, the relative risk of death for BMIs below the optimum were not statistically significant for men, although they were for women.[3] This study also found that height was inversely correlated with the risk of death except for the very tallest women, among whom the risk increased.

Studies in Japan, Puerto Rico, and Bangladesh show an increased risk of death at low BMIs. The low BMIs at which relative risk increased were very low indeed, <18.5 in the Japanese and Puerto Rican studies and <17.3 in the Bangladeshi study. The study in Puerto Rico also showed that at every level of

BMI, people who were physically active had lower risk of all-cause mortality than those who were inactive. Thus, the evidence suggests that the pattern of association between BMI and risk of death changes when other risk factors (e.g., smoking, activity level) are not controlled.[4] As noted in Appendix 2, mid-nineteenth century English data indicate that average BMIs for men in their 20s were 21 to 23, with an unknown proportion in the elevated risk range <18.5. It seems likely that in this population tobacco use was not as significant as it was a century later, that physical activity was greater, and that the prevailing diseases were different. In the face of these complications, and because contemporary studies of the association between BMI and mortality do not always agree, applying relative risks from the twentieth century to previous centuries in itself involves some risks, though not of premature death.

Appendix 4
Spatial Autocorrelation

Larry J. Layne

The association between the income inequality coefficient (the "Gini" coefficient) and mortality (age-adjusted death rate, infant mortality rate) is measured using the Pearson correlation, with varying strengths of the association appearing at different levels of geographic aggregation. Because the Pearson correlations are based on values averaged across differing geographic aggregations, it is reasonable to suspect that associations between the Gini coefficient and each of the mortality rates could be due purely to the presence of spatial autocorrelation in the data.

Spatial autocorrelation is the correlation of values within a single variable that appears to be due purely to location. Spatial autocorrelation found within a variable is similar in principle to the Pearson correlation between two variables in that spatial autocorrelation varies between $+1$ and -1, and a spatial autocorrelation coefficient value of 0 indicates no spatial autocorrelation. Positive spatial autocorrelation implies that adjacent areal units contain similar values found within a single variable. For instance, say that the distribution of mortality values across counties contains positive spatial autocorrelation. This means that if you encounter a mortality value of, say, 10 in a particular county, then you would expect the mortality values in all of the counties that are adjacent to (i.e., share a boundary with) this particular county to be near 10. If there were five counties adjacent to the particular county with a value of 10, the mortality values in the other five counties might be 12, 11, 14, 8, and 9, for example. Negative spatial autocorrelation indicates that high and low values alternate from one county to the next adjacent county, analogous to black and red squares alternating on a checkerboard. Finally, and to be complete, if no spatial autocorrelation were present in the data, then given the particular county with a mortality value of 10 and five adjacent counties, the mortality values in the adjacent counties would not be predictable. That is, they could be considered to be values drawn randomly from a set of values that range from, say, 1 to 100. Values for the surrounding counties might be 34, 8, 78, 21, and 3, for example.

The presence of spatial autocorrelation in data can have several interpretations.[1] For instance, one interpretation could be that some other variables have been left out of a regression model that would account for the presence of spatial autocorrelation. Another interpretation is the spatial autocorrelation parameter estimate gives an idea of how much the observations within a variable are violating the independence assumption. Irrespective of the interpretation of spatial autocorrelation, a primary result is that if significant positive spatial autocorrelation is present in data but unaccounted for in classical parametric statistical tests such as the Pearson correlation, the null hypotheses can be erroneously rejected at a higher rate than it should be. That is, more significance appears in the Pearson correlation coefficient than would be expected at a specified α level. Stated in yet another way, Type I error (rejecting a true null hypothesis) is increased when spatial autocorrelation is present but not accounted for.

There is also reason to predict that positive spatial autocorrelation will increase as smaller geographic units are aggregated into larger geographic units because of averaging effects in data values occurring during the process of geographic aggregation. Thus, spatial autocorrelation would be expected to become much more pronounced as smaller geographic units are aggregated into larger geographic units, resulting in the possibility of Pearson correlation coefficients becoming significant at higher aggregation levels due entirely to the unaccounted-for presence of spatial autocorrelation and not due to any real association between the variables in question. Since no mention has been made in the literature regarding the Pearson correlation between the Gini coefficient and mortality at varying levels of geography and the possibility of spatial autocorrelation being present, some very preliminary results are presented in this Appendix investigating the role of spatial autocorrelation and the Pearson correlation between the Gini coefficient and two measures of mortality.

Age-adjusted and infant mortality rates and Gini coefficients at the county level for the coterminous ("lower 48") states in the U.S. are used.[2] County boundaries were obtained from the 1999 Maptitude U.S. Geographic Data Disk ver. 4.2[3] and exported as a shape file. Further GIS layer and data manipulation were performed in ArcGIS ver. 9.1[4] and the SAS System ver. 9.1.3 software.[5] Counties were aggregated into increasing aggregate units that ranged from State Plane zone to Regions (see Figure A-4).

When data were aggregated from county level to another level of geography, weighted means were computed for the three analysis variables, where county population was used as the weight. While the State Plane Zone might

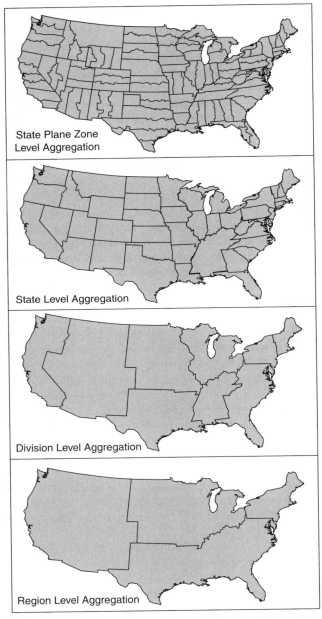

State Plane Zone
Level Aggregation

State Level Aggregation

Division Level Aggregation

Region Level Aggregation

Figure A-4. Levels of geographic aggregations used in combining counties for analyses.

be unfamiliar to those outside the geography/geodesy discipline, it provides a convenient method to aggregate counties together within a state. Larger states are usually divided into at least two zones, with boundaries between the zones coinciding with county boundaries. The use of State Plane zones provided a geographical aggregation level intermediate between the county level and the state level. Division and region geographies are the conventional ones defined by the Bureau of the Census. During aggregation from the county level to the state level, Washington, D.C., was considered to be a "county" of Maryland and therefore aggregated with Maryland counties. Also, spatially speaking, the upper peninsula of Michigan is adjacent (or "shares a boundary with") Wisconsin but not lower Michigan. Thus, at the state level of aggregation, the upper peninsula of Michigan was treated as a separate state, resulting in a total of 49 states at the state level of aggregation.

For each level of geographic aggregation, Moran's I coefficient, a spatial autocorrelation measure, was computed and plotted for each variable (Figure A-5). For this computation, the row stochastic definition of connectivity between adjacent areal units was applied. Pearson correlation coefficients were also computed between the Gini coefficient and age-adjusted death rate and infant mortality rate separately, and graphically displayed in the same plot as the Moran's I coefficient (see Figure A-5). The R software package was used to compute the Pearson correlation and Moran's I spatial autocorrelation coefficient values.[6] The SAS/GRAPH software system was used to create the plot of Moran's I and Pearson correlation coefficient values.[7] A significance level of 0.05 was used for all tests.

As seen in Figure A-5, the spatial autocorrelation values for both types of mortality increased from the county level to the state level, supporting the previous supposition, but then decreased quite dramatically from the state level to the region level of aggregation, and changed from positive to negative values. Additionally, the Moran's I coefficient values for both types of mortality were significant at the county, state plane zone, and state levels of aggregation but not at the division and region levels of aggregation. Spatial autocorrelation measures for the Gini coefficient did not follow the same pattern as the measures of mortality, in that measures for the Gini coefficient were highest at the county level, decreasing at each level to the region level of aggregation. However, similar to measures for the mortalities, Moran's I coefficient values were significant at the county, state plane zone, and state levels of aggregation but not at the division and region levels.

One explanation for the pattern of spatial autocorrelation observed for the two mortality rates is that homogenizing effects of values at increasing levels of aggregation occur up through the state level, but are lost at the division and region levels. That is, immediate neighbors of a state are similar to each other on average but differences among states appear when they are grouped into larger areal units. This same phenomenon should also be observed by examining spatial autocorrelation at higher-order spatial lags. On the other hand, Gini coefficient values are sufficiently heterogenous at the county level

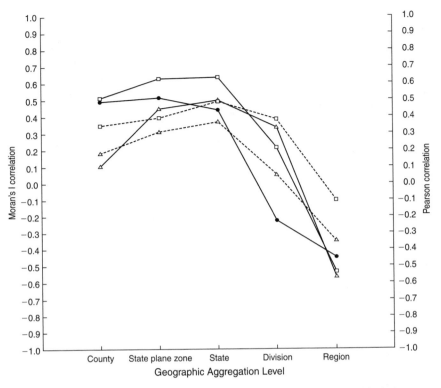

Figure A-5. Moran's I coefficient values (left vertical axis) for age-adjusted death rate, infant mortality rate, and income inequality at five different levels of geography. Moran's I coefficient values computed using the row-stochastic definition of areal unit connectivity. Pearson correlation coefficient values (right vertical axis) for the correlation between income inequality and age-adjusted death rate and infant mortality rate at five different levels of geography.

such that homogenization of aggregated means does not occur at higher levels of aggregation, resulting in steadily decreasing spatial autocorrelation values at higher levels of geographic aggregation.

The Pearson correlation coefficient values between the Gini coefficient and age-adjusted death rate, and the Gini coefficient and infant mortality rate, follow the same patterns observed for the spatial autocorrelation coefficient values of both types of mortality (Figure A-5). One explanation for this phenomenon is that spatial autocorrelation in the two measures of mortality is primarily driving the Pearson correlation values at differing levels of geographic aggregation.[8] Another explanation for the pattern is that the Pearson correlations between the Gini coefficient and the two measures of mortality are strongest in a particular area of the U.S. and different from other areas of the U.S.; this does not appear at the state level because this level of aggregation is at too fine a resolution, and is driving the Pearson correlation coefficient at the division and region levels of aggregation. This is more fully explained below.

As a preliminary examination of the effect of spatial autocorrelation on the Pearson correlation coefficient values, age-adjusted death rate was regressed on the Gini coefficient using first an ordinary least squares simple linear regression (OLS) and then a simultaneous autoregressive model (SAR). The same was done using infant mortality rate. The SAR model is specified as $Y = \rho WY + X\beta + \xi$, where ρ is the spatial autocorrelation coefficient parameter that is estimated only for the dependent variable. The R software package was used to compute the ordinary least squares and simultaneous autoregressive regression model coefficients, using the lm() and lagsarlm() functions, respectively. The results of these regressions are summarized in Table A-1.

Although the R^2 values for the OLS regressions are not shown in this table, they can be estimated from the plot of the Pearson correlation coefficients from Figure A-5. The highest R^2 value was found for the age-adjusted death rate regressed onto the Gini coefficient at the state level of aggregation— a value of about 0.23. Thus, using the OLS regression results, only 23% of the variation found in the age-adjusted death rate values was explained by the presence of the Gini coefficient. R^2 values at the other levels of aggregation were lower for age-adjusted death rate, and R^2 values for infant mortality regressed on the Gini coefficient were lower than for the age-adjusted death rate at the same level of geographic aggregation.

Examination of the summarized OLS regression results in Table A-1 reveals that the Gini coefficient was a significant regressor (i.e., independent variable) for both age-adjusted death rate and infant mortality at the county, state plane zone, and state levels of geographic aggregation, but not significant at the division and region levels. As seen in the SAR results, values for the spatial autocorrelation parameter, rho, are positive and highly significant from the county through state levels of aggregation, positive but not significant at the division level, and highly negative and significant at the region level.[9]

More important, however, is the pattern of the change in the P-values of the regressor (the Gini coefficient) in the presence of spatial autocorrelation. Comparing the P-values between the OLS regressions and the SAR regressions for the Gini coefficient, when spatial autocorrelation is taken into account the P-value is always greater (i.e., less significant) than its counterpart from the OLS regressions at the county through state levels of aggregation. This is expected for significant positive spatial autocorrelation.

In the case of age-adjusted death rates, the conclusions reached for the county through state levels remain unchanged even in the presence of significant positive spatial autocorrelation. However, because the relationship between infant mortality rate and the Gini coefficient is weaker than for age-adjusted death rate, the Gini coefficient becomes nonsignificant (speaking *sensu strictu*) in the presence of positive spatial autocorrelation. Thus, for the

Table A-1

Simple Linear Regressions of Age-Adjusted Death Rate and Infant Mortality Regressed on Income Inequality, Respectively, and the Same Two Variables Separately Regressed on Income Inequality and Adjusted for Spatial Autocorrelation[a]

Spatial Aggregation	Variable	OLS[b] model results				SAR[c] model results			
		Estimate	s.e.	t-value	Pr(>|t|)	Estimate	Log likelihood	LR statistic	Pr(>|z|)
Age-adjusted death rate regressed on income inequality									
County n = 3109	intercept	366.26	25.85	14.17	<0.0001	108.4	−18967.16	142.54	<0.0001
	inc. ineq.	1236.21	59.2	20.88	<0.0001	609.21	−18895.9	1040.6	<0.0001
	rho[d]					0.58792			
State Plane Zone n = 106	intercept	207.1	151	1.371	0.173	79.588	−598.81	13.714	0.0002
	inc. ineq.	1522.4	345.7	4.404	<0.0001	1152.571	−591.953	28.249	<0.0001
	rho					0.33314			
State n = 49	intercept	17.3	220.9	0.078	0.937925	−137.14	−265.48	6.6479	0.0099
	inc. ineq.	1969.2	506.5	3.888	0.000316	1026.14	−262.1542	23.617	<0.0001
	rho					0.64398			
Division n = 9	intercept	79.63	714.92	0.111	0.914	−731.059	−49.296	3.2843	0.0700
	inc. ineq.	1785.15	1614.18	1.106	0.305	2256.939	−47.65419	3.2878	0.0698
	rho					0.68714			
Region n = 4	intercept	1055.5	1379.8	0.765	0.524	1555.848	−18.702	0.1573	0.6917
	inc. ineq.	−440.8	3116.7	−0.141	0.9	403.476	−18.62352	4.6415	0.0312
	rho					−1.0000			

Infant mortality rate regressed on income inequality

County n = 3109	intercept	-2.6109	0.9264	-2.818	0.00486	-2.6987	-9077.1748	80.904	<0.0001
	inc. ineq.	22.5316	2.1218	10.619	<0.0001	19.2551	-9036.723	61.336	<0.0001
	rho					0.21015			
State Plane Zone n = 106	intercept	-2.122	2.693	-0.788	0.43252	-1.9805	-170.8034	5.9635	0.0146
	inc. ineq.	20.894	6.165	3.389	0.00099	13.5891	-167.8216	22.856	<0.0001
	rho					0.44213			
State n = 49	intercept	-4.25	4.071	-1.044	0.3018	-2.8252	-67.7567	2.7947	0.0946
	inc. ineq.	25.858	9.332	2.771	0.00798	11.7211	-66.3593	23.783	<0.0001
	rho					0.67483			
Division n = 9	intercept	4.873	12.922	0.377	0.717	-0.80859	-11.91498	0.1196	0.7295
	inc. ineq.	4.442	29.175	0.152	0.883	7.03983	-11.85519	2.647	0.1037
	rho					0.64502			
Region n = 4	intercept	19.3	24.18	0.798	0.509	16.0375	-2.2563	0.0902	0.7639
	inc. ineq.	-28.31	54.62	-0.518	0.656	-5.0268	-2.211209	5.1125	0.0238
	rho					-1.0000			

[a] Each type of regression was performed for each of 5 levels of geography, increasing from smallest geographical unit (county) to the largest (region).
[b] Ordinary least squares regression
[c] Simultaneous autoregressive model (spatial regression), implementing the row stochastic connectivity matrix
[d] Spatial autocorrelation coefficient

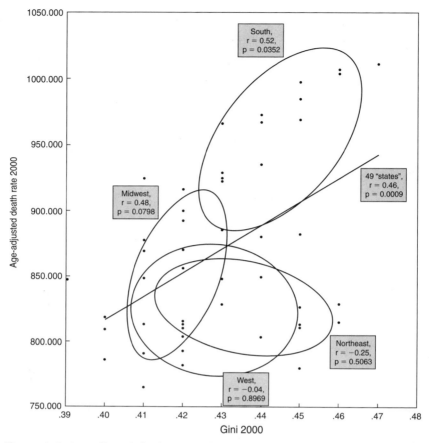

Figure A-6. Age-adjusted death rate and Gini coefficient, 2000, for the contiguous states and regions (50% density ellipses). (Michigan is divided into the Upper Peninsula and the rest of the state, and Washington, D.C., is combined with Maryland. Alaska and Hawaii are not included.)

state level of aggregation, the significant positive Pearson correlation between infant mortality rate and the Gini coefficient is merely an artifact of ignoring spatial autocorrelation.

Recall that at the regional level (see Table A-1) the spatial autocorrelation measure, rho, was negative and significant, meaning that the high and low values alternate like the black and red squares on a checkerboard. That is, the differences among regions are significant, whereas at lower levels of aggregation adjacent units of analysis are significantly similar. Regional boundaries therefore tend to encompass populations units that are more nearly similar to each other than they are to population units in other regions. This is important because, as Figures A-6 and A-7 illustrate, the South is very different from other parts of the country.

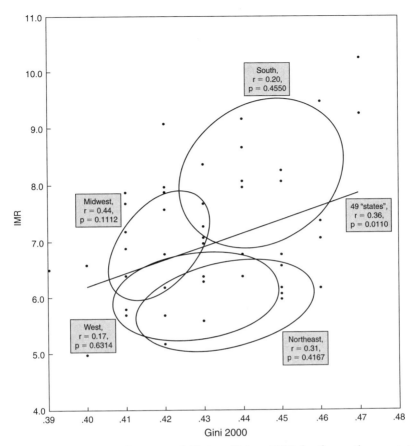

Figure A-7. Infant mortality rate and Gini coefficient, 2000, for the contiguous states and regions (50% density ellipses). (Michigan is divided into the Upper Peninsula and the rest of the state, Washington, D.C. is combined with Maryland, and Alaska and Hawaii are not included.)

Among the 49 states, the positive correlations between the Gini coefficient on the one hand and age-adjusted and infant mortality rates on the other result from regional differences between the South and the other three regions. Correlations between the Gini coefficient and each of the two death rates in those three regions combined are essentially zero (IMR and Gini, -0.008; AADR and Gini, -0.01). Moreover, as Table A-2 indicates, the South has higher mortality rates and income inequality than the other three regions, although among those regions the Midwest tends to have higher infant mortality and lower inequality than the other two.

Finally, when each mortality rate is regressed onto the Gini coefficient and region (South/non-South), region dominates the analyses (see Table A-3). This

Table A-2
Means[a] of Gini Coefficients, Infant Mortality, and Age-Adjusted Mortality among the Four Regions of the U.S., 2000

Variable	Midwest	Northeast	South	West
Gini coefficient	0.42	0.44	0.46	0.43
(s.e.)	(0.0043)	(0.0055)	(0.0041)	(0.0052)
p-value	0.0008			
Age-adjusted d.r.	851.2	826.9	954.4	824.4
(s.e.)	(13.657)	(17.034)	(12.775)	(16.160)
p-value	<0.001			
Infant mortality rate	6.9	5.9	8.2	6.0
(s.e.)	(0.2399)	(0.2992)	(0.2244)	(0.2838)
p-value	<0.0001			
No. of states	14	9	16	10

[a]State means are unweighted by population size to calculate regional means. They therefore differ from the results found on the CDC WONDER on-line database, which use the population of the region as the denominator and the number of deaths as the numerator.

suggests that region rather than income inequality is a significant determinant of mortality differences across the entire nation.

These preliminary analyses are meant to make two points, one methodological and the other substantive. The methodological point is that spatial effects are important and very likely account for many of the positive associations that have been observed, as well as for the high proportion of positive

Table A-3
Infant and Age-Adjusted Mortality Rates Regressed onto State Gini Coefficient and Region, 2000

	Estimate	Std. Error	t Ratio	p-value
A. Age-Adjusted Death Rate/100,000				
Intercept	643.8260	186.8062	3.45	0.0012
Gini coefficient	577.5779	428.5503	1.35	0.1843
Non-South/South	−53.4907	8.7218	−6.13	<0.0001
R^2: 0.57				
Adjusted R^2: 0.55				
B. Infant Mortality Rate				
Intercept	5.5144	3.6101	1.53	0.1335
Gini coefficient	4.0792	8.2819	0.49	0.6247
Non-South/South	−0.8827	0.1685	−5.24	<0.0001
R^2: 0.45				
Adjusted R^2: 0.43				

results at high levels of aggregation. The results suggest further that interpretation of the Pearson correlation between age-adjusted death rate and the Gini coefficient, and between infant mortality and the Gini coefficient, should be performed, taking into account the presence of spatial autocorrelation, particularly when the Pearson correlation coefficient is significant but low.

The substantive point is that spatial effects are important because places close to one another may share many features that distinguish them from other places. Such similarity violates the assumption of independence upon which most statistical analyses depend, and may reflect the importance of other unmeasured (i.e., latent) variables, such as social organization, cultural beliefs and practices, political institutions, the availability of health and social services, and, of course, income and income inequality. Although income inequality and mortality are on average higher in the South than elsewhere, the ranges in the non-southern states are adequate to detect an association if there were one. With such considerations in mind, it seems unwise to insist on the overwhelming significance of inequality, particularly when taken out of regional, historical, and sociocultural context.[10]

Appendix 5

Homicide in the 50 States
of the United States

Figure A-8 displays a regression of the homicide rate onto the Gini coefficient for all 50 states and excluding the District of Columbia.[1] The association between the two is significant: the greater the inequality, the greater the homicide rate. Like the analyses of the age-adjusted and infant mortality rates, however, the association is the result of high inequality and high homicide rates in the South. The correlation in the non-southern states is 0.33 ($p = 0.0583$), which is marginally significant at conventional levels.

Moreover, the average homicide level in the South is significantly higher than in the other regions of the country, and there is no significant difference among the other three regions (see Table A-4).

Finally, when the homicide rate is regressed onto the Gini coefficient, region (South vs. non-South), and average household income, only region is significant (see Table A-5, Panel A). When Washington, D.C., is included in the analysis (see Table a-5, Panel B), the Gini coefficient also becomes significant because Washington has such extremely high income inequality and homicide that it influences the entire analysis.

The point is, first, that homicide rates and inequality are higher in the South than elsewhere in the country, and that it is the South that accounts for the significant association between the two variables across all 50 states; and second, that as in the examples discussed in Appendix 4, it is important to attend to the significant regional differences in history, culture, and economy that shape behavior. Inequality is an important part of the difference, but it is part of a congeries of factors that shape differences among regions. It is misleading to give it pride of place among all the other causes that also contribute.

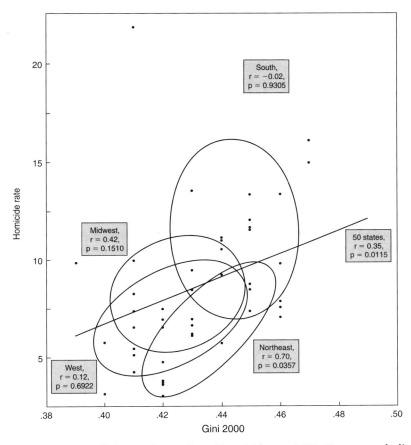

Figure A-8. Gini coefficient and age-adjusted homicide rate, 2000, 50 states, excluding Washington, D.C., and density ellipses for each region.

Table A-4

Homicide Rates in 50 States,[a] 2000, by Region

Variables	Midwest	Northeast	South	West
No. States	13	9	16	12
Unweighted average homicide rate[b]	7.0	6.4	11.5	8.3
(s.e.)	(0.8619)	(1.0358)	(0.7769)	(0.8971)
p-value all four regions		0.0004		
p-value three non-South regions		0.2703		

[a]Washington, D.C., is not included.
[b]The regional means are not weighted by the population of each state. They differ from the regional means obtainable for the same year from the CDC Wonder on-line site, which calculates them as the total number of homicides in a region divided by the total population of the region.

Table A-5

Homicide Rate/100,000 in 2000 Regressed onto Region, Gini Coefficient, and Income, 50 U.S. States, with and without Washington, D.C.

	Estimate	Standard error	t Ratio	P value
A. Excluding Washington, D.C.				
Intercept	−6.1140	11.3461	−0.54	0.5926
Non-South–South	−1.9852	0.5394	−3.68	0.0006
Gini 2000	28.7370	24.6732	1.16	0.2501
Household income 2000	0.00006	0.00006	1.02	0.3124
R-square: 0.3289				
Adjusted R-square: 0.2852				
B. Including Washington, D.C.				
Intercept	−34.8359	10.3630	−3.36	0.0015
Non-South–South	−1.8482	0.6232	−2.97	0.0047
Gini 2000	88.9156	23.0197	3.86	0.0003
Household income	0.00015	0.00006	1.76	0.0855
R-square: 0.4907				
Adjusted R-square: 0.4582				

Notes

Preface

1. I. Berlin, *The Hedgehog and the Fox,* New York: Simon & Schuster, 1953, p. 1.
2. A.N. Whitehead, *Science and the Modern World*. New York: The Free Press, [1925] 1967, p. 58.

Introduction

1. R.A. Nisbet, *The Sociological Tradition.* New York: Basic Books, 1966.
2. A.N. Whitehead, *Science and the Modern World*, New York: The Free Press, [1925] 1967.
3. T. Kuhn, *The Structure of Scientific Revolutions*. Chicago: The University of Chicago Press, 1962.

Chapter 1

1. G.B. Shaw, *The Doctor's Dilemma*. Baltimore: Penguin Books, [1913] 1965, pp. 107–108.
2. E.J. Hobsbawm, "The British standard of living 1790–1850." *The Economic History Review* New Series 10: 46–68, 1957, p. 47. See also R.M. Hartwell & S. Engerman, "Models of immiseration: the theoretical basis of pessimism." In A.J. Taylor, ed. *The Standard of Living in Britain in the Industrial Revolution*. London: Methuen & Co. Ltd., 1975; J.G. Williamson, "Was the industrial revolution worth it? Disamenities and death in 19th century British towns." *Explorations in Economic History* 19: 221–245, 1982; and C.H. Feinstein, "Pessimism perpetuated: real wages and the standard of living in Britain during the industrial revolution." *The Journal of Economic History* 58: 625–658, 1998.

3. K. Polanyi, *The Great Transformation: The Political and Economic Origins of our Times*. Boston: Beacon Press, [1944] 1957, p. 159.

4. Ibid., p. 157.

5. R.A. Nisbet, *The Sociological Tradition*. New York: Basic Books, 1966.

6. Polanyi's work is an interesting example of the similarity of the criticisms of market-driven society offered by both the political right and left. For his critique was adopted by the New Left but, in fact, as John Gerard Ruggie has pointed out, was "anchored in an organic conception of society that was . . . deeply conservative in the traditionalist sense of that term." J.G. Ruggie, "At home abroad, abroad at home: international liberalization and domestic stability in the new world economy." *Millennium: Journal of International Studies* 24: 507–526, 1994, p. 507. For more about Polanyi, see P.F. Drucker, *Adventures of a Bystander*. New York: Harper and Row, 1978.

7. J.H. Warner, *The Therapeutic Perspective: Medical Practice, Knowledge, and Identity in America, 1820–1885*. Cambridge, Mass.: Harvard University Press, 1986, p. 1.

8. C. Bernard, *An Introduction to the Study of Experimental Medicine*, translated by H.C. Greene. New York: Schuman, 1949, p. 139.

9. K.C. Carter, "Koch's Postulates in Relation to the Work of Jacob Henle and Edwin Klebs." *Medical History*, 29: 353–374, 1985.

10. S.J. Kunitz, "Explanations and ideologies of mortality patterns." *Population and Development Review*, 13: 380, 1987.

11. T.M. Brown, "The Holistic Elite: A Network of American Medical Humanists in the Early Twentieth Century," Lecture presented at the Institute of the History of Medicine, The Johns Hopkins University, Baltimore, Md., 2 Mar. 1989. See also S.J. Kunitz, "Holism and the idea of general susceptibility to disease." *International Journal of Epidemiology*, 31: 722–729, 2002.

12. G.C. Robinson, *The Patient as a Person*. New York: The Commonwealth Fund, 1939.

13. G. Rosen, *A History of Public Health*. New York: MD Publications, 1958, p. 314.

14. These several paragraphs are from S.J. Kunitz, "Explanations and ideologies of mortality patterns." *Population and Development Review* 13: 379–407, 1987.

15. J. Ettling, *The Germ of Laziness: Rockefeller Philanthropy and Public Health in the New South*. Cambridge: Harvard University Press, 1981.

16. C.V. Chapin, Originally published in 1902. "Dirt, disease, and the health officer." In *Papers of Charles Chapin, M.D.: A Review of Public Health Realities*. New York: Oxford University Press and the Commonwealth Fund, 1934.

17. B.G. Rosenkrantz, "Cart before horse: theory, practice and professional image in American Public Health, 1870–1920," *Journal of the History of Medicine and Allied Sciences* 29: 55–73, 1974.

18. C.V. Chapin, "Causes of deaths in Providence, 1856–1905." *American Journal of Hygiene and Journal of the Massachusetts Association of Boards of Health* 15: 529–541, 1905.

19. E. Fee and D. Porter, "Public health, preventive medicine, and professionalization: Britain and the United States in the nineteenth century." In E. Fee and R.M. Acheson, eds., *A History of Education in Public Health*. New York: Oxford University Press, 1991, p. 35.

20. H.W. Hill, *The New Public Health*. New York: The Macmillan Company, 1918,

p. 8. See also M. Warboys, *Spreading Germs: Disease Theories and Medical Practice in Britain, 1865–1900*. Cambridge: Cambridge University Press, 2000.

21. Hill, *The New Public Health*, p. 9.

22. Rosenkrantz, *Public Health and the State*, op. cit., pp. 98–99. Leavitt, *The Healthiest City*, op. cit., pp. 153–154.

23. Quoted by S.K. Schultz and C. McShane, "To engineer the metropolis: sewers, sanitation, and city planning in late-nineteenth-century America." *The Journal of American History* 65: 389–411, p. 395.

24. Leavitt, *The Healthiest City*, p. 244. See also N. Tomes, *The Gospel of Germs: Men, Women, and the Microbe in American Life*. Cambridge: Harvard University Press, 1998, p. 47.

25. Leavitt, *The Healthiest City*, p. 245.

26. R. Lubove, *The Progressives and the Slums: Tenement House Reform in New York City 1890–1917*. Pittsburgh: University of Pittsburgh Press, 1962, p. 88.

27. N. Tomes, *The Gospel of Germs*, op. cit., p. 211.

28. Ibid., p. 222.

29. Fee and Porter, "Public health, preventive medicine, and professionalization," op. cit., p. 33.

30. J.F. Kasson, *Rudeness and Civility: Manners in Nineteenth-Century Urban America*. New York: Hill and Wang, 1990, p. 124.

31. Ibid., p. 126.

32. Ibid., p. 34.

33. Ibid., p. 142.

34. Ibid., p. 162.

35. N. Rogers, "Germs with legs: flies, disease, and the new public health." *Bulletin of the History of Medicine* 63: 599–617, 1989.

36. S. Hoy, *Chasing Dirt: The American Pursuit of Cleanliness*. New York: Oxford University Press, 1995, pp. 140–141.

37. Tomes, *The Gospel of Germs*, op. cit., S. Hoy, *Chasing Dirt*.

38. E.R. Brown, *Rockefeller Medicine Men: Medicine and Capitalism in America*. Berkeley: University of California Press, 1979. J. Ettling, *The Germ of Laziness: Rockefeller Philanthropy and Public Health in the New South*. Cambridge: Harvard University Press, 1981.

39. One reader has written, "Historians of conspiracy once got away with claims that political machines were inimical to public health and that philanthropists . . . had industrial-strength agendas. Subsequent historians have documented, for example, the practical reasons Tammany Hall supported Hermann Biggs' reforms in policy for public health in New York City and State, and the effective work with politicians corrupt and otherwise conducted by the founders of [several] foundations." Clearly, politicians, corrupt and otherwise, often had an interest in civic improvements, as case studies in Milwaukee, Wisconsin and Newark, New Jersey demonstrate. Moreover, urban mortality began to decline in the last third of the nineteenth century, well before widespread acceptance of the germ theory and professionalization of public health. Nonetheless, as the discussion of Chapin's work and influence indicated, one attraction of the germ theory was precisely that it legitimated a focus on individuals rather than on social reform. J.W. Leavitt, *The Healthiest City*, op. cit.; S. Galishoff, *Safeguarding the Public Health: Newark, 1895–1918*. Westport, Conn.: Greenwood Press, 1975; S. Galishoff, *Newark: The Nation's Unhealthiest City, 1832–1895*. New Brunswick, N.J.: Rutgers University Press, 1988; F.L. Hoffman, "The general death-rate

of large American cities, 1871–1904." *Quarterly Publications of the American Statistical Association,* New Series, No. 73: 1–75, 1906.

40. The next several paragraphs are based upon S.J. Kunitz, "Hookworm and pellagra: exemplary diseases in the New South." *Journal of Health and Social Behavior* 29: 139–148, 1988.

41. T. Haskell, *The Emergence of Professional Social Science.* Urbana: University of Illinois Press, 1977, p. 43.

42. W.H. Allen, "Sanitation as social progress." *American Journal of Sociology* 8: 631–643, 1903, p. 632.

43. Ibid., p. 633.

44. Ibid., p. 643.

45. W. Coleman, *Death Is a Social Disease: Public Health and Political Economy in Early Industrial France.* Madison: University of Wisconsin Press, 1982.

46. G. Wright, *Old South, New South: Revolutions in the Southern Economy Since the Civil War.* New York: Basic Books, 1986, p. 139.

47. D.L. Carlton, *Mill and Town in South Carolina 1880–1920.* Baton Rouge: Louisiana State University Press, 1982.

48. Ettling, *The Germ of Laziness,* op. cit., p. 25.

49. H.M. Gilles, "Selective primary health care: strategies for control of disease in the developing world. XVII. Hookworm infection and anemia." *Reviews of Infectious Diseases* 7: 111–118, 1985.

50. D.L. Belding, *Basic Clinical Parasitology.* New York: Appleton-Century-Crofts, 1958, p. 161.

51. Quoted in Ettling, *Germ of Laziness,* op. cit., p. 35.

52. Ettling, *Germ of Laziness,* p. 44.

53. Gilles, "Hookworm," op. cit.

54. C.W. Stiles, *Hookworm Disease among Cotton-Mill Operatives.* Vol. XVII, *Report on Conditions of Woman and Child Wage-Earners in the United States.* 61st Congress, 2nd Session, Document 645. Washington, D.C.: U.S. Government Printing Office, 1912, pp. 36–37.

55. J.H. Cassedy, "The 'germ of laziness' in the South, 1900–1915: Charles Wardell Stiles and the Progressive paradox." *Bulletin of the History of Medicine* 45: 353–374, 1971. M. Boccaccio, "Ground itch and dew poison: the Rockefeller Sanitary Commission 1909–14," *Journal of the History of Medicine and Allied Sciences* 27: 30–53, 1972. Ettling, *Germ of Laziness,* op. cit.

56. Ettling, *Germ of Laziness,* pp. 206–207.

57. E.W. Etheridge, *The Butterfly Caste: A Social History of Pellagra in the South.* Westport, Conn.: Greenwood, 1972, pp. 10–11.

58. J. Goldberger, G.A. Wheeler, and E. Sydenstricker, "A study of the relation of diet to pellagra incidence in seven textile-mill communities of South Carolina in 1916." *Public Health Reports* 35: 648–713, 1920. Reprinted in M. Terris, ed. *Goldberger on Pellagra.* Baton Rouge: Louisiana State University Press, 1964, p. 185.

59. E.W. Etheridge, "Pellagra." In K.F. Kiple, ed. *The Cambridge World History of Human Disease.* Cambridge: Cambridge University Press, 1993, p. 918–919.

60. E. Sydenstricker, "The prevalence of pellagra. Its possible relation to the rise in the cost of food." *Public Health Reports* 30: 313231–48, 1915. Reprinted in M. Terris, ed., *Goldberger on Pellagra,* op. cit., p. 113.

61. J. Goldberger, G.A. Wheeler, and E. Sydenstricker, "A study of the relation of fam-

ily income and other economic factors to pellagra incidence in seven cotton-mill villages of South Carolina in 1916." *Public Health Reports* 35: 2673–2714, 1920. Reprinted in M. Terris, ed., *Goldberger on Pellagra,* pp. 241–242.

62. Ibid., p. 260.

63. Ibid., p. 263.

64. The following several paragraphs are adapted from S.J. Kunitz, "Explanations and ideologies of mortality patterns." *Population and Development Review* 13: 379–408, 1987.

65. R. Crawford, "Individual responsibility and health politics in the 1970s." In S. Reverby and D. Rosner, ed., *Health Care in America.* Philadelphia: Temple University Press, 1979.

66. R. Wilkinson, "Inequality and the social environment: a reply to Lynch et al." *Journal of Epidemiology and Community Health* 54: 411–413, 2000.

67. M. Feldstein, "Reducing poverty, not inequality." *The Public Interest* Fall, 1999, pp. 33–41.

68. T. McKeown, *The Modern Rise of Population.* New York: Academic Press, 1976. *The Role of Medicine.* London: Nuffield Provincial Hospitals Trust, 1976.

69. J. Farquhar, *The American Way of Life Need Not Be Hazardous to Your Health.* New York: W.W. Norton and Company, 1978.

70. M.B. Shimkin, "Preventive oncology." In J.F. Fraumeni, Jr. ed., *Persons at High Risk of Cancer: An Approach to Cancer Etiology and Control.* New York: Academic Press, 1975, pp. 441–446.

71. R. Doll, "Prevention: Some future perspectives." *Preventive Medicine* 7: 486–497, 1978, p. 486.

72. L. Breslow, "Prospects for improving health through reducing risk factors." *Preventive Medicine* 7: 449–458, 1978.

73. R.W. Fogel, "Secular trends in physiological capital: implications for equity in health care." *Perspectives in Biology and Medicine* 46 (supplement): S24–S38, 2003, pp. S34–S35.

74. E. Wynder, "Discussion." In J.F. Fraumeni, Jr., ed., *Persons at High Risk of Cancer: An Approach to Cancer Etiology and Control.* New York: Academic Press, 1975, p. 448.

75. G.B. Gori and B.J. Richter, "Macroeconomics of disease prevention in the United States." *Science* 200: 1124–1130, 1978, p. 1124.

76. R.W. Fogel, *The Escape from Hunger and Premature Death, 1700–2100.* Cambridge: Cambridge University Press, 2004, p. 57.

77. J.H. Knowles, "The responsibility of the individual." In J.H. Knowles, ed., *Doing Better and Feeling Worse: Health in the United States.* New York: W.W. Norton, 1977, pp. 58–59.

78. *Financial Times,* June 2, 1987.

79. *The Manchester Guardian Weekly,* October 5, 1986.

80. R.A. Epstein, "Let the shoemaker stick to his last: a defense of the 'old' public health." *Perspectives in Biology and Medicine* 46 (Supplement): S138–S159, 2003.

81. For a revealing recent contrast between these two approaches, see the following two books with the same title: L.A. Sagan, *The Health of Nations: True Causes of Sickness and Well-being.* New York: Basic Books, Inc., 1987, and I. Kawachi and B.P. Kennedy, *The Health of Nations: Why Inequality is Harmful to Your Health.* New York: The New Press, 2002. The first views individuals as largely responsible for what befalls them. The latter views social inequality as the most significant cause of mortality and morbidity.

82. E.J.M. Campbell, J.G. Scadding, and R.S. Roberts, "The concept of disease." *British Medical Journal* 2: 757–762, (Sept. 29) 1979.

Chapter 2

1. W.B. Yeats, *The Collected Poems of W.B. Yeats*. New York: The Macmillan Company, 1957, p. 214.

2. A. Harrington, *Reenchanted Science: Holism in German Culture From Wilhelm II to Hitler*. Princeton: Princeton University Press, 1996. A.N. Whitehead, *Science and the Modern World*. New York: The Macmillan Company, 1925. C.L. Morgan, *Emergent Evolution*. New York: Henry Holt, 1925. J.C. Smuts, *Holism and Evolution*. New York: The Macmillan Company, 1926. C.E. Russett, *The Concept of Equilibrium in American Social Thought*. New Haven: Yale University Press, 1966. L. von Bertalanffy, *General System Theory: Foundations, Development, Applications*. New York: George Braziller, 1968. J. Parascandola, "Organismic and holistic concepts in the thought of L.J. Henderson." *Journal of the History of Biology* 4: 63–118, 1971. D. Worster, *Nature's Economy*. Cambridge: Cambridge University Press, 1985. C. Lawrence and G. Weisz, eds., *Greater Than the Parts: Holism in Biomedicine, 1920–1950*. New York: Oxford University Press, 1998. M. Hau, "The holistic gaze in German medicine, 1890–1930." *Bulletin of the History of Medicine* 74: 495–524, 2000.

3. L. Dilworth, *Imagining Indians in the Southwest: Persistent Visions of a Primitive Past*. Washington, D.C.: Smithsonian Institution Press, 1996. L.P. Rudnick, *Utopian Vistas: The Mabel Dodge Luhan House and the American Counterculture*. Albuquerque, N.Mex.: The University of New Mexico Press, 1996.

4. S.J. Kunitz, "The social philosophy of John Collier." *Ethnohistory* 18: 213–229, 1971. S. Meacham, *Toynbee Hall and Social Reform 1880–1914: The Search for Community*. New Haven: Yale University Press, 1987.

5. E. Mayo, *The Social Problems of an Industrial Civilization*. Division of Research, Graduate School of Business Administration, Harvard University, Boston, Mass., 1945.

6. C.W. Mills, "The professional ideology of social pathologists." *American Journal of Sociology* 49: 165–180, 1943.

7. C.E. Rosenberg, "The therapeutic revolution: medicine, meaning, and social change in nineteenth century America." In M.J. Vogel and C.E. Rosenberg, eds., *The Therapeutic Revolution*. Philadelphia: University of Pennsylvania Press, 1979, pp. 3–26.

8. A. Jacobi, "Inaugural address delivered before the New York Academy of Medicine." *The Medical Record* 1885: 27: 69–74. H. Rolleston, "The classification and nomenclature of disease, with remarks on diseases due to treatment." *Lancet* May 22, 1909: 1437–1443. F.G. Crookshank, "First principles: and epidemiology." *Proceedings of the Royal Society of Medicine: Section of Epidemiology and State Medicine* 13: 159–184, 1920. S.J. Kunitz, "Classifications in medicine." In R.C. Maulitz and D.E. Long, eds., *Grand Rounds: One Hundred Years of Internal Medicine*. Philadelphia: University of Pennsylvania Press, 1987, pp. 279–296.

9. F.W. Peabody, "The care of the patient." *Journal of the American Medical Association* 80: 877–880, 1927.

10. S.W. Tracy, "An evolving science of man: the transformation and demise of American constitutional medicine, 1920–1950." In C. Lawrence and G. Weisz, eds., *Greater Than the Parts: Holism in Biomedicine, 1920–1950*. New York: Oxford University Press, 1988, pp. 161–188.

11. T.M. Brown, "George Canby Robinson and 'The Patient as a Person.' In

C. Lawrence and G. Weisz, eds., *Greater Than the Parts: Holism in Biomedicine, 1920–1950*. New York: Oxford University Press, pp. 135–160, 1998.

12. Committee on the Costs of Medical Care. *Medical Care for the American People: The Final Report of the Committee on the Costs of Medical Care*. Chicago: University of Chicago Press, 1932.

13. S.W. Tracy, "An evolving science of man: the transformation and demise of American constitutional medicine, 1920–1950." In C. Lawrence and G. Weisz, eds., *Greater Than the Parts: Holism in Biomedicine, 1920–1950*. New York: Oxford University Press, 1988, pp. 161–188, p. 161.

14. F.G. Crookshank "The importance of a theory of signs and a critique of language in the study of medicine." In C.K. Ogden and I.A. Richards, eds., *The Meaning of Meaning*. New York: Harcourt, Brace and Company, 1930, p. 343.

15. L.J. Henderson, Introduction to C. Bernard, *An Introduction to the Study of Experimental Medicine*. New York: Henry Schuman, Inc, 1927, pp. v–xii.

16. W.B. Cannon, *The Wisdom of the Body*. New York: W.W. Norton & Co, [1939] 1963.

17. J. Parascandola, J. "Organismic and holistic concepts in the thought of L.J. Henderson." *Journal of the History of Biology,* op. cit.

18. S.J. Cross, and W.R. Albury, "Walter B. Cannon, L.J. Henderson, and the organic analogy." *Osiris* 2nd series, 3: 165–192, 1987.

19. C.E. Russett, *The Concept of Equilibrium,* op. cit. L.J. Henderson, *Pareto's General Sociology: A Physiologist's Interpretation.* Cambridge: Harvard University Press, 1935. B.S. Heyl, "The Harvard 'Pareto Circle.' " *Journal of the History of Behavioral Sciences* 4: 316–334, 1968.

20. J. Parascandola, "Organismic and holistic concepts," op. cit. L.J. Henderson, "Physician and patient as a social system." *New England Journal of Medicine* 212: 819–823, 1935. L.J. Henderson, The practice of medicine as applied sociology. *Transactions of the Association of American Physicians* 51: 8–22, 1936.

21. W.B. Cannon, *The Wisdom of the Body*, op. cit.

22. W.B. Cannon, "The mechanism of emotional disturbance of bodily function." *New England Journal of Medicine* 198: 877–884, 1928.

23. J.E. Gordon, "The twentieth century—yesterday, today, and tomorrow (1920–)." In F.H. Top, ed., *The History of American Epidemiology*. St. Louis: C.V. Mosby, 1952, pp. 114–167, p. 115.

24. Ibid., pp. 115–116.

25. T.M. Brown, "Alan Gregg and the Rockefeller Foundation's support of Franz Alexander's psychosomatic research." *Bulletin of the History of Medicine* 61: 155–182, 1987. A. Young, "Walter Cannon and the psychophysiology of fear." In C. Lawrence and G. Weisz, eds., *Greater Than the Parts: Holism in Biomedicine, 1920–1950.* New York: Oxford University Press, 1998, pp. 234–256.

26. H. Selye, The general adaptation syndrome and the diseases of adaptation. *Journal of Clinical Endocrinology* 6: 117–230, 1946.

27. H. Selye, *The Stress of Life*. New York: McGraw-Hill, 1956.

28. Ibid.

29. Ibid., p. 204. Emphasis in original.

30. R. Dubos, R. *Man Adapting*. New Haven: Yale University Press, 1965, p. 164.

31. R.J. Haggerty, "Stress and illness in children." *Bulletin of the New York Academy of Medicine,* second series 62: 707–718, 1986. S.B. Friedman and L.A. Glasgow, "Psychologic factors and resistance to infectious disease." *Pediatric Clinics of North America* 13: 315–335, 1966.

32. G.L. Engel, "Homeostasis, behavioral adjustment and the concept of health and disease." In R.R. Grinker, ed., *Mid-Century Psychiatry: An Overview.* Springfield, Ill.: Charles C. Thomas, 1954, pp. 33–59. J. Romano, ed., *Adaptation.*, Ithaca, N.Y.: Cornell University Press, 1949.

33. Ibid. G.L. Engel, *Psychological Development in Health and Disease.* Philadelphia: W.B. Saunders, 1962.

34. T.M. Brown, "George Engel and Rochester's biopsychosocial tradition: historical and developmental perspectives." In R.M. Frankel, T.E. Quill, and S.H. McDaniel, eds., *The Biopsychosocial Approach: Past, Present, Future.* Rochester: University of Rochester Press, 2003, p. 208.

35. R.M. Frankel, T.E. Quill, and S.H. McDaniel, eds., *The Biopsychosocial Approach: Past, Present, Future.* Rochester: University of Rochester Press, 2003.

36. D. Levenson, *Mind, Body, and Medicine: A History of the American Psychosomatic Society.* McLean, Va.: American Psychosomatic Society, 1993, pp. 98–99.

37. L.W. Simmons and H.G. Wolff, *Social Science in Medicine.* New York: Russell Sage Foundation, 1954.

38. S. Wolf and H. Goodell, *Behavioral Science in Clinical Medicine.* Springfield, Ill.: Charles C. Thomas, 1976. L.E. Hinkle, R. Redmont, N. Plummer, and H.G. Wolff, "An examination of the relation between symptoms, disability and serious illness in two homogeneous groups of men and women." *American Journal of Public Health* 50, 1327–1336, 1960.

39. S. Wolf and H.G. Wolff, *Human Gastric Function.* 2nd edition. New York: Oxford University Press, 1947. H.G. Wolff and S. Wolf, *Pain.* Springfield, Illinois: Charles C. Thomas, 1948. T.H. Holmes, H. Goodell, S. Wolf, and H.G. Wolff, *The Nose.* Springfield, Illinois: Charles C. Thomas, 1950. S. Wolf, P.V. Cardon, E.M. Shepard, and H.G. Wolff, *Life Stress and Essential Hypertension.* Baltimore: Williams & Wilkins, 1955. H.G. Wolff, *Headache and Other Head Pain.* 2nd edition. New York: Oxford University Press, 1963.

40. K. Brodman et al., "Cornell Medical Index–Health Questionnaire." *Journal of the American Medical Association* 145: 152–157, 1951. K. Brodman et al., "Cornell Medical Index: adjunct to medical interview." *Journal of the American Medical Association* 140: 530–534, 1949. A.J. Erdman et al., "Cornell Medical Index," *Journal of the American Medical Association* 149: 550–551, 1952. S.D. Allison, "Dermatologist and the Cornell Medical Index." *AMA Archives of Dermatology and Syphilis* 65: 601–610, 1952. A.J. Ermann et al., "Health questionnaire use in industrial medical department." *Industrial Medicine* 22: 355–357, 1953. K. Brodman et al., "Cornell Medical Index-Health Questionnaire: III. The evaluation of emotional disturbances," *Journal of Clinical Psychology* 13: 119, 1952. K. Brodman et al, "The Cornell Medical Index-Health Questionnaire: The predictions of psychosomatic and psychiatric disabilities in army training." *American Journal of Psychiatry* 3: 37–40, 1954.

41. B.B. Berle, R.H. Pinsky, S. Wolf, and H.G. Wolff, "The Berle Index: a clinical guide to prognosis in stress disease." *Journal of the American Medical Association* 149: 1624–1628, 1952.

42. S. Wolf and H. Goodell, *Harold Wolff's Stress and Disease.* 2nd ed., revised and edited by S. Wolf and H. Goodell. Springfield, Ill.: Charles C. Thomas, 1968, pp. 8–9.

43. Ibid., p. 259.

44. T. H. Holmes, "It was in this setting . . ." In T.H. Holmes and E.M. David, eds., *Life Change, Life Events, and Illness. Selected Papers.* New York: Praeger, 1989, p. 5.

45. Ibid., p. 23.

46. A.R. Wyler, M. Masuda, and T.H. Holmes, "Magnitude of life events and seriousness of illness." In Holmes and David, eds., *Life Change, Life Events, and Illness*, p. 232.

47. G. de Araujo, P.P. Van Arsdel, Jr., T.H. Holmes, and D.L. Dudley, "Life change, coping ability, and chronic intrinsic asthma." N.G. Hawkins, R. Davies, and T.H. Holmes, "Evidence of psychosocial factors in the development of pulmonary tuberculosis." Both republished in Holmes and David, eds., *Life Change, Life Events, and Illness*.

48. T. H. Holmes, "It was in this setting . . ." In T.H. Holmes and E.M. David, eds., *Life Change, Life Events, and Illness*, p. 21.

49. L.E. Hinkle, Jr. and N. Plummer, "Life stress and industrial absenteeism: the concentration of illness and absenteeism in one segment of a working population." *Industrial Medicine and Surgery* 21: 365–373, 1952.

50. L.E. Hinkle et al., "Life stress and industrial absenteeism." *Industrial Medicine and Surgery* 21: 363, 1952. L.E. Hinkle, Jr. and H.G. Wolff, "The nature of man's adaptation to his total environment and the relation of this to illness." *Archives of Internal Medicine* 99: 442–460, 1957. L.E. Hinkle and H.G. Wolff, "Ecologic investigations of the relationship between illness, life experiences, and the social environment." *Annals of Internal Medicine* 49: 1373–1388, 1958.

51. L.E. Hinkle et al., "An investigation of the relation between life experience, personality characteristics, and general susceptibility to illness." *Psychosomatic Medicine* 20: 278–295, 1958.

52. J.G. Bruhn and S. Wolf, *The Roseto Story: An Anatomy of Health.* Norman: University of Oklahoma Press, 1979, p. vii.

53. H. Selye and T. McKeown, "Production of pseudo-pregnancy by mechanical stimulation of the nipples." *Proceedings of the Society of Experimental Biology* 31: 683, 1934.

54. S. Kark and E. Kark, *Promoting Community Health: From Pholela to Jerusalem.* Johannesburg, South Africa: Witwatersrand University Press, 1999. S.L. Kark and J. Cassel, "The Pholela health center: a progress report." *South African Medical Journal* 26: 101–104, 131–136, 1952. T.M. Brown and E. Fee, "Sidney Kark and John Cassel, social medicine pioneers and South African émigrés." *American Journal of Public Health* 92: 1744–1745, 2002. M. Susser, "A South African odyssey in community health: a memoir of the impact of the teachings of Sidney Kark." *American Journal of Public Health* 83: 1039–1042, 1993. M. Susser, "Pioneering community-oriented primary care." *Bulletin of the World Health Organization* 77: 436–438, 1999.

55. J. Cassel, "An epidemiological perspective on psychosocial factors in disease etiology." *American Journal of Public Health* 64: 1040–1043, 1974. J. Cassel, R. Patrick, and D. Jenkins, "Epidemiological analysis of the health implications of social change: a conceptual model." *Annals of the New York Academy of Science* 84: 938–949, 1960.

56. J. Cassel, "The contribution of the social environment to host resistance." *American Journal of Epidemiology* 104: 107–123, 1976.

57. Ibid., p. 110.

58. L.E. Hinkle, Jr. "The concept of 'stress' in the biological and social sciences." *Science, Medicine and Man* 1: 31–48, 1973, p. 45.

59. S.L. Syme, S.L. and L.F. Berkman, "Social class, susceptibility and sickness." *American Journal of Epidemiology* 104: 1–8, 1976. L.F. Berkman, L.F. and S.L. Syme, "Social network, host resistance, and mortality: a nine-year follow-up study of Alameda County residents." *American Journal of Epidemiology* 109: 186–204, 1979. M. Marmot, M.J. Shipley, and G. Rose, "Inequalities in death—specific explanations of a general pattern?" *The Lancet* 1984: 1 (8384): 1003–1006. J.M. Najman, "Theories of disease causation and the concept of a general susceptibility." *Social Science and Medicine* 14A: 231–237, 1980.

60. F.G. Crookshank, "The importance of a theory of signs and critique of language in the study of medicine," In C.K. Ogden and I.A. Richards, eds., *The Meaning of Meaning.* New York: Harcourt, Brace and Company, 1930. O. Temkin, "The scientific approach to disease: specific entity and individual sickness." In O. Temkin, *The Double Face of Janus and Other Essays in the History of Medicine.* Baltimore: Johns Hopkins University Press, 1977. R.A. Aronowitz, *Making Sense of Illness: Science, Society, and Disease.* New York: Cambridge University Press, 1998. C.E. Rosenberg, "Tyranny of diagnosis: specific entities and individual experience." *Milbank Quarterly* 80: 237–260, 2002. C.E. Rosenberg, "What is disease? In memory of Owsei Temkin." *Bulletin of the History of Medicine* 77: 491–505, 2003.

61. Aronowitz, *Making Sense,* p. 8.

62. R.M. Epstein, D.S. Morse, R.M. Frankel, L. Frarey, K. Anderson, and H.B. Beckman, "Awkward moments in patient-physician communication about HIV risk." *Annals of Internal Medicine* 128: 435–442, 1998.

63. M. Stewart, "Evidence for the patient-centered clinical method as a means of implementing the biopsychosocial approach." In R.M. Frankel, T.E. Quill, and S.H. McDaniel, eds., *The Biopsychosocial Approach: Past, Present, Future.* Rochester: University of Rochester Press, 2003. M. Stewart, J.B. Brown, A. Donner, I.R. McWhinney, J. Oates, W.W. Weston, and J. Jordan, "The impact of patient-centered care on outcomes." *The Journal of Family Practice* 49: 796–804, 2000.

64. R. Ader, "Psychoneuroimmunology: basic research in the biopsychosocial approach." In R.M. Frankel, T.E. Quill, and S.H. McDaniel, eds., *The Biopsychosocial Approach: Past, Present, Future.* Rochester: University of Rochester Press, 2003.

65. H. Weiner, *Perturbing the Organism: The Biology of Stressful Experience.* Chicago: University of Chicago Press, 1992. J.W. Mason, "A re-evaluation of the concept of 'nonspecificity' in stress theory." *Journal of Psychiatric Research* 8: 323–333, 1971. J.W. Mason. "A historical view of the stress field, part I." *Journal of Human Stress* 1: 6–12, 1975. J.W. Mason, "A historical view of the stress field, part II." *Journal of Human Stress* 1: 22–36, 1975.

66. B.S. McEwen, "Protective and damaging effects of stress mediators." *New England Journal of Medicine* 338: 171–179, 1998. B.S. McEwen, "The neurobiology of stress: from serendipity to clinical relevance." *Brain Research* 886: 172–189, 2000. E.M. Sternberg, *The Balance Within: The Science Connecting Health and Emotions.* New York: W.H. Freeman and Company, 2000.

67. H. Weiner, *Perturbing the Organism,* op. cit. R. Viner, "Putting stress in life: Hans Selye and the making of stress theory." *Social Studies of Science* 29, 391–410, 1999.

68. G. Davey Smith, D. Gunnell, and Y. Ben-Shlomo, "Life-course approaches to socio-economic differentials in cause-specific adult mortality." In D. Leon and G. Walt, eds., *Poverty, Inequality and Health: An International Perspective.* Oxford: Oxford University Press, 2000, pp. 88–124.

69. A. Kunst, F. Groenhof, A. Andersen, J-K Borgun et al., "Occupational class and ischemic heart disease mortality in the United States and 11 European countries." *American Journal of Public Health* 89: 47–53, 1999.

70. F.D. Miller, D.M. Reed, and C.J. MacLean, "Mortality and morbidity among blue and white collar workers in the Honolulu Heart Program cohort." *International Journal of Epidemiology* 22: 834–837, 1993.

71. See, for example, R. Anda, D. Williamson, D. Jones, C. Macera, E. Eaker, A. Glassman and J. Marks, "Depressed affect, hopelessness, and the risk of ischemic heart disease in a cohort of U.S. adults." *Epidemiology* 4: 285–294, 1993. S.G. Haynes,

M. Feinleib, and W.B. Kannel, "The relationship of psychosocial factors to coronary heart disease in the Framingham Study." *American Journal of Epidemiology* 111: 37–58, 1980. E.D. Eaker, J. Pinsky, and W.P. Castelli, "Myocardial infarction and coronary death among women: psychosocial predictors from a 20-year follow-up of women in the Framingham Study." *American Journal of Epidemiology* 135: 854–864, 1992.

72. D. Reed, D. McGee, and K. Yano, "Psychosocial processes and general susceptibility to chronic disease." *American Journal of Epidemiology* 119: 356–370, 1984.

73. V.J. Schoenbach, B.H. Kaplan, L. Fredman, L., and D.G. Kleinbaum, "Social ties and mortality in Evans County, Georgia." *American Journal of Epidemiology.* 123: 577–591, 1986.

74. L.F. Berkman, M. Melchior, J-F. Chastang, I. Niedhammer, A. Leclerc, and M. Goldberg, "Social integration and mortality: a prospective study of French employees of Electricity of France-Gas France: The GAZEL cohort." *American Journal of Epidemiology* 159: 167–174, 2004.

75. S. Cohen and T.B. Herbert, "Psychological factors and physical disease from the perspective of human psychoneuroimmunology." *Annual Review of Psychology* 7: 113–142, 1996.

76. M. Marmot, *The Status Syndrome.* New York: Times Books/Henry Holt, 2004, pp. 146–147.

77. S.J. Kunitz and J.E. Levy, *Drinking, Conduct Disorder, and Social Change: Navajo Experiences.* New York: Oxford University Press, 2000, p. 72.

78. P. Magnus and R. Beaglehole, "The real contribution of the major risk factors to the coronary epidemics: time to end the "only-50%" myth." *Archives of Internal Medicine* 161: 2657–2660, 2001.

79. C. Hajat, K. Tilling, J.A. Stewart, N. Lemic-Stojcevic, and C.D. Wolfe, "Ethnic differences in risk factors for ischemic stroke: a European case-control study." *Stroke* 35: 1562–1567, 2004. X.F. Zhang, J. Attia, K. D"este, X.H. Yu, and X.G. Wu, "Prevalence and magnitude of classical risk factors for coronary heart disease in a cohort of 4,400 Chinese steelworkers over 13.5 years follow-up." *European Journal of Cardiovascular Prevention & Rehabilitation* 11: 113–120, 2004. K.T. Knoops, L.C. de Groot, D. Kromhout, A.E. Perrin, O. Moreiras-Varela, A. Menotti, and W.A. van Staveren, "Mediterranean diet, lifestyle factors, and 10-year mortality in elderly European men and women: the HALE project." *Journal of the American Medical Association* 292: 1433–1439, 2004.

80. J.R. Emberson, P.H. Whincup, R.W. Morris, and M. Walker, "Social class differences in coronary heart disease in middle-aged British men: implications for prevention." *International Journal of Epidemiology* 33: 289–296, 2004. J. Lynch, G. Davey Smith, S. Harper, and K. Bainbridge, "Explaining the social gradient in coronary heart disease: comparing relative and absolute risk approaches." *Journal of Epidemiology and Community Health,* in press.

81. L.E. Hinkle, Jr. "The concept of 'stress' in the biological and social sciences." *Science, Medicine, and Man* 1: 31–48, 1973.

82. While in its present form the holistic approach to patients and populations may be understood as a reaction to forces unleashed in the nineteenth and twentieth centuries and as a challenge to the dominant disease-focused paradigm of the past century, these two ways of understanding afflictions and the afflicted are far older than 100 years. For the Western medical tradition has from its inception uneasily embraced two ways of thinking about diseases, patients, and populations: one emphasizing the importance of specific disease entities and their natural histories that are the same from one patient and population to another; the other emphasizing the importance of

knowing all that is wrong with a patient and less concerned with specific diseases and their specific causes. F.G. Crookshank, "Introductory essay on the relation of history and philosophy to medicine." In C.G. Cumston, ed., *An Introduction to the History of Medicine*. New York: Alfred A. Knopf, 1926, pp. xv–xxxii.

Chapter 3

1. William Blake, "London" in "Songs of Innocence and of Experience." In *The Complete Poetry and Selected Prose of John Donne and The Complete Poetry of William Blake*. New York: Modern Library/Random House, 1941. This is the first draft of the poem.

2. For a more detailed discussion, see S.J. Kunitz, "The personal physician and the decline of mortality." In R. Schofield, D. Reher, and A. Bideau, eds., *The Decline of Mortality in Europe*. Oxford: Oxford University Press, 1991.

3. R.W. Fogel, "The conquest of high mortality and hunger in Europe and America: Timing and mechanisms." In P. Higonnet, D.S. Landes, and H. Rosovsky, eds., *Favorites of Fortune: Technology, Growth and Economic Development Since the Industrial Revolution*. Cambridge: Harvard University Press, 1991, pp. 33–71, pp. 59–60.

4. For a review, see B. Harris, "Health, height, and history: an overview of recent developments in anthropometric history." *Social History of Medicine* 7: 297–320, 1994.

5. R.W. Fogel, "New sources and new techniques for the study of secular trends in nutritional status, health, mortality, and the process of aging." *Historical Methods* 26: 5–43, 1993, p. 19.

6. Ibid. pp. 20–21.

7. R. Floud, K. Wachter, and A. Gregory, *Height, Health and History: Nutritional Status in the United Kingdom, 1750–1980*. Cambridge: Cambridge University Press, 1990.

8. D.L. Kuh, C. Power, and B. Rodgers, "Secular trends in social class and sex differences in adult height." *International Journal of Epidemiology* 20: 1001–1009, 1991.

9. Life expectancy data are from E.A. Wrigley, R.S. Davies, J.E. Oeppen, and R.S. Schofield, *English Population from Family Reconstitution*, op. cit. p. 614. *Human Mortality Database*. University of California, Berkeley (USA), and Max Planck Institute for Demographic Research (Germany). Available at www.mortality.org. Data were downloaded on November 8, 2004.

10. G. Kearns, "The urban penalty and the population history of England." In A. Brandstrom and L-G Tedebrand, eds., *Society, Health and Population during the Demographic Transition*. Stockholm: Almqvist and Wiksell International, 1988.

11. D.J.P. Barker, C. Osmond, and J. Golding, "Height and mortality in the counties of England and Wales." *Annals of Human Biology* 17: 1–6, 1990.

12. H.T. Waaler, "Height, weight and mortality: the Norwegian experience." *Acta Medica Scandinavica*, Supplementum 679, 1984. G. Davey Smith et al., "Height and risk of death among men and women," op. cit. P. Allebeck and C. Bergh, "Height, body mass index and mortality: do social factors explain the association?" *Public Health* 106: 375–382, 1992. A.M. Nystrom Peck and D. H. Vagero, "Adult body height, self perceived health and mortality in the Swedish population." *Journal of Epidemiology and Community Health* 43: 380–384, 1989. G. Davey Smith, M.J. Shipley, and G. Rose, "Magnitude and causes of socioeconomic differentials in mortality: further evidence from the Whitehall Study." *Journal of Epidemiology and Community Health*, 44: 265–270, 1990.

13. G. Davey Smith et al., "Height and risk of death among men and women," op. cit., p. 102.

14. R.W. Fogel, "New sources and new techniques for the study of secular trends . . ." op. cit.

15. P.G. Lunn, "Nutrition, immunity, and infection." In R. Schofield, D. Reher, and A. Bideau, eds., *The Decline of Mortality in Europe*. Oxford: Oxford University Press, 1991, pp. 131–145.

16. J. C. Riley, "Height, nutrition, and mortality risk reconsidered." *Journal of Interdisciplinary History* 24: 465–492, 1994.

17. Unfortunately, published height data are not as readily available or plentiful for the last quarter of the nineteenth century as they are for earlier in the century. Using other kinds of data, however, Millward and Bell have argued that economic factors and maternal health are a better explanation of the decline of mortality in the last third of the nineteenth century than are public health interventions. They show that investments in public health, measured by local government finances and loans for capital improvements for water works, sewers, and roads, increased rapidly in the early twentieth century, after the decline in infant mortality had begun. Thus, they claim, improvements in the late nineteenth century could not have been sufficient to influence profoundly the decline of infant mortality in their selected cities that began so dramatically in the 1870s. They also argue that the gradual decline in infant mortality which occurred in the last 30 years of the nineteenth century were the result of improvements in maternal health and nutrition and declining fertility rates. See F. Bell and R. Millward, "Public health expenditures and mortality in England and Wales, 1870–1914." *Continuity and Change* 13: 221–249, 1998. R. Millward and F. Bell, "Economic factors in the decline of mortality in late nineteenth- and twentieth-century Britain." *European Review of Economic History* 2: 263–288, 1998. And R. Millward and F. Bell, "Infant mortality in Victorian Britain: the mother as medium." *Economic History Review* LIV: 699–733, 2001.

18. For a helpful review, see B. Harris, "Public health, nutrition and the decline of mortality: the McKeown thesis revisited." *Social History of Medicine* 17: 379–407, 2004. Harris offers a qualified defense of McKeown's thesis, concluding that it is difficult to precisely quantify the contribution of nutrition to the decline of mortality.

19. S. Szreter, "The importance of social intervention in Britain's mortality decline c. 1850–1914: a re-interpretation of the role of public health." *Social History of Medicine* 1: 1–37, 1988. I shall not deal with a critique of Szreter's paper, or with Szreter's reply. See S. Guha, "The importance of social intervention in England's mortality decline: the evidence reviewed." *Social History of Medicine* 7: 89–113, 1994. And S. Szreter, "Mortality in England in the eighteenth and nineteenth centuries: a reply to Sumit Guha." *Social History of Medicine* 7: 269–282, 1994.

20. S. Szreter, "Economic growth, disruption, deprivation, disease, and death: on the importance of the politics of public health for development." *Population and Development Review* 23: 693–728, 1997, p. 710.

21. e.g., Szreter, "The importance of social intervention," op. cit., p. 21.

22. A. Hardy, *The Epidemic Streets: Infectious Disease and the Rise of Preventive Medicine 1856–1900*. Oxford: Oxford University Press, 1993.

23. F. Bell and R. Millward, "Public health expenditures and mortality in England and Wales, 1870–1914." op. cit.

24. R. Woods, *The Demography of Victorian England and Wales*. Cambridge: Cambridge University Press, 2000. pp. 355–356.

25. G. Davey Smith and J. Lynch, "Social capital, social epidemiology and disease aetiology." *International Journal of Epidemiology* 33: 691–700, 2004.

26. S. Szreter, "Debating mortality trends in 19th century Britain." *International Journal of Epidemiology* 33: 705–709, 2004.

27. S. Szreter and G. Mooney, "Urbanization, mortality, and the standard of living debate: new estimates of the expectation of life at birth in nineteenth-century British cities." *Economic History Review* 51: 84–112, 1998, p. 107. For a slightly earlier period, see P. Huck, "Infant mortality and living standards of English workers during the Industrial Revolution." *The Journal of Economic History* 55: 528–550, 1995.

28. J. Vogele, *Urban Mortality Change in England and Germany, 1870–1913*. Liverpool: Liverpool University Press, 1998, p. 93.

29. Ibid., p. 213. See also the earlier paper by J.C. Brown, "Public reform for private gain? Public health and sanitary infrastructure in German cities 1877–1910." Paper presented at the annual meeting of the Social Science History Association, Chicago, November, 1988. And J.C. Brown, "Coping with crisis? The diffusion of waterworks in late nineteenth-century German towns." *The Journal of Economic History* XLVIII (No. 2): 307–318, 1988.

30. For a somewhat different explanation of the differences between England and Germany, see E.P. Hennock, "The urban sanitary movement in England and Germany, 1838–1914: a comparison." *Continuity and Change* 15: 269–296, 2000.

31. A.S. Wohl, *Endangered Lives*, op. cit., pp. 170–171. G. Kearns, "Private property and public health reform in England 1830–70." *Social Science and Medicine* 26: 187–199, 1988. Szreter, "Economic growth, disruption, deprivation, disease, and death," op. cit.

32. A. Hardy, *The Epidemic Streets*, op. cit., p. 268.

33. J.C. Brown, "Public health reform and the decline of urban mortality: the case of Germany, 1876–1912." Paper presented at the annual meeting of the Population Association of America, March, 1989.

34. W.R. Lee and J.P. Vogele, "The benefits of federalism? The development of public health policy and health care systems in nineteenth-century Germany and their impact of mortality reduction." *Annales de Demographie Historique* No. 1, pp. 65–96, 2001. Similar differences have been observed among French cities. S.H. Preston and E. van de Walle, "Urban French mortality in the nineteenth century." *Population Studies* 32: 275–297, 1978.

35. R.J. Evans, *Death in Hamburg: Society and Politics in the Cholera Years 1830–1910*. Oxford: Oxford University Press, 1987.

36. M.R. Haines and H.J. Kintner, "The mortality transition in Germany, 1860–1935. Evidence by region." *Historical Methods* 33: 83–104, 2000.

37. The Swedish data come from: L.G. Sandberg and R.H. Steckel, "Was industrialization hazardous to your health? Not in Sweden!," and R.H. Steckel and R. Floud, "Conclusions," both in R.H. Steckel and R. Floud, eds., *Health and Welfare during Industrialization*. Chicago: The University of Chicago Press, 1997.

38. Sandberg and Steckel, "Was industrialization hazardous to your health?" p. 143. See also P. Skold, "The key to success: the role of local government in the organization of smallpox vaccination in Sweden." *Medical History* 45: 201–226, 2000.

39. This occurred in France as well as Germany. J.-P. Goubert, *The Conquest of Water: The Advent of Health in the Industrial Age*. Princeton: Princeton University Press, 1986.

40. Steckel and Floud, "Conclusions," op. cit. p. 424.

41. P.W. Ewald, "The evolution of virulence." *Scientific American* April, 1993, pp. 86–93. And *Evolution of Infectious Disease*. New York: Oxford University Press, 1993.

42. D.M. Fox, "Populations and the law: the changing scope of health policy." *Journal of Law, Medicine & Ethics* 31: 607–614, 2003, p. 608.

43. F.B. Smith, *The People's Health 1830–1910*. Canberra: The Australian National University Press, 1979, pp. 414–415.

44. R. Haines and R. Shlomowitz, "Explaining the modern mortality decline: what can we learn from sea voyages?" *Social History of Medicine* 11: 15–48, 1998.

45. R. Spree, *Health and Social Class in Imperial Germany*. Oxford: Berg Publishers, 1988, p. 151

46. G.V. Rimlinger, *Welfare Policy and Industrialization in Europe, America, and Russia*. New York: John Wiley & Sons., 1971.

47. International Labour Office, *Compulsory Sickness Insurance: Comparative Analysis of National Laws and Statistics*. Studies and Reports, Series M (Social Insurance) No. 6, Geneva, 1927.

48. C.R. Winegarden and J.E. Murray, "The contributions of early health-insurance programs to mortality declines in pre-World War I Europe: Evidence from fixed-effects models." *Explorations in Economic History* 35: 431–446, 1998.

49. For two specific diseases (typhoid and diphtheria), Jorge Vogele has failed to find significant correlations between the availability of medical practitioners per 1000 population and mortality rates. See Vogele, *Urban Mortality Change in England and Germany,* op. cit. pp. 195–196.

50. D.T. Rogers, *Atlantic Crossings: Social Politics in a Progressive Age.* Cambridge: Harvard University Press, 1998, p. 61.

51. W.H. Dawson, *Social Insurance in Germany, 1883–1911: Its History, Operation, Results.* London: T. Fisher Unwin, [1912] 1979, p. 202.

52. Ibid., pp. 183–185.

53. Ibid., p. 254.

54. Ibid., p. 203.

55. J.P. Mackenbach, "The contribution of medical care to mortality decline: McKeown revisited." *Journal of Clinical Epidemiology* 49: 1207–1213, 1996.

56. E. Sydenstricker and W. I. King, "A method of classifying families according to incomes in studies of disease prevalence." *Public Health Reports* 35: 2829–2846, 1920, p. 2829,

57. Ibid., p. 2830, italics in original. See also S.D. Collins, *Economic Status and Health: A Review and Study of the Relevant Morbidity and Mortality Data*. Treasury Department, United States Public Health Service, Public Health Bulletin No. 165. Washington, D.C.: U.S. Government Printing Office, 1927.

58. E. Sydenstricker, *Health and Environment*. New York: McGraw-Hill, 1933, pp. 13–15.

59. C.K. Wu and C.-E. A. Winslow, "Mortality, prosperity and urbanization in United States Counties," *American Journal of Hygiene* 18: 491–542, 1933. J.H. Watkins and A.G. Evans, "Mortality changes as related to prosperity and urbanization in United States counties." *American Journal of Hygiene* 26: 449–471, 1936.

60. G. St.J. Perrott and S.D. Collins, "Sickness and the Depresssion: a preliminary report upon a survey of wage-earning families in Birmingham, Detroit, and Pittsburgh." *Milbank Memorial Fund Quarterly* 11: 281–298, 1933, and "Sickness and the Depression: a preliminary report upon a survey of wage-earning families in Baltimore, Cleveland, and Syracuse." *Milbank Memorial Fund Quarterly* 12: 28–34, 1934. G. St. J. Perrott, E. Sydenstricker, and S.D. Collins, "Medical care during the Depression: a preliminary report upon a survey of wage-earning families in seven large cities." *Milbank Memorial Fund Quarterly*

12: 99–114, 1934. G. St.J. Perrott and S.D. Collins, "Relation of sickness to income and income change in 10 surveyed communities." *Public Health Reports* 50: 595–622.

61. L.P. Herrington and I.M. Moriyama, "The relation of mortality from certain metabolic diseases to climatic and socio-economic factors." *American Journal of Hygiene* 28: 396–422, 1938. I.W. Moriyama and L.P. Herrington, "The relation of diseases of the cardiovascular and renal systems to climatic and socio-economic factors." *American Journal of Hygiene* 28: 423–436, 1938. L.P. Herrington and I.M. Moriyama, "The relation of mortality from certain respiratory diseases to climatic and socio-economic factors." *American Journal of Hygiene* 29: 111–120, 1939. C.A. Mills, "Climate and metabolic stress." *American Journal of Hygiene* 29: 147–164, 1939.

62. S. H. Preston, "The changing relation between mortality and level of economic development." *Population Studies* 29: 213–248, 1975. See also R.A. Easterlin, "Industrial revolution and mortality revolution: two of a kind?" *Journal of Evolutionary Economics* 5: 393–408, 1995 and R.A. Easterlin, *Growth Triumphant: The Twenty-first Century in Historical Perspective.* Ann Arbor: University of Michigan Press, 1996, p. 77.

63. D.D. Rutstein, W. Berenbert, T.C. Chalmers, C.G. Child, 3rd, A.P. Fishman, and E.B. Perrin, "Measuring the quality of medical care: a clinical method." *New England Journal of Medicine* 294: 582–588, 1976, p. 582. Italics in original.

64. Ibid., p. 583.

65. E. Nolte and M. McKee, *Does Healthcare Save Lives? Avoidable Mortality Revisited.* London: The Nuffield Trust, 2004, p. 30. Much of the discussion in the following paragraphs is based upon the literature reviewed in this publication.

66. Ibid., p. 43.

67. Ibid., p. 42.

68. J. Billings, L. Zeitel, J. Lukomnik, T.S. Carey, A.E. Blank, and L. Newman, "Impact of socioeconomic status on hospital use in New York City." *Health Affairs* 12: 162–173, 1993. A.B. Bindman, K. Grumbach, D. Osmond, M. Komaromy, K. Vranizan, N. Lurie, J. Billings, and A. Stewart, "Preventable hospitalizations and access to health care." *Journal of the American Medical Association* 274: 305–311, 1995. J. Billings, G.M. Anderson, and L.S. Newman, "Recent findings on preventable hospitalizations." *Health Affairs* 15: 239–250, 1996.

69. See, for example, P. Braverman, R. Oliva, M.G.G. Miller, R. Reiter, and S. Egerter, "Adverse outcomes and lack of health insurance among newborns in an eight-county area of California, 1982 to 1986." *New England Journal of Medicine* 321: 508–513, 1989. G.L. Lindberg, N. Lurie, S. Bannick-Mohrland, R.E. Sherman, and P.A. Farseth, "Health care cost containment measures and mortality in Hennepin County's Medicaid elderly and all elderly." *American Journal of Public Health* 79: 1481–1485, 1989. D.R. Calkins, L.A. Burns, and T.L. Delbanco, "Ambulatory care and the poor: tracking the impact of changes in federal policy." *Journal of General Internal Medicine* 1: 109–115, 1986. C.A. Miller, "Infant mortality in the U.S." *Scientific American* 253: 31–37, 1985. N. Lurie, N.B. Ward, M.F. Shapiro, and R.H. Brook, "Termination from Medi-Cal—does it affect health?" *New England Journal of Medicine* 311: 480–484, 1984. N. Lurie, N.B. Ward, M.F. Shapiro, C. Gallego, R. Vaghaiwalla, and R.H. Brook, "Termination of Medi-Cal benefits: a follow-up study one year later." *New England Journal of Medicine* 314: 1266–1268, 1986.

70. J.E. Wennberg, J.L. Freeman, R.M. Shelton, and T.A. Bubolz, "Hospital use and mortality among Medicare beneficiaries in Boston and New Haven." *New England Journal of Medicine* 321: 1168–1173, 1989.

71. E.M. Sloss, E.B. Keeler, R.H. Brook, B.H. Ooperskalski, G.A. Goldberg, and

J.P. Newhouse, "Effect of a health maintenance organization on physiologic health." *Annals of Internal Medicine* 106: 130–138, 1987.

72. E.B. Keeler, R.H. Brook, G.A. Goldberg, C.J. Kamberg, and J.P. Newhouse, "How free care reduced hypertension in the Health Insurance Experiment." *Journal of the American Medical Association* 254: 1926–1931, 1985.

73. J. McKinlay and S. McKinlay, "The questionable contribution of medical measures to the decline of mortality in the U.S. in the twentieth century." *Milbank Memorial Fund Quarterly* 53: 405–428, 1977. S. Wing, "The role of medicine in the decline of hypertension-related mortality." *International Journal of Health Services* 14: 649–665, 1984. J.B. McKinlay, S.M. McKinlay, and R. Beaglehole, "A review of the evidence concerning the impact of medical measures on recent mortality and morbidity in the United States." *International Journal of Health Services* 19: 181–208, 1989.

74. Nolte and McKee, *Healthcare,* op. cit., p. 56.

75. W.H. Barker and J.P. Mullooly, "Stroke in a defined elderly population, 1967–1985: a less lethal and disabling but no less common disease." *Stroke* 28: 284–290, 1997.

76. W.H. Barker, J.P. Mullooly, and K.L.P. Linton, "Trends in hypertension prevalence, treatment, and control in a well-defined older population." *Hypertension* 31 [part 2]: 552–559, 1998.

77. In terms of purchasing power parity, the figures have been more nearly similar.

Year	Canada	United States	Canada as a % of the U.S.
1980	$11,500	$13,020	88%
1990	$19,400	$23,440	82.7%
2000	$27,170	$34,100	79%

Source: The World Bank, *World Development Report, 2002.* CD-ROM.

78. A more complete discussion of the differences in mortality reported in this section is to be found in S.J. Kunitz, with I. Pesis-Katz, "Mortality of White Americans, African Americans, and Canadians: the causes and consequences for health of welfare state institutions and policies. *Milbank Quarterly* 83: 5–39, 2005.

79. M.R. Haines and R.H. Steckel, eds., *A Population History of North America.* New York: Cambridge University Press, 2000, pp. 696–697.

80. Comparison of racial differences in avoidable deaths have been the subject of several previous articles. See, for instance, S. Woolhandler, D.U. Himmelstein, R. Silber, M. Bader, M. Harnly, and A.A. Jones, "Medical care and mortality: racial differences in preventable deaths." *International Journal of Health Services* 15: 1–22, 1985.

81. W.W. Holland, ed., *European Community Atlas of "Avoidable Death"*, Vol.1, Oxford: Oxford University Press, 1991, p. 1. Italics added.

82. M.D. Wong, M.F. Shapiro, W.J. Boscardin, and S.L. Ettner. "Contribution of major diseases to disparities in mortality." *New England Journal of Medicine* 347: 1585–1592, 2002.

83. All the mortality data come from the Centers for Disease Control (http://wonder.cdc.gov) with the exception of perinatal mortality. D. Hoyert, "Perinatal mortality in the United States." *Vital and Health Statistics* 20 (25), 1995.

84. R. Farley and W.R. Allen, *The Color Line and the Quality of Life in America.* New York: The Russell Sage Foundation, 1987, pp. 42–43.

85. M.B. Wenneker and A.M. Epstein, "Racial inequalities in the use of procedures for patients with ischemic heart disease in Massachusetts." *Journal of the American Medical*

Association 261: 253–257, 1989. A.M. Gittelsohn, J. Halpern, and R.L. Sanchez, "Income, race, and surgery in Maryland." *American Journal of Public Health* 81: 1435–1441, 1991.

86. Farley and Allen, *The Color Line,* op. cit., pp. 42–43. Ewbank, "History of Black mortality and health before 1940," op. cit., p. 123.

87. L. Tabar, M-F Yen, B. Vitak, H-H. T. Chen, R.A. Smith, and S.W. Duffy, "Mammography service screening and mortality in breast cancer patients: 20-year follow-up before and after introduction of screening." *The Lancet* 361: 1405–1410, 2003.

88. B.A. Jones, E.A. Patterson, and L. Calvocoressi, "Mammography screening in African American women: evaluating the research." *Cancer* 97 (supplement): 258–272, 2003.

89. K.M. McConnochie, M.J. Russo, J. McBride, P. Szilagy, A.M. Brooks, and K.J. Roghmann, "Socioeconomic variations in asthma hospitalization: excess utilization or greater need?" *Pediatrics* 103: e75, 1999.

90. M.D. Wong et al. "Contribution of major diseases to disparities in mortality," op. cit.

91. M.D. Wong et al. "Contribution of major diseases to disparities in mortality," op. cit.

92. A.M. Gittelsohn, J. Halpern, and R.L. Sanchez, "Income, race, and surgery in Maryland," op. cit.

93. P.B. Bach, H.M. Pham, D. Schrag, R.C. Tate, and J.L. Hargraves, "Primary care physicians who treat Blacks and Whites." *New England Journal of Medicine* 351: 575–584, 2004.

94. T.R. Marmor, "Review essay of *Atlantic Crossings* and *Shifting the Color Line.*" *Public Opinion Quarterly* 64: 110–113, 2000.

95. B.A. Virnig, N. Lurie, Z. Huang, D. Musgrave et al., "Racial variations in quality of care among Medicare + Choice enrollees." *Health Affairs,* 21: 224–230, 2002.

96. D.B. Smith, "Addressing racial inequality in health: civil rights monitoring and report cards." *Journal of Health Politics, Policy, and Law,* 23: 75–105, 1998.

97. R.T. Kuderle and T.R. Marmor. "The Development of Welfare States in North America." In P. Flora and A.J. Heidenheimer, eds. *The Development of Welfare States in Europe and America.* New Brunswick, N.J.: Transaction Books, 1982, pp. 83–85.

98. M. Wolfson, "Income inequality in Canada and the United States." *The Daily,* Statistics Canada, July 28, 2000, http://www.statcan.ca/Daily/English/000728/d000728a. htm. M. Wolfson and B. Murphy, "Income inequality in North America: does the 49th parallel still matter?" *Canadian Economic Observer* August 2000, pp. 1–24.

99. E. Wood, A.M. Sallar, M.T. Schechter, and R.S. Hogg, "Social inequalities in male mortality amenable to medical intervention in British Columbia." *Social Science and Medicine* 48: 1751–1758, 1999. J.R. Dunn and M.V. Hayes, "Social inequality, population health, and housing: a study of two Vancouver neighborhoods." *Social Science and Medicine* 51: 563–587, 2000. S. Dunlop, P.C. Coyte, and W. McIsaac, "Socio-economic status and the utilization of physicians' services: results from the Canadian National Population Health Survey." *Social Sciences and Medicine* 51: 123–133, 2000. R. Wilkins, J-M Berthelot, and E. Ng, *Trends in Mortality by Neighbourhood Income in Urban Canada from 1971 to 1996.* Supplement to Health Reports, Vol. 13. Ottawa: Statistics Canada, 2002.

100. L. Munan, J. Vobecky, and A. Kelly, "Population health care practices: an epidemiologic study of the immediate effects of a universal health insurance plan." *International Journal of Health Services* 2: 285–295, 1974. A.D. McDonald, J.C. McDonald, V. Salter, and P.E. Enterline, "Effects of Quebec Medicare on physician consultation for selected symptoms." *New England Journal of Medicine* 291: 649–652, 1974. J. Siemiatycki, L. Richardson, and I.B. Pless, "Equality in medical care under national health insurance in Montreal." *New England Journal of Medicine* 303: 10–15, 1980.

101. C.D. Naylor, "Health care in Canada: incrementalism under fiscal duress." *Health Affairs* 18: 9–26, 1999.

102. Billings et al., "Recent findings on preventable hospitalizations," op. cit.

103. S.J. Katz, J.R.W. Armstrong, and J.P. LoGerfo, "The adequacy of prenatal care and incidence of low birthweight among the poor in Washington State and British Columbia." *American Journal of Public Health* 84: 986–991, 1994.

104. J.C. Hornberger, A.M. Garver, and J.R. Jeffery, "Mortality, hospital admissions, and medical costs of end-stage renal disease in the United States and Manitoba, Canada." *Medical Care* 35: 686–700, 1997.

105. G.M. Anderson, J.P. Newhouse, and L.L. Roos, "Hospital care for elderly patients with diseases of the circulatory system: a comparison of hospital use in the United States and Canada." *New England Journal of Medicine* 321: 1443–1448, 1989. J.V. Tu, C.L. Pashos, C.D. Naylor, E. Chen, S-L Normand, J.P. Newhouse, and B.J. McNeil, "Use of cardiac procedures and outcomes in elderly patients with myocardial infarction in the United States and Canada." *New England Journal of Medicine* 336: 1500–1505, 1997.

106. L.L. Roos, E.S. Fisher, S.M. Sharp, J.P. Newhouse, G.Anderson, and T.A. Bubolz, "Postsurgical mortality in Manitoba and New England." *Journal of the American Medical Association* 263: 2453–2458, 1990.

107. R. Wilkins, J-M Berthelot, and E. Ng, *Trends in Mortality by Neighbourhood Income in Urban Canada from 1971 to 1996.* Supplement to Health Reports, Vol. 13. Ottawa: Statistics Canada, 2002.

108. S.J. Katz, K. Cardiff, M. Pascali, M.L. Barer, and R.G. Evans. 2002. "Phantoms in the snow: Canadians' use of health care service in the United States." *Health Affairs* 21: 19–31.

109. K.M. Gorey, E.J. Holowaty, G. Fehringer, E. Laukkanen, A. Moskowitz, D.J. Webster, and N.L. Richter, "An international comparison of cancer survival: Toronto, Ontario, and Detroit, Michigan, metropolitan areas." *American Journal of Public Health* 87: 1156–1163, 1997. K.M. Gorey, E.J. Holowaty, E. Laukkanen, G. Fehringer, and N.L. Richter, "An international comparison of cancer survival: advantage of Toronto's poor over the near poor of Detroit." *Canadian Journal of Public Health* 89: 102–104, 1998. K.M. Gorey, E.J. Holowaty, G. Fehringer, E. Laukkanen, N.L. Richter, and C.M. Meyer, "An international comparison of cancer survival: Toronto, Ontario and three relatively resourceful United States metropolitan areas." *Journal of Public Health Medicine* 22: 343–348, 2000. K.M. Gorey, E.J. Holowaty, G. Fehringer, E. Laukkanen, N.L. Richter, and C.M. Meyer, "An international comparison of cancer survival: metropolitan Toronto, Ontario, and Honolulu, Hawaii." *American Journal of Public Health* 90: 1866–1872, 2000. K.M Gorey, E. Kliewer, E.J. Holowaty, E. Laukkanen, and E.Y. Ng, "An international comparison of breast cancer survival: Winnipeg, Manitoba and Des Moines, Iowa, metropolitan areas." *Annals of Epidemiology* 13: 32–41, 2003.

110. D. Manuel, and Y. Mao, "Avoidable mortality in the United States and Canada, 1980–96." *American Journal of Public Health* 92: 1481–1484, 2002.

111. The data are from Statistics Canada 1987–1999.

112. D. Blumenthal, C. Vogeli, L. Alexander, and M. Pittman, *A Five-Nation Hospital Survey: Commonalities, Differences, and Discontinuities.* New York: The Commonwealth Fund, 2004.

113. U.E. Reinhardt, P.S. Hussey, and G.F. Anderson, "U.S. health care spending in an international context: why is U.S. spending so high, and can we afford it?" *Health Affairs* 23: 10–25, 2004.

114. *World Development Indicators 2002*, CD-ROM. Washington, D.C.: The World Bank, 2002. Health expenditures are defined as follows: "Total health expenditure is the

sum of public and private health expenditure as a ratio of total population. It covers the provision of health service (preventive and curative), family planning activities, nutrition activities, and emergency aid designated for health but does not include provision of water and sanitation."

115. E. Sydenstricker, *Health and Environment*, op. cit., p. 13–15.

Chapter 4

1. W.S. Gilbert and A. Sullivan, *The Gondoliers* [1889]. In *Martyn Green's Treasury of Gilbert & Sullivan*. New York: Simon and Schuster, 1961, p. 660.

2. N.E. Adler, T. Boyce, M.A. Chesney, S. Cohen, S. Folkman, R.L. Kahn, and S.L. Syme, "Socioeconomic status and health: the challenge of the gradient." *American Psychologist* 49: 15–24, 1994, p. 15. Emphasis added.

3. M. Marmot and A. Feeney, "General explanations for social inequalities in health." In M. Kogevinas, N. Pearce, M. Susser, and P. Boffetta, eds., *Social Inequalities and Cancer*. ARC Scientific Publications No. 138. Lyon: International Agency for Research on Cancer, 1997, p. 207. Emphasis added.

4. J.C. Phelan, B.G. Link, A. Diez-Roux, I. Kawachi, and B. Levin, "Fundamental causes of social inequalities in mortality: a test of the theory." *Journal of Health and Social Behavior* 45: 265–285, 2004, p. 280. Emphasis added.

5. See Coleman, W. *Death is a Social Disease: Public Health and Political Economy in Early Industrial France*. Madison: The University of Wisconsin Press, 1982, Chapter 9.

6. F. Engels, *The Condition of the Working Class in England*. Oxford: Oxford University Press, [1845] 1993.

7. R. Taylor and A. Riegier, "Medicine as social science: Rudolf Virchow on the typhus epidemic in Upper Silesia." *International Journal of Health Services* 15: 547–559, 1985.

8. D.S. Smith, "Differential mortality in the United States before 1900." *Journal of Interdisciplinary History* 13: 735–759, 1983.

9. S.H. Preston and M.R. Haines, *Fatal Years: Child Mortality in Late Nineteenth-Century America*. Princeton: Princeton University Press, 1991, pp. 177–198.

10. S. Hautaniemi, personal communication, March 22, 2000.

11. A. Reid, "Locality or class? Spatial and social differentials in infant and child mortality in England and Wales, 1895–1911." In C.A. Corsini and P.P. Viazzo, eds., *The Decline of Infant and Child Mortality: The European Experience 1750–1990*. Florence, Italy: UNICEF, 1997.

12. A. Blum and J. Houdaille, "Les inequalities devant la mort dans le passe." *Cahiers de Sociologie et de Demographie Medicales* 39: 5–20, 1989.

13. A. Antonovsky, "Social class, life expectancy and overall mortality." *Milbank Memorial Fund Quarterly* 45: 31–73, 1967.

14. Period life expectancy estimates for the total population from 1541 to 1871 are from E.A. Wrigley and R.S. Schofield, *The Population History of England 1541–1871, A Reconstruction*. London: Edward Arnold, 1981, p. 230. Subsequently, these estimates have been revised in E.A. Wrigley, R.S. Davies, J.E. Oeppen, and R.S. Schofield, *English Population History from Family Reconstitution 1580–1837*. Cambridge: Cambridge University Press, 1997. I have compared estimates published there (Table A9.1) with those from the first volume. While there are differences, for my purposes they are not significant since both illustrate equally well the point I wish to make in Figure 4–1: that the life expectancy of the total population diverged from that of peerage in the second half of the

eighteenth century. For the sake of clarity, I have not included both curves in the figure. Period life expectancy figures since 1871 are from the *Human Mortality Database*, University of California, Berkeley (USA), and Max Planck Institute for Demographic Research (Germany). Available at www.mortality.org or www.humanmortality.de (data downloaded on November 10, 2004). Life expectancy data for the peerage are from T.H. Hollingsworth, *The Demography of the British Peerage*, Supplement to *Population Studies* Vol. 18, No. 2, November, 1964. These are cohort life expectancies based upon births with 25-year intervals. I have centered them on the approximate mid-point of each interval. The figures are for males and females combined.

15. S.J. Kunitz, "Making a long story short: Men's height and mortality in England 1st–19th centuries," *Medical History*, 31: 269–280, 1987.

16. S.R. Johansson, *Death and the Doctors: Medicine and Elite Mortality in Britain from 1500 to 1800*. Cambridge: Cambridge Group for the History of Population and Social Structure, Working Paper Series, No. 7, 1999.

17. J. Oeppen, "Mortality and marital status in the British peerage: 1603–1938." Paper presented at the annual meeting of the Social Science History Association, Chicago, 1998.

18. A. Perrenoud, "L'Inegalite social devant la mort a Geneve au XVIIe siecle." *Population* 30 (numero speciale): 221–243, 1975.

19. R. Woods and N. Williams, "Must the gap widen before it can be narrowed? Long-term trends in social class mortality differentials." *Continuity and Change* 10: 105–137, 1995.

20. R.T. Vann and D. Eversley, *Friends in Life and Death: The British and Irish Quakers in the Demographic Transition, 1650–1900*. Cambridge: Cambridge University Press, 1992, pp. 228–229.

21. Ibid., p. 237.

22. U.O. Schmelz, *Infant and Early Childhood Mortality among the Jews of the Diaspora*. Jewish Population Studies, The Institute of Contemporary Jewry, The Hebrew University of Jerusalem, 1971, see Tables 1 and 3.

23. Ibid., Table 6.

24. R.M. Woodbury, *Infant Mortality and its Causes*. Baltimore: Williams & Wilkins, 1926. G.A. Condran and E.A. Kramarow, "Child mortality among Jewish immigrants to the United States." *Journal of Interdisciplinary History* 22: 223–254, 1991.

25. Schmelz, *Infant and Early Childhood Mortality,* Tables 3 and 15.

26. Schmelz, *Infant and Early Childhood Mortality,* Table 14.

27. J. Sundin, "Culture, class, and infant mortality during the Swedish mortality transition, 1750–1850." *Social Science History* 19: 117–145, 1995.

28. J.E. Knodel, *Demographic Behavior in the Past: A Study of Fourteen German Village Populations in the Eighteenth and Nineteenth Centuries*. Cambridge: Cambridge University Press, 1988. S. Scott and C.J. Duncan, "Interacting effects of nutrition and social class differentials on fertility and infant mortality in a pre-industrial population." *Population Studies* 54: 71–87, 2000.

29. R. Woods and N. Williams, "Must the gap widen," op. cit., p. 127.

30. M. Haines, "Socio-economic differentials in infant and child mortality during mortality decline: England and Wales, 1890–1911." *Population Studies* 49: 297–315, 1995.

31. B. Burstrom and E. Bernhardt, "Social differentials in the decline of child mortality in nineteenth century Stockholm." *European Journal of Public Health* 11: 29–34, 2001.

32. D.C. Ewbank and S.H. Preston, "Personal health behaviour and the decline in in-

fant and child mortality: the United States, 1900–1930." In J. Caldwell, S. Findley, P. Caldwell, G. Santow, W. Cosford, J. Braid, and D. Broers-Freeman, eds. *What We Know about Health Transition: The Cultural, Social and Behavioural Determinants of Health.* The Health Transition Centre, The Australian National University. Canberra: ANUTECH Pty Ltd., 1990, Vol. 1, pages 116–149.

33. H. Kaelble, *Industrialization and Social Inequality in 19th-Century Europe.* Leamington Spa/Heidelberg: Berg, 1986, p. 135.

34. J.R. Hollingsworth, "Inequality in levels of health in England and Wales, 1891–1971." *Journal of Health and Social Behavior* 22: 268–283, 1981. E.R. Pamuk, "Social class inequality in mortality from 1921 to 1972 in England and Wales." *Population Studies* 39: 17–31, 1985. *Report of the Working Group on Inequalities in Health*, republished as the *Black Report* in *Inequalities in Health.* London: Penguin Books, 1988. G.D. Smith, D. Dorling, D. Gordon, and M. Shaw, "The widening health gap: what are the solutions?" *Critical Public Health* 9: 151–170, 1999.

35. J.P. Mackenbach, M.J. Bakker, A.E. Kunst, and F. Diderichsen, "Socioeconomic inequalities in health in Europe." In J. Mackenbach and M. Bakker, eds., *Reducing Inequalities in Health: A European Perspective.* London: Routledge, 2002, p. 11.

36. D. Mechanic, "Disadvantage, inequality, and social policy." *Health Affairs* 21: 48–59, 2002. Of course, many such environmental improvements do not benefit everyone equally. The affluent are better able to protect their neighborhoods from polluting industries than the poor, for instance.

37. J.C. Phelan, B.G. Link, A. Diez-Roux, I. Kawachi, and B. Levin, " 'Fundamental causes' of social inequalities in mortality," op. cit.

38. P. Bourdieu, *Distinction: A Social Critique of the Judgement of Taste.* Translated by R. Nice. London: Routledge & Kegan Paul, 1984, p. 179.

39. Ibid., pp. 182–183.

40. Ibid., p. 196.

41. Ibid., p. 214. See also M.R. Gillick, "Health promotion, jogging, and the pursuit of the moral life." *Journal of Health Politics, Policy and Law.* 9: 369–387, 1984.

42. W.F. Ogburn, *Social Change with Respect to Culture and Original Nature.* Gloucester, Mass.: Peter Smith, [1922] 1964.

43. G. Simmel, "Fashion." *American Journal of Sociology* 62: 541–558, 1957 (reprint).

44. N. Elias, *The Civilizing Process: The Development of Manners.* New York: Urizen Books, 1978. And N. Elias, *The Civilizing Process: State Formation and Civilization.* Oxford: Blackwell, 1982.

45. H. Blumer, "Fashion: from class differentiation to collective selection." *The Sociological Quarterly* 10: 275–291, 1969.

46. Blumer, "Fashion," p. 278.

47. T. Williams and W. Kornblum, *The Uptown Kids: Struggle and Hope in the Projects.* New York: G.P. Putnam's Sons, 1994, pp. 82–84. F. Davis, *Fashion, Culture, and Identity.* Chicago: The University of Chicago Press, 1992. D. Crane, "Diffusion models and fashion: a reassessment." *Annals of the American Academy of Political and Social Sciences* 566: 13–24, 1999.

48. Blumer, "Fashion," pp. 286–287.

49. C. Kadushin, "The friends and supporters of psychotherapy: on social circles in urban life." *American Sociological Review* 31: 786–802, 1966.

50. J.R. Gusfield, "The social symbolism of smoking and health." In R.C. Rabin and S.D. Sugarmen, eds., *Smoking Policy: Law, Politics, and Culture.* New York: Oxford University Press, 1993, pp. 49–68.

51. R. G. Ferrence, *Deadly Fashion: The Rise and Fall of Cigarette Smoking in North America*. New York: Garland Publishing, 1989. J.P. Pierce, M.C. Fiore, T.E. Novotny, E.J. Hatziandreu, and R.M. Davis, "Trends in cigarette smoking in the United States." *Journal of the American Medical* Association 261: 56–60, 1989. F.C. Pampel, "Inequality, diffusion, and the status gradient in smoking." *Social Problems* 49: 35–57, 2002.

52. M.G. Marmot, A.M. Adelstein, N. Robinson, and G.A. Rose, "Changing social class distribution of heart disease." *British Medical Journal* 2: 1109–1112, 1978.

53. S. Wing, C. Hayes, G. Heiss, E. John, M. Knowles, W. Riggan, and H.A. Tyroler, "Geographic variation in the onset of decline of ischemic heart disease mortality in the United States." *American Journal of Public Health*, 76: 1404–1408, 1986.

54. S. Wing, M. Casper, W. Riggan, C. Hayes, and H.A. Tyroler, "Socioenvironmental characteristics associated with the onset of decline of ischemic heart disease mortality in the United States." *American Journal of Public Health* 78: 923–926, 1988, p. 925.

55. T.A. Pearson, D.T. Jamison, and J. Trejo-Gutierrez, "Cardiovascular disease." In D.T. Jamison, ed., *Disease Control Priorities in Developing Countries.* New York: Oxford University Press, 1993. T.A. Pearson, "Cardiovascular diseases as a growing health problem in developing countries: the role of nutrition in the epidemiologic transition." *Public Health Reviews* 24: 131–144, 1995. T.A. Pearson, "Global perspectives on cardiovascular disease." *Evidence-Based Cardiovascular Medicine* April, 1997, pp. 4–6.

56. J.F. Burnum, "Medical practice a la mode: how medical fashions determine medical care." *New England Journal of Medicine* 317: 1220–1222, 1987.

57. T.J. Philipson and R.A. Posner, "The long-run growth in obesity as a function of technological change." *Perspectives in Biology and Medicine* 46 (supplement): S87-S107, 2003.

58. J. Frykman and O. Lofgren, *Culture Builders: A Historical Anthropology of Middle-Class Life.* Translated by A. Crozier. New Brunswick, N.J.: Rutgers University Press, 1987, p. 177.

59. N. Elias, *The Civilizing Process: The Development of Manners.* New York: Urizen Books, [1939] 1978. And *State Formation and Civilization.* Oxford: Basil Blackwell, [1939] 1982.

60. See also J. Goudsblom, "Public health and the civilizing process." *Milbank Quarterly* 64: 161–188, 1986. P. Pinell, "Modern medicine and the civilising process." *Sociology of Health & Illness* 18: 1–16, 1996.

61. J.F. Kasson, *Rudeness and Civility: Manners in Nineteenth-Century Urban America.* New York: Hill and Wang, 1990, pp. 11–12.

62. M. Marmot, *The Status Syndrome: How Social Standing Affects our Health and Longevity.* New York: Times Books/Henry Holt and Company, 2004.

63. M. Marmot and A. Feeney, "General explanations for social inequalities in health," op. cit., p. 219. See also N.E. Adler et al., "Socioeconomic status and health: the challenge of the gradient," op. cit., p. 21.

64. M. Marmot, C.D. Ryff, L.L. Bumpass, M. Shipley, and N.F. Marks, "Social inequalities in health: next questions and converging evidence." *Social Science and Medicine* 44: 901–910, 1997.

65. M.D. Hayward, A. M. Pienta, and D.K. McLaughlin, "Inequality in men's mortality: the socioeconomic status gradient and geographic context." *Journal of Health and Social Behavior* 38," 313–330, 1997.

66. M.L. Kohn, A. Naoi, C. Schoenbach, C. Schooler, and K.M. Slomczynski, "Position in the class structure and psychological functioning in the United States, Japan, and Poland." *American Journal of Sociology* 95: 964–1008, 1990, p. 982. See also

M.L. Kohn, *Class and Conformity: A Study in Values*. Chicago: The University of Chicago Press, 1977.

67. Ibid., p. 1005.

68. M. Marmot, M. Shipley, E. Brunner, and H. Hemingway, "Relative contribution of early life and adult socioeconomic factors to adult mortality in the Whitehall II study." *Journal of Epidemiology and Community Health* 55: 301–307, 2001.

69. F.D. Miller, D.M. Reed, and C.J. MacLean, "Mortality and morbidity among blue and white collar workers in the Honolulu Heart Program cohort." *International Journal of Epidemiology* 22: 834–837, 1993.

70. L.E. Hinkle, Jr., L.H. Whitney, E.W. Lehman, J. Dunn, B. Benjamin, R. King, A. Plakum, and B. Flehinger, "Occupation, education, and coronary heart disease: risk is influenced more by education and background than by occupational experiences in the Bell System." *Science* 161: 238–245, 1968. See also H. Bosma, R. Peter, J. Siegrist, and M. Marmot, "Two alternative job stress models and the risk of coronary heart disease." *American Journal of Public Health* 88: 68–74, 1998.

71. N.E. Adler et al., "Socioeconomic status and health: the challenge of the gradient," op. cit., p. 21. R.M. Sapolsky, "Hormonal correlates of personality and social contexts: from non-human to human primates." In C. Panter-Brick and C.M. Worthman, eds., *Hormones, Health, and Behavior: A Socio-Ecological and Lifespan Perspective*. Cambridge: Cambridge University Press, 1999.

72. E. Mayo, *The Social Problems of an Industrial Civilization*. Boston, Mass.: Division of Research, Harvard Business School, 1945, pp. 90–91.

73. C.R. Janes and G.M. Ames, "Ethnographic explanations for the clustering of attendance, injury, and health problems in a heavy machinery assembly plant." *Journal of Occupational Medicine* 34: 993–1003, 1992. Similar observations have been told to me of the highly paid white-collar sales representatives of an industrial firm, half of whom regularly engaged in abuse of alcohol, cocaine, and marijuana at company sales meetings.

74. R.G. Wilkinson, *Unhealthy Societies: The Afflictions of Inequality*. New York: Routledge, 1996, pp. 3–4.

75. R. Wilkinson, "Inequality and the social environment: a reply to Lynch *et al.*" *Journal of Epidemiology and Community Health* 54: 411–413, 2000.

76. J.E. Levy and S.J. Kunitz, "Indian reservations, anomie, and social pathologies." *Southwestern Journal of Anthropology* (now *Journal of Anthropological Research*) 27: 97–128, 1971.

77. J. Savishinsky, "Mobility as an aspect of stress in an arctic community." *American Anthropologist* 73: 604–618, 1971. P. Sutton, "The politics of suffering: indigenous policy in Australia since the seventies." *Anthropological Forum* 11: 125–173, 2001.

78. I. Clendinnen, *Dancing with Strangers: Europeans and Australians at First Contact*. Cambridge: Cambridge University Press, 2005, p. 166.

79. S. Webb, *Palaeopathology of Aboriginal Australians: Health and Disease Across a Hunter-Gatherer Continent*. Cambridge: Cambridge University Press, 1995, pp. 205–207.

80. J. Lynch, G.D. Smith, S. Harper, M. Hillemeier, N. Ross, G.A. Kalan, and M. Wolfson, "Is income inequality a determinant of population health? Part 1. A systematic review." *The Milbank Quarterly*. 82: 5–99, 2004. J. Lynch, G.D. Smith, S. Harper, and M. Hillemeier, "Is income inequality a determinant of population health? Part 2. U.S. national and regional trends in income inequality and age- and cause-specific mortality." *The Milbank Quarterly* 82: 355–400, 2004. See also A. Wagstaff and E. van Doorslaer, "Income inequality and health: what does the literature tell us?" *Annual Review of Public*

Health 21: 543–567, 2000. S.V. Subramanian and I. Kawachi, "Income inequality and health: what have we learned so far?" *Epidemiologic Reviews* 26: 78–91, 2004.

81. Other combinations of rich countries give different results for the association of GDP per capita and life expectancy, but because I have limited this part of my discussion to western Europe to retain some historical and cultural consistency, I have focused on countries of the European Union. See J. Lynch, P. Due, C. Muntaner, and G. Davey Smith, "Social capital—Is it a good investment strategy for public health?" *Journal of Epidemiology and Community Health* 54: 404–408, 2000.

82. V. Navarro and L. Shi, "The political context of social inequalities and health." *Social Science and Medicine* 52: 481–491, 2001. See also J.A. Macinko, L. Shi, and B. Starfield, "Wage inequality, the health system, and infant mortality in wealthy industrialized countries, 1970–1996." *Social Science and Medicine* 58: 279–292, 2004.

83. *World Development Indicators.* CD-ROM. Washington, D.C.: The World Bank, 2002. Ireland is excluded due to missing data. Using Analysis of Variance (ANOVA), the differences are significant: F ratio 9.0959, p = 0.0017.

84. T. Blakely, J. Atkinson, and D. O'Dea, "No association of income inequality with adult mortality within New Zealand: a multi-level study of 1.4 million 25–64 year olds." *Journal of Epidemiology and Community Health* 57: 279–284, 2003. G. Veenstra, "Income inequality and health—Coastal communities in British Columbia, Canada." *Canadian Journal of Public Health* 95: 374–379, 2002.

85. J.P. Mackenbach, "Income inequality and population health: evidence favoring a negative correlation between income inequality and life expectancy has disappeared." *British Medical Journal* 324: 1–2, 2002.

86. D.K. McLaughlin and C.S. Stokes, "Income inequality and mortality in U.S. counties: does minority racial concentration matter?" *American Journal of Public Health* 92: 99–104, 2002.

87. A. Shmueli, "Population health and income inequality: new evidence from Israeli time-series analyses." *International Journal of Epidemiology* 33: 311–317, 2004.

88. J. Lynch et al., "Is income inequality a determinant of population health? Part 2," op. cit.

89. R. Wilkinson, *The Impact of Inequality: How to Make Sick Societies Healthier.* New York and London: The New Press, 2005, p. 140. The study of violence is by C-C Hsieh and M.D. Pugh, "Poverty, income inequality, and violent crime: a meta-analysis of recent aggregate data studies." *Criminal Justice Review* 18: 182–202, 1993, p. 195. See also a more recent review of the literature on level of aggregation and the association between inequality and mortality: R.G. Wilkinson and K.E. Pickett, "Income inequality and population health: a review and explanation of the evidence." *Social Science and Medicine* 62: 1768–1784, 2006.

90. A. Forbes and S.P. Wainwright, "On the methodological, theoretical and philosophical context of health inequalities research: a critique." *Social Science and Medicine* 53: 801–816, 2001, p. 807.

91. S.J. Kunitz, H.D. Delaney, L.J. Layne, D.R. Wheeler, E.M. Rogers, and W.G. Woodall, "Small-area variations in conviction rates for DWI: the significance of contextual variables in a Southwestern state." *Accident Analysis & Prevention* 38: 600–609, 2006.

92. G.A. Kaplan, E.R. Pamuk, J.W. Lynch, R.D. Cohen, and J.L Balfour, "Inequality in income and mortality in the United States: analysis of mortality and potential pathways." *British Medical Bulletin* 312: 999–1003, 1996.

93. J. Lynch, et al., "Is income inequality a determinant of population health? Part 2," op. cit.

94. S.L. Engerman, S.H. Haber, and K.L. Sokoloff, "Inequality, institutions, and differential growth among New World economies." In C. Menard, ed., *Institutions, Contracts and Organizations: Perspectives from the New Institutional Economics.* Cheltenham, UK and Northampton, Mass.. U.S.A.: E. Elgar, 2000, S.L. Engerman and K.L. Sokoloff, 2002. *Factor Endowments, Inequality, and Paths of Development among New World Economies.* Working paper 9259, National Bureau of Economic Research, Cambridge, Mass.., 2002.

95. A.M. Schlesinger, "Biography of a nation of joiners." *The American Historical Review* 50: 1–25, 1944, p. 12.

96. G.A. Kaplan et al., "Inequality in income and mortality in the United States." A. Alesina and E.L. Glaeser, *Fighting Poverty in the US and Europe: A World of Difference.* Oxford: Oxford University Press, 2004, p. 147.

97. E.H. Monkkonen, *Murder in New York City.* Berkeley: University of California Press, 2001, p. 197. See also R. Lane, *Murder in America: A History.* Columbus: Ohio State University Press, 1997.

98. G. McWhiney, *Cracker Culture: Celtic Ways in the Old South.* Tuscaloosa: The University of Alabama Press, 1988, p. 268.

99. D.H. Fischer, *Albion's Seed: Four British Folkways in America.* New York: Oxford University Press, 1989, pp. 403–405.

100. S. Hackney, "Southern violence." *The American Historical Review* 74: 906–935, 1969. J.S. Reed, "To live—and die—in Dixie: a contribution to the study of southern violence." *Political Science Quarterly* 86: 429–443, 1971. R.D. Gastil, "Homicide and a regional culture of violence." *American Sociological Review,* 36: 412–427, 1971. L. Baron and M.A. Straus, "Cultural and economic sources of homicide in the United States." *The Sociological Quarterly* 29: 371–390, 1988. D. Cohen and R.E. Nisbett, "Self-protection and the culture of honor: explaining southern violence." *Personality and Social Psychology Bulletin* 20: 551–567, 1994.

101. D. Cohen and R.E. Nisbett, "Self-protection and the culture of honor," p. 552.

102. R.J. Sampson and W.J.Wilson, "Toward a theory of race, crime, and urban inequality." In J. Hagan and R.D. Peterson, eds., *Crime and Inequality.* Stanford, CA: Stanford University Press, 1995.

103. C.E. Kubrin and R. Weitzer, "Retaliatory homicide: concentrated disadvantage and neighborhood culture." *Social Problems* 50: 157–180, 2003. See also R.J. Sampson and W.J. Wilson, "Toward a theory of race, crime, and urban inequality." In J. Hagan and R.D. Peterson, eds., *Crime and Inequality.* Stanford: Stanford University Press, 1995.

104. A. Blumstein, F.P. Rivara, and R. Rosenfeld, "The rise and decline of homicide—and why." *Annual Review of Public Health* 21: 505–541, 2000.

105. C. Cubbin, L.W. Pickle, and L. Fingerhut, "Social context and geographic patterns of homicide among US Black and White males." *American Journal of Public Health* 90: 579–587, 2000.

106. E. H. Monkkonen, *Homicide in New York,* op. cit., pp. 152–170.

107. D. Bramley, P. Herbert, L. Tuzzio, and M. Chassin, "Disparities in indigenous health: a cross-country comparison between New Zealand and the United States." *American Journal of Public Health* 95: 844–850, 2005.

108. Indian Health Service, *1996 Trends in Indian Health.* Rockville, MD: Office of Planning, Department of Health and Human Services, 1996.

109. R.C. Gregory, A.C. Abello, and J. Johnson, "The individual economic well-being of native American men and women during the 1980s: a decade of moving backwards." In

G.D. Sandefur, R.R. Rindfuss, and B. Cohen, eds., *Changing Numbers, Changing Needs: American Indian Demography and Public Health*. Washington D.C.: National Academy Press, 1996.

110. J. Taylor, *Changing numbers, changing needs? A preliminary assessment of Indigenous population growth 1991–96*. Canberra: Centre for Aboriginal Economic Policy Research, The Australian National University, 1997.

111. (New Zealand Income Survey 1996). Statistics New Zealand, *Incomes*. Wellington, N.Z.: Statistics New Zealand, 1999.

112. S.J. Kunitz, "The history and politics of health care policy for American Indians." *American Journal of Public Health* 86: 1464–1473, 1996. See also J.J. Hisnanick and D.A. Coddington, "Measuring human betterment through avoidable mortality: a case for universal health care in the USA." *Health Policy* 34: 9–19, 1995.

113. S.J. Kunitz, *Disease and Social Diversity*. New York: Oxford University Press, 1994.

114. B. Milanovic, *True World Income Distribution, 1988 and 1993: First Calculations, Based on Household Surveys Alone*. Policy Research Working Paper No. 2244, Washington, D.C.: The World Bank, Development Research Group, Poverty and Human Resources, November, 1999. J. Flemming and J. Micklewright, *Income Distribution, Economic Systems and Transition*. Innocenti Occasional Papers, Economic and Social Policy Series, No. 70. Florence: UNICEF International Child Development Centre, 1999. B. Gustafsson and M. Johansson, "In search of smoking guns: what makes income inequality vary over time in different countries?" *American Sociological Review* 64: 585–605. 1999. C. Kenny, "Why are we worried about income? Nearly everything that matters is converging." *World Development* 33: 1–19, 2005.

115. R.A. Epstein, "Let the shoemaker stick to his last: a defense of the 'old' public health." *Perspectives in Biology and Medicine* 46 (supplement): S138–S159, 2003.

116. M. Marmot, "Understanding social inequalities in health." *Perspectives in Biology and Medicine* 46 (supplement): S9–S23, 2003.

117. R.A. Epstein, "Let the shoemaker stick to his last," op. cit., pp. 156–157.

118. R.A. Epstein, "Let the shoemaker stick to his last," op. cit., p. 157.

119. P.D. Curtin, *Death by Migration: Europe's Encounter with the Tropical World in the Nineteenth Century*. Cambridge: Cambridge University Press, 1989, p. 99.

120. P.D. Curtin, *Death by Migration,* op. cit., p. 99.

121. M. Marmot, *The Status Syndrome,* op. cit., p. 27.

122. R.M. Sapolsky, "Hormonal correlates of personality and social contexts: from non-human to human primates," op. cit.

123. R.A. Epstein, "Let the shoemaker stick to his last," op. cit.

124. R. Klein, "Acceptable inequalities." In D. Green, ed., *Acceptable Inequalities? Essays on the Pursuit of Equality in Health Care*. London: Institute of Economic Affairs Health Unit, 1988. R. Klein, "Making sense of inequalities: a response to Peter Townsend." *International Journal of Health Services* 21: 175–181, 1991.

125. P. Townsend, "Individual or social responsibility for premature death? Current controversies in the British debate about health." *International Journal of Health Services* 20: 373–392, 1990. And P. Townsend, "Evading the issue of widening inequalities of health in Britain: a reply to Rudolf Klein." *International Journal of Health Services* 21: 183–189, 1991.

126. A.M. Pollock, *NHS plc: The Privatisation of Our Health Care*. London: Verso, 2004.

127. E. Huber and J. D. Stephens, *Development and Crisis of the Welfare State: Parties and Policies in Global Markets*. Chicago: The University of Chicago Press, 2001.

128. A. Kunst, *Cross-National Comparisons of Socio-Economic Differences in Mortality.* Department of Public Health, Erasmus University, Rotterdam, The Netherlands: 1997.

Chapter 5

1. T. Hardy, "The Curate's Kindness: A Workhouse Irony." *Selected Poems of Thomas Hardy.* London, Macmillan and Co., 1958. Italics in original.

2. R.D. Putnam, *Bowling Alone: The Collapse and Revival of American Community.* New York: Simon and Schuster, 2000.

3. R.D. Putnam, "Bowling alone: America's declining social capital." *Journal of Democracy,* 6: 65–78, 1995, p. 67.

4. R.D. Putnam, *Making Democracy Work: Civic Traditions in Modern Italy.* Princeton: Princeton University Press, 1993, p. 182.

5. R.D. Putnam, *Bowling Alone: The Collapse and Revival of American Community,* op. cit. P. Hawe and A. Shiell, "Social capital and health promotion: a review." *Social Science and Medicine* 51: 871–885, 2000.

6. J.S. Coleman, "Social capital in the creation of human capital." *American Journal of Sociology* (Supplement), 94: S-95-S120, 1988, p. S98.

7. Ibid., pp. S95–S96

8. Putnam, *Making Democracy Work,* op. cit., p. 87.

9. E. Cox, *A Truly Civil Society.* The 1995 Boyer Lectures, Sydney, Australia: ABC Books, 1995, pp. 1, 8.

10. A. Portes, "Social capital: its origins and applications in modern sociology." *Annual Review of Sociology* 24: 1–24, 1988.

11. B. Wellman, P.J. Carrington, and A. Hall, "Networks as Personal Communities." In B. Wellman and S.D. Berkowitz, eds., *Social Structures: A Network Approach.* New York: Cambridge University Press, 130–184, 1988.

12. See, for instance, I. Kawachi, B.P. Kennedy, and K. Lochner, "Long live community: social capital and public health." *The American Prospect.* November-December, 1997.

13. D.H. Fischer, *Albion's Seed: Four British Folkways in America.* New York: Oxford University Press, 1989.

14. A. de Tocqueville, *Democracy in America.* Translated by Henry Reeve. New York: Schocken Books, 2 Vols., 1961, pp. 16–18.

15. Ibid., Vol. 1, p. 19.

16. Quoted in G. McWhiney, *Cracker Culture: Celtic Ways in the Old South.* Tuscaloosa: The University of Alabama Press, 1988, pp. 268–269. See also P. Smith, *As a City Upon a Hill: The Town in American History.* New York: Alfred A. Knopf, 1966, pp. 248–252.

17. de Tocqueville, *Democracy in America,* op. cit., Vol. 1, pp. 77–78.

18. R.D. Putnam, *Making Democracy Work,* op. cit.

19. de Tocqueville, *Democracy in America,* op. cit., Vol. 1, pp. 16–18.

20. H.M. Caudill, *Night Comes to the Cumberlands: A Biography of a Depressed Area.* Boston: Little, Brown and Company, 1963.

21. R.D. Gastil, "Homicide and a regional culture of violence." *American Sociological Review,* 36: 412–427, 1971. D. Lester, *Patterns of Suicide and Homicide in America.* Commack, N.Y.: Nova Science Publisher, Inc., 1994. S. Hackney, "Southern violence."

The American Historical Review 74: 906–925, 1969. J.S. Reed, "To live—and die—in Dixie: a contribution to the study of southern violence." *Political Science Quarterly* 86: 429–443, 1971.

22. L.W. Pickle, M. Mungiole, G.K. Jones, and A.A. White, *Atlas of United States Mortality*. Hyattsville, MD: National Center for Health Statistics, 1996.

23. K. Hart, S.J. Kunitz, D. Mukamel, and R. Sell, "Metropolitan governance, residential segregation, and mortality among African Americans." *American Journal of Public Health,* 88: 434–438, 1998.

24. K. Jackson, *Crabgrass Frontier*. New York: Oxford University Press, 1985.

25. D. Rusk, *Cities Without Suburbs*. Washington, D.C.: Woodrow Wilson Center Press, 1993.

26. A.M. Schlesinger, "Biography of a nation of joiners." *The American Historical Review* 50: 1–25, 1944, pp. 24–25.

27. Ibid., p. 21.

28. Tocqueville, *Democracy in America,* op. cit., Vol. 2, pp. 387–388.

29. B. Turner, "Social capital, inequality and health: the Durkheimian revival." *Social Theory & Health* 1: 4–20, 2003. H. Kushner and C.E. Sterk, "The limits of social capital: Durkheim, suicide, and social cohesion." *American Journal of Public Health* 95: 1139–1143, 2005.

30. Durkheim, *Suicide,* pp. 388–389.

31. Ibid., p. 389.

32. Ibid., pp. 389–390. Emphasis in original.

33. *Rerum Novarum, On Capital and Labor,* Encyclical of Pope Leo XIII, May 15, 1891, St. Peter's, Rome.

34. H. Pesch, *Ethics and the National Economy*. Norfolk, VA: I H S Press, [originally published in German in 1918] 2004, p. 171. Emphasis in the original.

35. M.P. Ryan, "Civil society as democratic practice: North American cities during the nineteenth century." In R.I. Rotberg, ed., *Patterns of Social Capital: Stability and Change in Historical Perspective*. Cambridge: Cambridge University Press, 2001.

36. R.D. Brown, "The emergence of voluntary associations in Massachusetts, 1760–1830." *Journal of Voluntary Action Research* 2: 64–73, 1973, p. 68.

37. Ibid., p. 68.

38. Ryan, "Civil society," op. cit., p. 246.

39. K. Whittington, "Revisiting Tocqueville's America: society, politics, and association in the nineteenth century." In B. Edwards, M.W. Foley, and M. Diani, eds., *Beyond Tocqueville: Civil Society and the Social Capital Debate in Comparative Perspective*. Hanover, NH: University Press of New England, 2001, p. 22.

40. Ryan, "Civil society," op. cit.

41. G. Gamm and R.D. Putnam, "The growth of voluntary associations in America, 1840–1940." *Journal of Interdisciplinary History* 29: 511–557, 1999. Reprinted in R.I. Rotberg, ed., *Patterns of Social Capital: Stability and Change in Historical Perspective*. Cambridge: Cambridge University Press, 2001. Page references are to the original journal article.

42. M. Weber, *Max Weber: A Biography*. H. Zohn, ed. and trans. New York: John Wiley & Sons, 1975, p. 299.

43. R.V. Hine, *Community on the American Frontier: Separate But Not Alone*. Norman: University of Oklahoma Press, 1980, p. 18.

44. Ibid., pp. 137–142.

45. P. Smith, *As a City Upon a Hill,* op. cit. p. 174.

46. R.S. and H.M. Lynd, *Middletown: A Study in American Culture.* New York: Harcourt, Brace and Company, 1929, pp. 286, 303–312. J. West (Psuedonym for C. Withers), *Plainville, U.S.A.* New York: Columbia University Press, 1945, pp.81–85, 134. M. Meeker, "The joiners—male and female." In W.L. Warner, *Democracy in Jonesville: A Study in Quality and Inequality.* New York: Harper & Brothers, 1949, pp. 115–131. A.B. Hollingshead, *Elmtown's Youth.* New York: John Wiley and Sons,1949, pp. 87–109.

47. Lynd and Lynd, *Middletown,* pp. 303–305.

48. T. Caplow, H.M. Bahr, B.A. Chadwick, R. Hill, and M.H. Holmes, *Middletown Families: Fifty Years of Change and Continuity.* Minneapolis: University of Minnesota Press, 1982, p. 84.

49. R.D. Putnam, *Bowling Alone: The Collapse and Revival of American Community.* New York: Simon & Schuster, 2000, pp. 52 and 54. There has been explosive growth in voluntary associations since World War II, but it has for the most part been growth of what Robert Putnam has called "tertiary" organizations, Washington-based groups with a mass membership and professional staff, but without the face-to-face contact that locally based organizations require, what are usually considered secondary associations. D.L. Costa and M.E. Kahn, "Understanding the American decline in social capital, 1952–1998." *KYKLOS* 56: 17–46, 2003.

50. S.V. Subramanian, D.J. Kim, and I. Kawachi, "Social trust and self-rated health in US communities: a multilevel analysis." *Journal of Urban Health* 79 (Supplement 4): S21–S34, 2002, p. S21.

51. I. Kawachi, B.P. Kennedy, K. Lochner, and D. Prothrow-Stith, "Social capital, income inequality, and mortality." *American Journal of Public Health* 87: 1491–1498, 1997. I. Kawachi, B.P. Kennedy, and K. Lochner, "Long live community: social capital as public health." *The American Prospect* No. 35 (November-December) 1997, pp. 56–59. S.V. Subramanian et al., "Social trust."

52. G. Veenstra, "Social capital, SES and health: an individual-level analysis. *Social Science and Medicine* 50: 619–629, 2000.

53. G.T.H. Ellison, "Income inequality, social trust, and self-reported health in high-income countries." *Annals of the New York Academy of Sciences* 896: 325–328, 1999.

54. J. Lynch, G. Davey Smith, M. Hillemeier, M. Shaw, T. Raghunathan, and G. Kaplan, "Income inequality, the psychosocial environment, and health: comparisons of wealthy nations." *The Lancet* 358: 194–200, 2001.

55. Georgia, Kentucky, North Carolina, South Carolina, Louisiana, Virginia, Texas, Tennessee, West Virginia, Mississippi, Alabama, and Arkansas. See the figures in Kawachi et al., "Social capital," op. cit. and "Long live community," op. cit.

56. M. Woolcock, "Social capital and economic development: toward a theoretical synthesis and policy framework." *Theory and Society* 27: 151–208, 1998, pp. 156–157.

57. J.E. Curtis, E.G. Grabb, and D.E. Baer, "Voluntary association membership in fifteen countries: a comparative analysis." *American Sociological Review* 57: 139–152, 1992.

58. B. Rothstein, "Social capital in the social democratic welfare state." *Politics & Society* 29: 207–241, 2001, p. 232.

59. S. Berman, "Civil society and political institutionalization." *American Behavioral Scientist* 40: 562–574, 1997.

60. P. Evans, "Government action, social capital, and development: reviewing the evidence on synergy." In P. Evans, ed., *State-Society Synergy: Government and Social Capital in Development.* International and Area Studies, Research series No. 94. Berkeley: University of California, 1997, pp. 180–181.

61. See L.C. Kelly, *The Assault on Assimilation: John Collier and the Origins of Indian Policy Reform*. Albuquerque: University of New Mexico Press, 1983, various pages.

62. S. Szreter, "The state of social capital: bringing back in power, politics, and history." *Theory and Society* 31: 573–621, 2002.

63. E.T. Devine, "Social ideals implied in present American programs of voluntary philanthropy." *American Journal of Sociology* 18: 784–795, 1913, p. 785.

64. Woolcock, "Social capital and economic development," op. cit.

65. The description of the function of clubs and associations in Jonesville appears to represent one version of this type of social capital. Jonesville was full of clubs and associations in the early 1940s, one for every 35 citizens, and authors of this study took a much less skeptical attitude toward the functioning of these organizations than had the Lynds. They wrote:

> Touching all major spheres of group life, they bind the community together. As activities of any association overlap those of other associations and other groups, they unify the interests and the aims of discrete elements. They cut across the major divisions which exist, causing individuals from different groups and different segments of the society to meet, talk, and act together.

This description of the unifying effects of associational life is, however, somewhat at odds with the description of club life as it actually existed. In Jonesville, as in Middletown and Plainville, lodges were dying out. As in Middletown, lodges were being replaced by civic clubs with exclusive memberships. Rotary included the most prominent members of the business community, and the Lions Club was "just a notch lower." Indeed, the authors wrote, "It is possible . . . to distinguish the pattern of associational behavior of the various classes and to show how this pattern maintains and strengthens the class structure of the community." The types of organizations to which members of the different classes belonged differed very considerably, as did the average number of memberships per family: upper class, 3.6; upper-middle class, 3.5; lower-middle class, 2.4; upper-lower class, 1.1; lower-lower class, 0.66. As in Middletown, socially ambitious people used clubs as a means of upward social mobility, joining those (if they could) that gave them access to people above them in status. Considering the great differences in memberships, the differences among clubs and associations, and their utility for reinforcing class boundaries, it is hard to know just how unifying these associations could be. M. Meeker, "Status aspirations and the social club," op. cit, pp. 115–116, 121, 130–131, 134, 139, 143.

66. Szreter, "The state of social capital," op. cit., pp. 576, 579.

67. J. Kaufman, *For the Common Good? American Civic Life and the Golden Age of Fraternity*. New York: Oxford University Press, 2002, Chapter 7.

68. For a brief description of "iron triangles," see Y. Yishai, "From an iron triangle to an iron duet? Health policy making in Israel." *European Journal of Political Research* 21: 91–108, 1992, esp. p. 92.

69. H. Johnson and D. Broder, *The System: The American Way of Politics at the Breaking Point*. New York: Little, Brown & Co., 1996.

70. C. Perrow and M.F. Guillen, *The AIDS Disaster: The Failure of Organizations in New York and the Nation*. New Haven: Yale University Press, 1990, Chapter 6.

71. Putnam, *Bowling Alone: The Collapse and Revival of American Community,* op. cit., p. 331, emphasis in original.

72. Coleman, "Social capital," op. cit., p. S98.

73. Some of the articles that address this issue are: J. Cassel, 1976, "The contribution of the social environment to host resistance." *American Journal of Epidemiology*, 104: 107–123, 1976. S. Cobb, "Social support as a moderator of life stress." *Psychosomatic Medicine*, 38: 300–314, 1976. W.E. Broadhead, R. Grimson, S. Heyden, et al., "The epidemiologic evidence for a relationship between social support and health." *American Journal of Epidemiology*, 117: 521–537, 1983. P.A. Thoits, "Stress coping, and social support processes: where are we? what next?." *Journal of Health and Social Behavior, Extra Issue*: 53–79, 1995. P.A. Thoits, "Conceptual, methodological and theoretical problems in studying social support as a buffer against life stress." *Journal of Health and Social Behavior*, 23: 145–159, 1982.

74. L.F. Berkman, M. Melchior, J-F. Chastang, I. Niedhammer, A. Leclerc, and M. Goldberg, "Social integration and mortality: a prospective study of French employees of Electricity of France-Gas France: The GAZEL cohort." *American Journal of Epidemiology* 159: 167–174, 2004.

75. V.J. Schoenbach, B.H. Kaplan, L. Fredman, D.G. Kleinbaum, "Social ties and mortality in Evans County, Georgia." *American Journal of Epidemiology*, 123: 577–591, 1986.

76. D. Reed, D. McGee, K. Yano, "Psychosocial processes and general susceptibility to chronic disease." *American Journal of Epidemiology*, 119: 356–370, 1984.

77. S.J. Kunitz and J.E. Levy, "A prospective study of isolation and mortality in a cohort of elderly Navajo Indians." *Journal of Cross-Cultural Gerontology* 3: 71–85, 1988. S.J. Kunitz and J.E. Levy, *Navajo Aging: The Transition from Family to Institutional Support*. Tucson: University of Arizona Press, 1991.

78. Some of the relevant publications are: L.F. Berkman and S.L. Syme, "Social networks, host resistance, and mortality: a nine-year follow-up study of Alameda County residents." *American Journal of Epidemiology*, 104: 186–204, 1979. J.S. House, H.L. Metzner, and C. Robbins, "The association of social relationships and activities with mortality: prospective evidence from the Tecumseh Community Study." *American Journal of Epidemiology*, 116: 123–140, 1982. J.S. House, K.R. Landis, and D. Umberson, "Social relationships and health." *Science*, 241: 540–545, 1988. B.S. Hanson, S.O. Isacsson, L. Janzon, and S.E. Lindell, "Social network and social support influence mortality in elderly men." *American Journal of Epidemiology*, 130: 100–111, 1989. L. Welin, B. Larsson, K. Svardsudd, B. Tibblin, and G. Tibblin, "Social network and activities in relation to mortality from cardiovascular diseases, cancer and other causes: a 12 year follow-up of the study of men born in 1913 and 1923." *Journal of Epidemiology and Community Health*, 46: 127–132, 1992. D. Blazer, "Social support and mortality in an elderly community population." *American Journal of Epidemiology*, 115: 684–694, 1982. T.E. Seeman, G.A. Kaplan, L. Knudsen, R. Cohen, and J. Guralnik, "Social network ties and mortality among the elderly in the Alameda County Study." *American Journal of Epidemiology*, 126: 714–723, 1987. D.M. Zuckerman, S.V. Kasl, and A.M. Ostfeld, "Psychosocial predictors of mortality among the elderly poor." *American Journal of Epidemiology*, 119: 410–423, 1984.

79. L.F. Berkman, "Social networks, support, and health: taking the next forward step." *American Journal of Epidemiology*, 123: 59–62, 1986. See also I. Kawachi and L. Berkman, "Social cohesion, social capital, and health." In L.F. Berkman and I. Kawachi, eds., *Social Epidemiology*. New York: Oxford University Press, 2000, p. 185.

80. D.S. Strogatz, and S.A. James, "Social support and hypertension among blacks and whites in a rural, Southern community." *American Journal of Epidemiology*, 124: 949–956, 1986.

81. D.R. Williams and T.B. Fenton, "The mental health of African-Americans: findings, questions, and directions." In I.L.Livingston, ed., *Handbook of Black American*

Health: The Mosaic of Conditions, Issues, Policies, and Prospects. Westport, Conn.: Greenwood Press, 1994, pp. 262–263.

82. B.R. Sarason, I.G. Sarason, and R.A.R. Gurung, "Close Personal Relationships and Health Outcomes: A Key to the Role of Social Support." In S. Duck et al., *Handbook of Personal Relationships: Theory, Research, and Interventions*, 2nd ed. New York: John Wiley and Sons, 1997, p. 553.

83. D. Dyck, R. Short, and P.P. Vitaliano, "Predictors of burden and infectious illness in schizophrenia caregivers." *Psychosomatic Medicine,* 61: 411–419, 1999. H. Wu, J. Wang, J.T. Cacioppo, R. Glaser, J.K. Kiecolt-Glaser, and W.B. Malarkey, "Chronic stress associated with spousal caregiving of patients with Alzheimer's dementia is associated with downregulation of B-lymphocyte GH mRNA." *Journals of Gerontology,* Series A, Biological Sciences and Medical Sciences, 54: M212–M215, 1999. K. Vedhara, N.K. Cox, G.K. Wilcock, P. Perks, M. Hunt, S. Anderson, S.L. Lightman, and N.M. Shanks, "Chronic stress in elderly carers of dementia patients and antibody response to influenza vaccination." *Lancet,* 353: 627–631, 1999. L. Fredman, M.P. Daly, and A.M. Lazur, "Burden among white and black caregivers to elderly adults." *Journals of Gerontology,* Series B, Psychological Sciences and Social Sciences 50: S110-S118, 1995. A.C. King, R.K. Oka, and D.R. Young, "Ambulatory blood pressure and heart rate responses to the stress of work and caregiving in older women." *Journals of Gerontology,* 49: M239–M245, 1994.

84. B. Wellman and S. Wortley, "Different strokes from different folks: community ties and social support." *American Journal of Sociology,* 96: 558–588, 1990, pp. 583–584.

85. M. Granovetter, "The strength of weak ties: a network theory revisited." In R. Collins, ed., *Sociological Theory,* San Francisco: Jossey-Bass, 1983.

86. A. Portes and J. Sensenbrenner, "Embeddedness and immigration: notes on the social determinants of economic action." *American Journal of Sociology* 98: 1320–1350, 1993. A. Portes and P. Landolt, "The downside of social capital." *American Prospect* 26: 18–22, 1996. A. Portes, "Social capital: its origins and applications in modern sociology." *Annual Review of Sociology* 24: 1–24, 1998.

87. F. Hollinger and M. Haller, "Kinship and social networks in modern societies: a cross-cultural comparison among seven nations." *European Sociological Review,* 6: 103–124, 1990, p. 104. B. Wellman, "Which types of ties and networks provide what kinds of social support?" *Advances in Group Processes,* 9: 207–235, 1992.

88. M. Granovetter, "The strength of weak ties." *American Journal of Sociology* 78: 1360–1380, 1973.

89. W.J. Wilson, *The Truly Disadvantaged: The Inner City, the Underclass and Public Policy.* Chicago: The University of Chicago Press, 1987.

90. D.F. Aberle, "A Plan for Navajo Economic Development." In *Toward Economic Development for Native American Communities.* A compendium of papers submitted to the Sub-Committee on Economy in Government of the Joint Economic Committee of the Congress of the United States. Washington, D.C.: U.S. Government Printing Office, 1969, pp. 243–245. S.J. Kunitz, *Disease Change and the Role of Medicine: The Navajo Experience.* Berkeley: University of California Press, 1983, pp. 53–54.

91. Kunitz and Levy, *Navajo Aging,* op. cit.

92. S.J. Kunitz and M. Tsianco, "Kinship dependence and contraceptive use among Navajo women." *Human Biology,* 53: 439–452, 1981.

93. S. J. Kunitz and J.E.Levy, *Drinking Careers: A Twenty-five Year Follow-up of Three Navajo Populations.* New Haven: Yale University Press, 1994.

94. E.B. Henderson, S.J. Kunitz, and J.E. Levy, "The origins of Navajo youth gangs."

American Indian Culture and Research Journal, 23: 243–264, 1999. S.J. Kunitz and J.E. Levy *Drinking, Conduct Disorder, and Social Change: Navajo Experiences.* New York: Oxford University Press, 2000.

95. G.A. Kaplan, "People and places: contrasting perspectives on the association between social class and health." *International Journal of Health Services* 26: 507–519, 1996. M. Lindstrom, J. Merlo, and P-O Ostergren, "Social capital and sense of insecurity in the neighbourhood: a population-based multilevel analysis in Malmo, Sweden." *Social Science and Medicine* 56: 1111–1120, 2003. S.V. Subramanian, K.A. Lochner, and I. Kawachi, "Neighbourhood differences in social capital: a compositional artifact or a contextual construct?" *Health and Place* 9: 33–44, 2003. P. Martikainen, T.M. Kauppinen, and T. Valkonen, "Effects of the characterics of neighbourhood and the characteristics of people on cause specific mortality: a register based follow up study of 252,000 men." *Journal of Epidemiology and Community Health* 57: 210–217, 2003.

96. J.G. Bruhn and S. Wolf, *The Roseto Story: An Anatomy of Health.* Norman: University of Oklahoma Press, 1979. S. Wolf and J.G. Bruhn, *The Power of Clan: The Influence of Human Relationships on Heart Disease.* New Brunswick, N.J.: Transaction Publishers, 1993.

97. S. Wolf and J.G. Bruhn, *The Power of Clan,* p. 121.

98. Ibid., p. 91.

99. Ibid., p. 127.

100. C. Bianco, *The Two Rosetos.* Bloomington: Indiana University Press, 1974, p. 141.

101. C.L. Valletta, *A Study of Americanization in Carneta: Italian-American Identity through Three Generations.* New York: Arno Press, 1975.

102. Ibid., p. 151.

103. Ibid., p. 418.

104. Ibid., p. 405.

105. G. Foster, "Peasant society and the image of limited good." *American Anthropologist* 67: 293–315, 1965, p. 296. Italics in original.

106. Ibid., p. 301.

107. Ibid., p. 303.

108. J. Blum, "The European village as community: origins and functions." *Agricultural History* 45: 757–778, 1971.

109. P. Kutsche, "Introduction: atomism, factionalism and flexibility." In P. Kutsche, ed., *The Survival of Spanish American Villages.* Colorado College Studies, No. 15. The Colorado College, Colorado Springs, Colorado, 1979.

110. A. Keys, "Arteriosclerotic heart disease in Roseto, Pennsylvania." *Journal of the American Medical Association* 195: 137–139, 1966.

111. B. Egolf, J. Lasker, S. Wolf, and L. Potvin, "The Roseto effect: a 50-year comparison of mortality rates." *American Journal of Public Health* 82: 1089–1092, 1992. J.N. Lasker, B.P. Egolf, and S. Wolf, "Community social change and mortality." *Social Science and Medicine* 39: 53–62, 1994.

112. J. Lynch and G.D. Smith, "Rates and states: reflections on the health of nations." *International Journal of Epidemiology* 32: 663–670, 2003.

113. Valletta, *Carneta,* op. cit., p. 410.

114. J. Lynch and G.D. Smith, "Rates and states," op. cit., p. 668.

115. R. Nisbet, *The Sociological Tradition.* New York: Basic Books, 1966.

116. S. Berman, "Civil society and political institutionalism." *The American Behavioral Scientist* 40: 562–574, 1997, pp. 569–570.

117. Ibid., pp. 570–571.

118. C.D. Merrett, "Declining social capital and nonprofit organizations: consequences for small towns after welfare reform." *Urban Geography* 22: 407–423, 2001.

119. Fischer, *Albion's Seed,* op. cit.

120. S. Wolf and J.G. Bruhn, *The Power of Clan,* op. cit., p. 127.

121. I. Kawachi and L. Berkman, "Social cohesion, social capital, and health," op. cit. S. Szreter and M. Woolcock, "Health by association? Social capital, social theory, and the political economy of public health." *International Journal of Epidemiology* 33: 65–67, 2004. R.D. Putnam, *Bowling Alone,* op. cit., Chapter 22.

Chapter 6

1. G.B. Shaw, *John Bull's Other Island*. Collected Plays, Vol. II. New York: Dodd, Mead & Company, [1906] 1971, p. 914.

2. The use of this measure has been criticized by some but for my purposes is useful. For a justification, see B. Milanovic, "Can we discern the effect of globalization on income distribution? Evidence from household surveys." *The World Bank Economic Review* 19: 21–44, 2005, p. 26.

3. D. Held, A. McGrew, D. Goldblatt, and J. Perraton, *Global Transformations: Politics, Economics and Culture* Stanford, CA: Stanford University Press, 1999.

4. J. Mander, "Facing the rising tide." In J. Mander and E. Goldsmith, eds., *The Case against the Global Economy and for a Turn Toward the Local*. San Francisco: Sierra Club Books, 1996, pp. 3–5.

5. P. Bourdieu, *Firing Back: Against the Tyranny of the Market 2*. New York: The New Press, 2003, p. 68.

6. J. Mazur, "Labor's new internationalism." *Foreign Affairs* 79: 79–93, 2000.

7. S.A. Aaronson, *Taking Trade to the Streets: The Lost History of Public Efforts to Shape Globalization*. Ann Arbor: The University of Michigan Press, 2001, p. 135.

8. Ibid., p. 4.

9. P.J. Buchanan, *The Great Betrayal: How American Sovereignty and Social Justice are Being Sacrificed to the Gods of the Global Economy*. Boston: Little, Brown and Company, 1998, pp. 62–68.

10. P. Krugman, *Pop Internationalism*. Cambridge: MIT Press, 1997. D. Dollar and A. Kraay, "Spreading the wealth." *Foreign Affairs* 81: 120–133, 2002. J. Bhagwati, *In Defense of Globalization*. New York: Oxford University Press, 2004. M. Wolf, *Why Globalization Works*. New Haven: Yale University Press, 2004.

11. D. Dollar and A. Kray, "Growth is good for the poor." Policy Research Working Paper No. WPS 2587. Washington, D.C.: The World Bank, April, 2001. Also published in the *Journal of Economic Growth* 7: 195–225, 2002.

12. "Does inequality matter?" pp. 9–10, and Supplement "The new wealth of nations." *The Economist,* June 16, 2001.

13. "Globalisation and its critics: a survey of globalisation." Supplement to *The Economist*, September 29, 2001, p. 4.

14. Bhagwati, *In Defense of Globalization,* op. cit., p. 32.

15. D. Dollar, "Is globalization good for your health?" *Bulletin of the World Health Organization* 79: 827–833, 2001, pp. 829–830.

16. F. Fukuyama, "Bring back big government." *The Guardian Weekly* July 9–15, 2004, p. 3.

17. Wolf, *Why Globalization Works,* op. cit., p. 61.

18. For example, fearing passage of legislation in the United States that would ban imports of textiles made by child laborers, Bangladeshi employers "dismissed an estimated fifty thousand children from factories." Some of the girls turned to, or were forced by their parents into, prostitution. Bhagwati, *In Defense of Globalization*, op. cit., p. 71.

19. H.E. Daly and J.B. Cobb, Jr. *For the Common Good: Redirecting the Economy Toward Community, the Environment, and a Sustainable Future.* Boston: Beacon Press, 1989, pp. 8–9.

20. The idea of the nation as a community of communities is from Martin Buber. See P. Smith, *As a City Upon a Hill: The Town in American History*. New York: Alfred A. Knopf, 1966, p. 303.

21. I am grateful to Stanley Engerman for suggesting this distinction to me.

22. S.P. Huntington, "Dead souls: the denationalization of the American elite." *The National Interest*, Number 75, Spring, 2004, pp. 5–18, p. 5.

23. J.D. Hunter and J. Yates, "In the vanguard of globalization: the world of American globalizers." In P.L. Berger and S.P. Huntington, eds., *Many Globalizations: Cultural Diversity in the Contemporary World*. New York: Oxford University Press, 2002.

24. Ibid., p. 334.

25. Ibid., p. 337.

26. Ibid., pp. 338–339, emphasis in original.

27. Huntington, "Dead souls," op. cit., p. 7.

28. Quoted in Buchanan, *The Great Betrayal*, op. cit., p. 99.

29. *Quadragesimo Anno*. Encyclical of Pope Pius XI On Reconstruction of the Social Order. Given at Rome, at Saint Peter's, 15 May, 1931.

30. Buchanan, *The Great Betrayal*, p. 57.

31. W. Berry, "Conserving communities." In. Mander and Goldsmith, eds., *The Case Against the Global Economy*, op. cit., p. 412.

32. P. Temin, *Lessons from the Great Depression*. Cambridge: The MIT Press, 1989, p. 108.

33. Ibid., p. 111, emphasis in original.

34. Temin, *Lessons*, p. 111.

35. J.G. Ruggie, "Trade, protectionism and the future of welfare capitalism." *Journal of International Affairs* 48: 1–11, 1994, pp 4–5. See also J.G. Ruggie, "At home abroad, abroad at home: international liberalization and domestic stability in the new world economy." *Millennium: Journal of International Studies* 24: 507–526, 1994.

36. Ruggie, "Trade, protectionism and the future," and "At home abroad."

37. Ruggie, "Abroad at home," p. 512.

38. Ibid., pp. 513–515.

39. Ibid., p. 518.

40. Organisation for Economic Co-operation and Development, *Societal Cohesion and the Globalising Economy: What does the Future Hold?* Paris: Organisation for Economic Co-operation and Development, 1997. G. Esping-Andersen, "The sustainability of welfare states into the twenty-first century." *International Journal of Health Services* 30: 1–12, 2000. F.G. Castles, "The future of the welfare state: crisis myths and crisis realities." *International Journal of Health Services* 32: 255–277, 2002.

41. D.M Fox "Health policy and the politics of research in the United States." *Journal of Health Politics, Policy & Law*. 15: 481–499, 1990. E. Melhado, "Economists, public provision, and the market: changing values in policy debate." *Journal of Health Politics, Policy and Law* 23: 215–263, 1998.

42. R.E. Feinberg, "The adjustment imperative and U.S. policy." In R.E. Feinberg and V. Kallab, eds., *Adjustment Crisis in the Third World*. U.S.–Third World Policy Perspectives, No. 1, Overseas Development Council, Washington, D.C.. New Brunswick, N.J.: Transaction Books, 1984, pp. 3–4.

43. Ibid., p. 7.

44. J.E. Stiglitz, *The Roaring Nineties*. New York: W.W. Norton, 2003, p. 39.

45. S.J. Kunitz, "The making and breaking of Yugoslavia and its impact on health." *American Journal of Public Health* 94: 1894–1904, 2004.

46. G.A. Cornia, "Adjustment policies 1980–1985: effects on child welfare." In G.A. Cornia, R. Jolly, and F. Stewart, eds., *Adjustment with a Human Face: Protecting the Vulnerable and Promoting Growth, Vol. 1*. New York: Oxford University Press, 1987, p. 49.

47. C. Jayarajah, W. Branson, and B. Sen, *Social Dimensions of Adjustment: World Bank Experience, 1980–93*. Washington, D.C.: The World Bank, 1996.

48. This section is based upon S.J. Kunitz, "Explanations and ideologies of mortality patterns." *Population and Development Review* 13: 379–408, 1987.

49. F.L. Soper, "Eradication versus control in communicable disease prevention." *Journal of the American Veterinary Medical Association* 137: 234–238, 1960. Reprinted in J. A. Kerr, ed., *Building the Health Bridge: Selections from the Work of Fred L. Soper, M.D.* Bloomington: Indiana University Press, 1970, p. 334.

50. F.L. Soper, "Rehabilitation of the eradication concept in prevention of communicable disease." *Public Health Reports* 80: 855–869, 1965. Reprinted in J. A. Kerr, ed., *Building the Health Bridge*, p. 338.

51. A. Cockburn, ed., *Infectious Diseases: Their Evolution and Eradication*. Springfield, Illinois: Charles C. Thomas, 1967, p. 128.

52. R. Packard, "Visions of postwar health and development and their impact on public health interventions in the developing world." In F. Cooper and R. Packard, eds., *International Development and the Social Sciences: Essays on the History and Politics of Knowledge*. Berkeley: University of California Press, 1997, p. 111. T.M. Brown, M. Cueto, and E. Fee, "The World Health Organization and the transition from international to global public health." *American Journal of Public Health* 96: 62–72, 2006.

53. It was in this same context that vertically organized family planning programs were also advocated by demographers and development specialists. See J. Sharpless, "World population growth, family planning, and American foreign policy." In D.T. Crichlow, ed., *The Politics of Abortion and Birth Control in Historical Perspective*. University Park, PA: The Pennsylvania State University Press, 1995.

54. J. Bryant, *Health and the Developing World*. Ithaca: Cornell University Press, 1969, pp. 96–98.

55. R. Packard, "Visions of postwar health and development," op. cit., p. 98.

56. J.E. Gordon, "The twentieth century—yesterday, today, and tomorrow (1920–)." In F.H. Top, ed., *The History of American Epidemiology*. St. Louis: C.V. Mosby, 1952, p. 118.

57. N.S. Scrimshaw, C.E. Taylor, and J.E. Gordon, *Interactions of Nutrition and Infection*. Geneva: World Health Organization, 1986.

58. W. McDermott, "Modern medicine and the demographic–disease pattern of overly traditional societies: a technologic misfit." In H. van Zile Hyde, ed., *Manpower for the World's Health*. Evanston, Ill: Association of American Medical Colleges, 1966.

59. K. Lee and A. Mills, "Developing countries, health, and health economics." In K. Lee and A. Mills, eds., *The Economics of Health in Developing Countries*. Oxford: Oxford University Press, 1983.

60. N.S. Scrimshaw, C.E. Taylor, and J.E. Gordon, *Interactions of Nutrition and Infection*, op. cit., p. 13. See also C. Taylor, "Health and population," *Foreign Affairs* (April) 475–486, 1965. C. Taylor and M-F. Hall, "Health, population, and economic development," *Science* 157: 651–657, 1967. N.S. Scrimshaw, "Myths and realities in international health planning," *American Journal of Public Health,* 64: 792–798, 1974.

61. S. Litsios, "The long and difficult road to Alma-Ata: a personal reflection." *International Journal of Health Services* 32: 709–732, 2002. S. Litsios, "The Christian Medical Commission and the development of the World Health Organization's primary health care approach." *American Journal of Public Health* 94: 1884–1893, 2004. M. Cueto, "The origins of primary health care and selective primary health care." *American Journal of Public Health* 94: 1864–1874, 2004.

62. V. Djukanovic and E.P. Mach, eds., *Alternative Approaches to Meeting Basic Health Needs in Developing Countries.* Geneva: World Health Organization, 1975, p. 7.

63. World Health Organization (WHO)-United Nations Children's Fund (UNICEF), *Report of the International Conference on Primary Health Care, Alma-Ata, USSR, 6–12 September 1978.* Geneva: World Health Organization, 1978.

64. Ibid., p. 17.

65. R. Packard, "Visions of postwar health and development," op. cit., p. 111.

66. J.A. Walsh and K.S. Warren, "Selective primary health care." *New England Journal of Medicine,* 301: 967–974, 1979, p. 967.

67. Ibid., p. 972.

68. S.B. Halstead, J.A. Walsh, and K.S. Warren, eds., *Good Health at Low Cost.* New York: The Rockefeller Foundation, 1985. See also J.C. Caldwell, "Routes to low mortality in poor countries." *Population and Development Review,* 12: 171–220, 1986.

69. Ibid., p. 246.

70. P.A. Berman, "Selective primary health care: is efficient sufficient?" *Social Science and Medicine* 16: 1054–1059, 1982. O. Gish, "Selective primary health care: old wine in new bottles." *Social Science and Medicine* 16: 1049–1063, 1982. J.-P. Unger and J.R. Killingworth, "Selective primary health care: a critical review of methods and results." *Social Science and Medicine* 22: 1001–1013, 1986.

71. W.H. Mosley, "Will primary health care reduce infant and child mortality? A critique of some current strategies with special reference to Asia and Africa." Seminar on Social Policy, Health Policy and Mortality Prospects, Paris, 28 February–4 March, 1983. Paris: Institut National d'Etudes Demographiques (INED), p. 5.

72. Ibid., p. 7.

73. World Bank, *World Development Report 1993: Investing in Health.* New York: Oxford University Press, 1993.

74. Ibid., pp. 7–8.

75. Ibid., p. 8.

76. Ibid., pp. 9–10.

77. Ibid., p. 119.

78. Report of the Commission on Macroeconomics and Health, Jeffrey D. Sachs, Chair. *Macroeconomics and Health: Investing in Health for Economic Development.* Geneva: World Health Organization, 2001.

79. D. Werner and D. Sanders, *Questioning the Solution: The Politics of Primary Health Care and Child Survival.* Palo Alto, CA: Healthwrights, 1997. M. Turshen, *Privatizing Health Services in Africa.* New Brunswick, N.J.: Rutgers University Press, 1999. K. Stocker, H. Waitzkin, and C. Iriart, "The exportation of managed care to Latin

America." *The New England Journal of Medicine* 340: 1131–1136, 1999. N. Homedes and A. Ugalde, "Why neoliberal health reforms have failed in Latin America." *Health Policy* 30: 1–14, 2004. H. Waitzkin, "Report of the WHO Commission on Macroeconomics and Health: a summary and critique." *The Lancet* 361: 523–526, 2003. C. Thomas and M. Weber, "The politics of global health governance: whatever happened to 'Health for All by the Year 2000'?" *Global Governance* 10: 187–205, 2004. M. Rao, ed., *Disinvesting in Health: The World Bank's Prescriptions for Health.* New Delhi: Sage Publications, 1999.

80. World Bank, *World Development Report 1993*, op. cit.

81. M. Rao, "Introduction." In M. Rao, ed., *Disinvesting in Health,* op. cit., p. 13.

82. Ibid., p. 20.

83. S.A. Aaronson, *Taking Trade to the Streets*, op. cit.

84. K. Stocker, H. Waitzkin, and C. Iriart, "The exportation of managed care to Latin America," op. cit. D. Price, A.M. Pollock, and J. Shaoul, "How the World Trade Organisation is shaping domestic policies in health care." *The Lancet* 354: 1889–1892, 1999. A.M. Pollock and D. Price, "Rewriting the regulations: how the World Trade Organisation could accelerate privatization in health-care systems." *The Lancet* 356: 1995–2000, 2000. D.J. Lipson, "The World Trade Organization's health agenda." *British Medical Journal* 323: 1139–1140, 2001.

85. J. Orbinski, "Health, equity, and trade: a failure in global governance." In G.P. Sampson, ed., *The Role of the World Trade Organization in Global Governance.* Tokyo: United Nations University Press, 2001. P. Cullett, "Patents and medicines: the relationship between TRIPS and the human right to health." *International Affairs* 79: 139–160, 2003. E. Hong, *Globalisation and the Impact on Health: A Third World View.* Penang: Third World Network, http://www.twnside.org.sg. Prepared for The Peoples' Health Assembly, December 4–8, 2000, Savar, Bangladesh.

86. R.G.A. Feachem, "Globalisation is good for your health, mostly." *British Medical Journal* 323: 504–506, 2001, p. 505. I have made a similar argument in S.J. Kunitz, "Globalization, states, and the health of indigenous peoples." *American Journal of Public Health*, 90: 1531–1539, 2000.

87. Feachem, "Globalisation is good," p. 505.

88. D. Dollar and A. Kray, "Trade, growth, and poverty." *The Economic Journal* 114: F22–F49, 2004.

89. Dollar and Kray, "Growth *is* good for the poor," op. cit. Dollar, "Is globalization good for your health?" op. cit. Dollar and Kraay, "Spreading the wealth," op. cit.

90. B. Milanovic, "Can we discern the effect of globalization on income distribution?" op. cit.

91. L. Pritchett and L.H. Summers, "Wealthier is healthier." *The Journal of Human Resources* 31: 841–68, 1996. D. Filmer and L. Pritchett, "Child mortality and public spending on health: how much does money matter." The World Bank, Washington, D.C. October 17, 1997.

92. C. Hippert, "Multinational corporations, the politics of the world economy, and their effects on women's health in the developing world: a review." *Health Care for Women International* 23: 861–869, 2002. A.M. Jaggar, "Vulnerable women and neoliberal globalization: debt burdens undermine women's health in the global South." *Theoretical Medicine* 23: 425–440, 2002.

93. S. Amin, I. Diamond, R.T. Naved, and M. Newby, "Transition to adulthood of female garment-factory workers in Bangladesh." *Studies in Family Planning* 29: 185–200, 1998.

94. Ibid., p. 199.

95. R.E. Feinberg, "The adjustment imperative and U.S. policy." In R.E. Feinberg and V. Kallab, eds., *Adjustment Crisis in the Third World*. U.S.–Third World Policy Perspectives, No. 1, Overseas Development Council, Washington, D.C. New Brunswick: Transaction Books, pp. 3–4.

96. G. Tapinos, A. Mason, J. Bravo, eds., *Demographic Responses to Economic Adjustment in Latin America*. Oxford: Oxford University Press, 1997.

97. A. Palloni and K. Hill, "The effects of economic changes on mortality by age and cause: Latin America, 1950–90." In Tapinos et al., eds., *Demographic Response*.

98. F. Abdala, R.N. Geldstein, and S.M. Mychaszula, "Economic restructuring and mortality changes in Argentina: is their any connection?" In G.A. Cornia and R. Paniccia, eds., *The Mortality Crisis in Transition Economies*. Oxford: Oxford University Press, 2000, p. 347.

99. F. Diop, K. Hill, and I. Sirageldin, *Economic Crisis, Structural Adjustment, and Health in Africa*. Working Paper 766, Population and Human Resources Department, The World Bank, Washington, D.C., September, 1991.

100. R. Sell and S.J. Kunitz, "The debt crisis and the end of an era in mortality", *Studies in Comparative International Development*, 21: 3–30, 1986–1987.

101. S.J. Kunitz, S. Simic, and C.L. Odoroff, "Infant mortality and economic instability in Yugoslavia," *Social Science and Medicine*, 24: 953–960, 1987. S.J. Kunitz, "The making and breaking of federated Yugoslavia, and its impact on health." *American Journal of Public Health*, 94: 1894–1904, 2004. Mortality increased in the Soviet Union before it collapsed, but the situation worsened very substantially afterwards.

102. G.A. Cornia, "Globalization and health: results and options." *Bulletin of the World Health Organization* 79: 834–841, 2001, p. 839.

103. G.A. Cornia and R. Paniccia, "The transition mortality crisis: evidence, interpretation and policy responses." In G.A. Cornia and R. Paniccia, eds., *The Mortality Crisis in Transition Economies*, op. cit., pp. 5–7.

104. P. Desai, *Financial Crisis, Contagion, and Containment: From Asia to Argentina*. Princeton: Princeton University Press, 2003, p. 1.

105. L.A. Cameron, *The Impact of the Indonesian Financial Crisis on Children: Data from 100 Villages Survey*. Department of Economics, University of Melbourne, Parkville, Victoria, Australia, March, 2002.

106. S.A. Block, L. Kiess, P. Webb, S. Kosen, R. Moench-Pfanner, M.W. Bloem, and C.P. Timmer, "Macro shocks and micro outcomes: child nutrition during Indonesia's crisis." *Economics and Human Biology* 2: 21–44, 2004.

107. Cornia, "Globalization and health," op. cit., p. 839.

108. The World Bank, *World Development Indicators 2002*. CD-ROM. Washington, D.C.: The International Bank for Reconstruction and Development, 2002. The results are essentially the same, though IMR estimates often differ widely, using infant mortality rates for 1990, 1995, and 2000 as reported in the United Nations *Statistical Yearbook, Forty-seventh issue, CD-ROM* (ST/ESA/STAT/SER.S/CD/23). New York: Statistics Division, Department of Economic and Social Affairs, The United Nations.

109. Cornia, "Globalization and health," p. 836.

110. Ibid., pp. 834–835. See also T. Collins, "Globalization, global health, and access to healthcare." *International Journal of Health Planning and Management* 18: 97–104, 2003.

111. The World Bank, *World Development Indicators 2002*. CD-ROM. Washington, D.C.: The International Bank for Reconstruction and Development, 2002.

112. P.J. Katzenstein, *Small States in World Markets: Industrial Policy in Europe.* Ithaca: Cornell University Press, 1985.

113. Openness is measured as Exports + Imports as percent of GDP. A log transformation of population size was used.

114. Population in 1980 was significantly correlated with the percent change in openness between 1980 and 2000 (r = 0.28, p = 0.0016).

115. The correlation between percent change in openness and percent change in GDP per capita 1980–2000 is 0.35, p = 0.0002, N = 105.

116. L. Pritchett and L.H. Summers, "Wealthier is healthier." *The Journal of Human Resources* 31: 841–868, 1996.

117. R = −0.50, p <0.0001, N = 133.

118. Percent change in infant mortality 1980–2000 regressed onto change in openness and GDP 1980–2000 and GDP/capita in 1980.

Term	Estimate	Standard Error	T-ratio	p
Intercept	−75.4816	9.0609	−8.33	<0.0001
% change openness	−0.1715	0.1532	−1.12	0.2658
% change GDP/cap	−0.2207	0.1234	−1.79	0.0769
GDP/cap 1980	−0.0035	0.0010	−3.29	0.0014

N = 100

119. R = −0.22, p = 0.0284, N = 92.

120. R = 0.37, p = 0.0003, N = 84.

121. Dollar and Kraay considered several categories of globalizers: those that primarily reduced tariffs, those that increased their imports and exports, and those that did both. Table 8-1 combines all three types into one category. In similar analyses with the three types considered separately, the numbers in each category become quite small, but again there is no difference in mortality rates and life expectancy among them.

122. D.T. Jamison, M.D. Sandbu, and J. Want, "Why has infant mortality decreased at such different rates in different countries?" Working Paper No. 21, Disease Control Priorities Project. Bethesda, MD: National Institutes of Health, Feb. 6, 2004. A. Case and A. Deaton, "Health and wealth among the poor: India and South Africa compared." Research Program in Development Studies and Center for Health and Wellbeing. Princeton, N.J.: Princeton University, April, 2005.

123. R = −0.56, p = 0.0131, N = 18.

124. Cornia, "Globalization and health," op. cit., pp. 834–835.

125. E. Huber and J.D. Stephens, *Development and Crisis of the Welfare State: Parties and Policies in Global Markets.* Chicago: University of Chicago Press, 2001, pp. 228–229. The countries are classified as follows. Social Democratic welfare states: Sweden, Norway, Denmark, Finland. Christian Democratic welfare states: Austria, Belgium, Netherlands, Germany, France, Italy, Switzerland. Liberal welfare states: Canada, Ireland, United Kingdom, United States. Wage earner welfare states: Australia and New Zealand. The trade and spending data are from 1990–1994. Life expectancy and infant mortality are for 1995 and are from the *World Development Report 2002*.

126. Alberto Alesina and Edward Glaeser observe in their study of the United States and European welfare states that openness is not associated with the size of the welfare state when political variables are controlled. A. Alesina and E.L. Glaeser, *Fighting*

Poverty in the US and Europe: A World of Difference. Oxford: Oxford University Press, 2004, pp. 85–86. A study of wealthy industrialized countries also indicates that trade openness is not associated with infant mortality rates and is inversely correlated with income inequality as measured by the Gini coefficient. See J.A. Macinko, L. Shi, and B.Starfield, "Wage inequality, the health system, and infant mortality in wealthy industrialized countries, 1970–1996." *Social Science and Medicine* 58: 279–292, 2004. This same study showed that the funding and organization of health care systems attenuated the association between income inequality and infant mortality.

127. The World Bank, *World Development Indicators 2002*, op. cit.

128. M. Ramesh and I. Holliday, "The health care miracle in East and Southeast Asia: activist state provision in Hong Kong, Malaysia and Singapore." *Journal of Social Policy* 30: 637–651, 2001.

129. Ibid., p. 640.

130. Ibid., p. 644.

131. Ibid., p. 645.

132. L. Taylor, "Outcomes of external liberalization and policy implications." In L. Taylor, ed., *External Liberalization, Economic Performance, and Social Policy.* New York: Oxford University Press, 2001.

133. The World Bank includes estimates of GDP per capita for Russia from 1980 but not for Cuba. The U.N. provides estimates for Cuba from 1980 and for Russia from 1990. Using the U.N. data, Cuba had GDP per capita that was roughly the same as was estimated for Colombia. The estimates for Cuban GDP are displayed in Figure 8-4.

134. L. Taylor, "Outcomes of external liberalization and policy implications," pp. 7–8.

135. Ibid., p. 9.

136. The data are from The World Bank, *World Development Indicators 2002*, op. cit. Results using estimates from the United Nations are similar.

137. As a result of the American military occupation of Cuba during the war with Spain in 1898, there was a substantial decline in mortality due to the sanitary improvements made by the U.S. Army. During the first half of the twentieth century, life expectancy in Cuba was better than in Brazil, Guatemala, and Mexico, worse than in Argentina, and roughly comparable to Chile and Costa Rica. See S. Diaz-Briquets, *The Health Revolution in Cuba.* Austin: The University of Texas Press, 1983, pp. 119–121.

138. For recent reviews, see A. Chomsky, " 'The threat of a good example': health and revolution in Cuba." In J.Y. Kim, J.V. Millen, A. Irwin, and J. Gershman, eds., *Dying for Growth: Global Inequality and the Health of the Poor.* Monroe, Maine: Common Courage Press, 2000. J.M. Spiegel and A. Yassi, "Lessons from the margins of globalization: appreciating the Cuban health paradox." *Journal of Public Health Policy* 25: 85–110, 2004.

139. A.F. Muruaga, "Cuba: external opening, labor market and inequality of labor incomes." In L. Taylor, ed., *External Liberalization, Economic Performance, and Social Policy.* New York: Oxford University Press, 2001.

140. United Nations *Statistical Yearbook, Forty-seventh issue, CD-ROM* (ST/ESA/STAT/SER.S/CD/23). New York: Statistics Division, Department of Economic and Social Affairs, The United Nations.

141. J.C. Caldwell, "Routes to low mortality in poor countries," op. cit.

142. Inter-American Development Bank, *Facing up to Inequality in Latin America.* Economic and Social Progress in Latin America, 1998–1999 Report. Washington, D.C.: Inter-American Development Bank, 1998, p. 25.

143. The World Bank, *World Development Indicators 2002*, op. cit. Because of differences

in data collection, these figures should only be regarded as indicative of the magnitude of differences and similarities among nations.

144. The following section is adapted from S.J. Kunitz, "The making and breaking of Yugoslavia and its impact on health." *American Journal of Public Health* 94: 1894–1904, 2004.

145. A.R. Johnson, *The Transformation of Communist Ideology: The Yugoslav Case, 1945–1953*. Cambridge: MIT Press, 1972.

146. B. Denitch, *The Legitimation of a Revolution*. New Haven: Yale University Press, 1976. R. Supek, "Problems and perspectives of workers' self-management in Yugoslavia," in M.J. Broekmeyer, ed., *Yugoslav Workers' Self-Management*. Dordrecht: D. Reidel Publishing Company, 1970.

147. *Statistical Yearbook of Yugoslavia*, Vols. 27 and 31, Beograd: Savezni Zavod za Statistiku, 1980 and 1984.

148. J. Stiglitz, *The Roaring Nineties*. New York: W.W. Norton, 2003, p. 39.

149. The World Bank, *Yugoslavia: Adjustment Policies and Development Perspectives*. Washington, D.C.: The International Bank for Reconstruction and Development/ World Bank, 1983.

150. Much of the detail provided in these paragraphs is from S.J. Kunitz, S. Simic, and C.L. Odoroff, "Infant mortality and economic instability in Yugoslavia," *Social Science and Medicine* 24: 953–960, 1987. The data on inflation during the decades 1970–1980 and 1979–1989 are from The World Bank, *World Development Report: Investing in Health*. New York: Oxford University Press, 1993. The figures for the end of the decade are from S.P. Ramet, *Nationalism and Federalism in Yugoslavia, 1962–1991*. Bloomington: Indiana University Press, 1992, p. 239. See also J.R. Lampe, *Yugoslavia as History: Twice There was a Nation*, 2nd ed. Cambridge: Cambridge University Press, 2000.

151. V. Vugacic and V. Zaslavsky, "The causes of disintegration in the USSR and Yugoslavia," *Telos* 88: 120–140, 1991.

152. R. Brubaker, *Nationalism Reframed: Nationhood and the National Question in the New Europe*. Cambridge: Cambridge University Press, 1996.

153. For useful histories of this period, see the following: B. Denitch, *Limits and Possibilities: The Crisis of Yugoslav Socialism and State Socialist Systems*. Minneapolis: University of Minnesota Press, 1990; B. Denitch, *Ethnic Nationalism: The Tragic Death of Yugoslavia*. Minneapolis: University of Minnesota Press, 1994; M. Glenny, *The Fall of Yugoslavia: The Third Balkan War*. New York: Penguin Books, 1992.

154. The following several paragraphs are adapted from S.J. Kunitz, "Mortality of White Americans, African Americans, and Canadians: the causes and consequences for health of welfare state institutions and policies." *The Milbank Quarterly* 83: 5–39, 2005.

155. S.P. Huntington, "Political modernization: America vs. Europe." *World Politics* 18: 378–414, 1966, p. 397.

156. Ibid., p. 396.

157. A. Maioni, *Parting at the Crossroads*. Princeton: Princeton University Press, 1998, p. 23.

158. Ibid., p. 24.

159. J. Quadagno, *The Color of Welfare: How Racism Undermined the War on Poverty*. New York: Oxford University Press, 1994.

160. J. Quadagno, *The Color of Welfare*, p. 21. R.C. Lieberman, *Shifting the Color Line: Race and the American Welfare State*. Cambridge: Harvard University Press, 1998.

161. Ibid., p. 23.

162. Ibid.

163. M. Oliver, and T. Shapiro, *Black Wealth/White Wealth: A New Perspective on Racial Inequality*. New York: Routledge, 1995. T.M. Shapiro, *The Hidden Cost of Being African American: How Wealth Perpetuates Inequality*. New York: Oxford University Press, 2004.

164. I. Katznelson, K. Geiger, and D. Kryder, "Limiting liberalism: the southern veto in Congress, 1933–1950." *Political Science Quarterly* 108: 283–306, 1993, p. 297.

165. In the first decades of the twentieth century, for instance, 79% of white women in rural Mississippi had their deliveries done by a physician, compared to only 8% of African American women. A third of white women but only 12% of African American women had some prenatal care. Similar patterns were found elsewhere in the rural South. And despite major changes, even by the last decade of the twentieth century, among regions of the United States, income inequality was greatest and spending on libraries, schools, hospitals, Medicaid programs, and other services was least in the South. D. C. Ewbank, "History of Black mortality and health before 1940." In D.P. Willis, ed., *Health Policies and Black Americans*. New Brunswick: Transaction Publishers, 1994, p. 123. R.J. Blendon, L.H. Aiken, H.E. Freeman, and C.R. Corey, "Access to medical care for black and white Americans," *Journal of the American Medical Association* 261: 278–281, 1989, p. 280. G.A. Kaplan, E.R. Pamuk, J.W. Lynch, R.D. Cohen, and J.L. Balfour, "Inequality in income and mortality in the United States: analysis of mortality and potential pathways." *British Medical Journal* 312: 999–1003, 1996.

166. D. Rusk, *Cities Without Suburbs*. Washington, D.C.: Woodrow Wilson Center Press, 1993.

167. For instance, such towns often refuse to allow low-cost housing, while the inner cities have welcomed such projects as a way to replace decayed housing stock. Mandated minimum lot and house sizes also make it difficult for poor people to acquire homes in these communities. Legal enforcement of fair housing practices is difficult, for individuals must bear the costs of lawsuits.

168. D.G. Whiteis, "Third world medicine in first world cities: capital accumulation, uneven development and public health." *Social Science & Medicine* 47: 795–808, 1998.

169. R.J. Blendon, L.H. Aiken, H.E. Freeman, and C.R. Corey, "Access to medical care for black and white Americans", op. cit.. J. Hadley, E.P. Steinberg, and J. Feder, "Comparison of uninsured and privately insured hospital patients: condition on admission, resource use, and outcome." *Journal of the American Medical Association* 265: 374–379, 1991. D.W. Baker, J.J. Sudano, J.M. Albert, E.A. Borawski, and A. Dor, "Loss of health insurance and the risk for a decline in self-reported health and physical functioning." *Medical Care* 40: 1126–1131, 2002.

170. W.J. Wilson, *The Truly Disadvantaged: the Inner City, the Underclass and Public Policy*. Chicago: The University of Chicago Press, 1987.

171. Maioni, *Parting*, J.S. Hacker, "The historical logic of national health insurance: structure and sequence in the development of British, Canadian and U.S. medical policy." *Studies in American Political Development* 12: 57–130, 1998.

172. S.M. Lipset and G. Marks, *It Didn"t Happen Here: Why Socialism Failed in the United States*. New York: W.W. Norton, 2000, pp. 79–81. W. Sombart, *Why Is There No Socialism in the United States?* London: Macmillan, 1976. H.G. Gutman, *Work, Culture, and Society in Industrializing America*. New York: Alfred A. Knopf, 1976.

173. Lipset and Marks, *It Didn"t Happen Here*, pp. 79–81.

174. S.M. Lipset, *Continental Divide: The Values and Institutions of the United States and Canada*. New York: Routledge, 1990, p. 225. A.J. Hall, *The American Empire and the Fourth World*. Montreal and Kingston: McGill-Queens University Press, 2003.

175. In the case of English Canada, the development of socialism was also encouraged by the immigration of British socialists, who were not foreign in their new country as European socialists were alleged to be foreign in the United States. G. Horowitz, *Canadian Labour in Politics.* Toronto: University of Toronto Press, 1968, Chap. 1. That Canadian society has remained more hierarchical—more "English," in fact—than American is widely agreed. There is no agreement concerning the causes. See, for instance, D. Harrison, *The Limits of Liberalism: The Making of Canadian Sociology.* Montreal: Black Rose Books 1981.

176. J. Myles, "When markets fail: social welfare in Canada and the United States." In G. Esping-Andersen, ed., *Welfare States in Transition: National Adaptations in Global Economies.* London: Sage Publcations,1996, p. 128.

177. Quoted in Lipset, *Continental Divide,* op. cit., p. 173.

178. Lipset, *Continental Divide,* p. 197.

179. R.T. Kuderle and T.R. Marmor, "The development of welfare states in North America." In P. Flora and A.J. Heidenheimer, eds., *The Development of Welfare States in Europe and America.* New Brunswick, N.J.: Transaction Books, 1982, p. 112.

180. Ibid., p. 89.

181. M.J. Brodie and J. Jenson, *Crisis, Challenge and Change: Party and Class in Canada.* Toronto: Methuen, 1980. Kuderle and Marmor, "The development of welfare states," p. 111.

182. S.M. Lipset, *Agrarian Socialism.* Berkeley: University of California Press, 1950. F.B. Roth, G.W. Meyers, F.D. Mott, and L.S. Rosenfield, "The Saskatchewan experience in payment for hospital care," *American Journal of Public Health* 43: 752–756, 1953. R.F. Badgley and S. Wolfe, *Doctors' Strike: Medical Care and Conflict in Saskatchewan.* Toronto: Macmillan of Canada, 1967.

183. J. Porter, *The Vertical Mosaic.* Toronto: University of Toronto Press, 1965, p. 378. M.G. Taylor, *Health Insurance and Canadian Public Policy: The Seven Decisions That Created the Canadian Health Insurance System.* Montreal: McGill-Queens University Press, 1978. G. Gray, *Federalism and Health Policy: The Development of Health Systems in Canada and Australia.* Toronto: University of Toronto Press, 1991. Hacker, "The historical logic of national health insurance," op. cit.

184. Opposition from the Canadian Medical Association, though very stiff, never reached the level of invective or red-baiting achieved by the American Medical Association in its opposition to any form of government support of health insurance from the 1930s through the 1960s. C.D. Naylor, *Private Practice, Public Payment: Canadian Medicine and the Politics of Health Insurance 1911–1966.* Montreal: McGill-Queens University Press, 1986, p. 252.

185. G. Esping-Andersen, "The sustainability of welfare states into the twenty-first century." *International Journal of Health Services* 30: 1–12, 2000.

186. A. Alesina and E.L. Glaeser, *Fighting Poverty in the US and Europe: A World of Difference.* New York: Oxford University Press, 2004, pp. 136–146.

187. W. Lutz, B.C. O'Neill, and S. Scherbov, "Europe's population at a turning point." *Science* 299: 1991–1992, 2003.

Chapter 7

1. W.B. Yeats, *The Collected Poems of W.B. Yeats.* New York: Macmillan, 1957.

2. Robert Gall, as quoted in A. Mosley, "Does HIV or poverty cause AIDS? Biomedical and epidemiological perspectives." *Theoretical Medicine* 25: 399–421, 2004, p. 406.

3. L. Thomas, "Science and health—possibilities, probabilities, and limitations." *Social Research* 55: 379–395, 1988, pp. 381–382.

4. P.A. Treichler, "AIDS, gender, and biomedical discourse: current contests for meaning." In E. Fee and D.M. Fox, eds., *AIDS and the Burdens of History*. Berkeley: University of California Press, 1988. W.E. Marshall, "AIDS, race and the limits of science." *Social Science and Medicine* 60: 2515–2525, 2005.

5. I. Woffers, "Biomedical and development paradigms in AIDS prevention." *Bulletin of the World Health Organization* 78: 267–271, 2000.

6. E. Kalipeni, "Health and disease in southern Africa: a comparative and vulnerability perspective." *Social Science and Medicine* 50: 965–983, 2000. S.M. Kawewe and R. Dibie, "The impact of economic structural adjustment programs [ESAPs] on women and children: implications for social welfare in Zimbabwe." *Journal of Social Work and Social Welfare* 27: 79–107, 2000. L. Gilbert and L. Walker, "Treading the path of least resistance: HIV/AIDS and social inequalities—a South African case study." *Social Science and Medicine* 54: 1095–1110, 2002.

7. D. Fassin and H. Schneider, "The politics of AIDS in South Africa: beyond the controversies." *British Medical Journal* 326: 495–497, 2003. See also C. Butler, "HIV and AIDS, poverty and causation." *The Lancet* 356: 1445–1446, 2000; N. O'Farrell, "Poverty and HIV in sub-Saharan Africa." *The Lancet* 357: 636–637, 2001; and S. Basu, K. Mate, and P.E. Farmer, "Debt and poverty turn a disease into an epidemic." *Nature* 407: 13, 2000.

8. For example, P. Duesberg, "Retroviruses as carcinogens and pathogens: expectations and reality." *Cancer Research* 47: 1199–1220, 1987, and "HIV is not the cause of AIDS." *Science* 241: 514, 1988.

9. A. Mosley, "Does HIV or poverty cause AIDS? Biomedical and epidemiological perspectives." *Theoretical Medicine* 25: 399–421, 2004.

10. T. McKeown, *The Role of Medicine: Dream, Mirage or Nemesis?* Oxford: Basil Blackwell, 1979.

11. N.L. Letvin, "Progress towards an HIV vaccine." *Annual Review of Medicine* 56: 213–223, 2005.

12. S. Lindenbaum, "Knowledge and action in the shadow of AIDS." In G. Herdt and S. Lindenbaum, eds., *The Time of AIDS: Social Analysis, Theory, and Method*. Newbury Park, CA: Sage Publications, 1992, p. 325.

13. A. Quinton, "Plagues and morality." *Social Research* 55: 477–489, 1988, pp. 485–486.

14. M. Fumento, "The political uses of an epidemic." *The New Republic* August 8 & 15, 1988, pp. 19–23.

15. S. Basu, "AIDS, empire, and public health behaviourism." *International Journal of Health Services* 34: 155–167, 2004.

16. W.E. Marshall, "AIDS, race and the limits of science," op. cit., p. 2518.

17. P.W. Setel, *A Plague of Paradoxes: AIDS, Culture, and Demography in Northern Tanzania*. Chicago: The University of Chicago Press, 1999, p. 203.

18. In addition to the contextual features outlined above, John C. Caldwell and his coauthors have argued that there is "a distinct and internally coherent African pattern embracing sexuality, marriage and much else, and that it is no more right or wrong, progressive or unprogressive than the western model," and, they say, denying the difference will impede, not enhance, understanding of ways to intervene in the epidemic. The pattern they describe is broadly different from the so-called Eurasian model that, they continue (based upon the work of anthropologist Jack Goody), derives from a very different ecology and adaptation to it. In the African system, the lineage and reproduction

were paramount and sexual abstinence and virginity of brides did not have the same high value that it had in Eurasian countries. J.C. Caldwell, P. Caldwell, and P. Quiggan, *Disaster in an Alternative Civilization: The Social Dimension of AIDS in Sub-Saharan Africa.* Working paper No. 2, National Centre for Epidemiology and Population Health, Health Transition Centre, The Australian National University, Canberra, 1989, p. 2. See also J.C. Caldwell, P. Caldwell, and P. Quiggan, "The social context of AIDS in Sub-Saharan Africa." *Population and Development Review* 15: 185–234, 1989 and "The African sexual system: reply to Le Blanc et al." *Population and Development Review* 17: 506–515, 1991. See also A. Larson, "Social context of human immunodeficiency virus transmission in Africa: historical and cultural bases of East and Central African sexual relations." *Reviews of Infectious Diseases* 11: 716–731, 1989. J.C. Caldwell, "Rethinking the African AIDS epidemic." *Population and Development Review* 26: 117–135, 2000.

19. H. Dilger, "Sexuality, AIDS, and the lures of modernity: reflexivity and morality among young people in rural Tanzania." *Medical Anthropology* 22: 23–52, 2003.

20. B.G. Schoepf, "Women at risk: case studies from Zaire." In G. Herdt and S. Lindenbaum, eds., *The Time of AIDS: Social Analysis, Theory, and Method.* Newbury Park, CA: Sage Publications, 1992. P. Farmer, *Infections and Inequalities: The Modern Plagues.* Berkeley: University of California Press, 1999.

21. M. Ainsworth and M. Over, "AIDS and African development." *The World Bank Research Observer.* 9: 203–241, 1994.

22. World Bank, *Confronting AIDS: Public Priorities in a Global Epidemic.* New York: Oxford University Press, 1997, Tables 3.2 and 3.3.

23. B.G. Schoepf, "Women at risk: case studies from Zaire," op. cit., p. 272.

24. L. Garrett, "Gaps between rich and poor." EMBO Reports 4: S15-S19, 2003.

25. S. Basu, "AIDS, empire, and public health behaviourism," op. cit.

26. L. Garrett, "The Lessons of HIV/AIDS." *Foreign Affairs* 84: 51–64, 2005.

27. World Bank, *Confronting AIDS,* op. cit., Figures 1-7a and 1-7b.

28. A.S. Klovdahl, "Social networks and the spread of infectious diseases: the AIDS example." *Social Science and Medicine* 21: 1203–1216, 1985. S. Fergus, M.A. Lewis, L.A. Darbes, and R.M. Butterfield, "HIV risk and protection among gay male couples: the role of gay community integration." *Health Education & Behavior* 32: 151–171, 2005.

29. C. Perrow and M.F. Guillen, *The AIDS Disaster: The Failure of Organizations in New York and the Nation.* New Haven: Yale University Press, 1990.

30. R.G. Wight, C.S. Aneshensel, and A.J. LeBlanc, "Stress buffering effects of family support in AIDS caregiving." *AIDS Care* 15: 595–613, 2003. K.E. Stewart, L.R. Cianfrini, and J.F. Walker, "Stress, social support and housing are related to health status among HIV-positive persons in the Deep South of the United States." *AIDS Care* 17: 350–358, 2005.

31. K.E. Mosack, M. Abbott, M. Singer, M.R. Weeks, and L. Rohena, "If I didn't have HIV, I'd be dead now: illness narratives of drug users living with HIV/AIDS." *Qualitative Health Research* 15: 586–605, 2005.

32. T. Barnett and A. Whiteside, *AIDS in the Twenty-First Century: Disease and Globalization.* London: Macmillan Palgrave, 2002, p. 94.

33. Ibid., p. 99.

34. Ibid., p. 105.

35. N.S. Karnik, "Locating HIV/AIDS and India: cautionary notes on the globalization of categories." *Science, Technology, & Human Values* 26: 322–348, 2001.

36. National Research Council, *Demographic Effects of Economic Reversals in Sub-Saharan Africa.* Washington, D.C.: National Academy Press, 1993.

37. B.G. Schoepf, "Women at risk: case studies from Zaire," op. cit., p. 263.

38. J.G. Ruggie, "Reconstituting the global public domain—Issues, actors, and practices." *European Journal of International Relations* 10: 499–531, 2004.

39. Ibid., p. 510.

40. R. Jenkins, "Globalization, corporate social responsibility and poverty." *International Affairs* 81: 525–540, 2005.

41. This paragraph is based upon D.F. Aberle, "What kind of science is anthropology?" *American Anthropologist* 89: 551–566, 1987.

42. P.E. Tetlock, *Expert Political Judgment: How Good Is It? How Can We Know?* Princeton: Princeton University Press, 2005.

43. Ibid., p. 73.

44. Ibid., p. 81.

45. Ibid., pp. 73–75.

46. Ibid., p. 118.

47. Ibid., p. 75.

48. A.N. Whitehead, *Science and the Modern World*. New York: The Free Press, [1925] 1967, p. 58.

49. Ibid., p. 59.

50. T. Kuhn, *The Structure of Scientific Revolutions*. Chicago: The University of Chicago Press, 1962. T.M. Brown, "Putting paradigms into history." *Marxist Perspectives* 9: 34–63, 1980.

Appendix 1

1. *Human Mortality Database.* University of California, Berkeley (USA), and Max Planck Institute for Demographic Research (Germany). Available at www.mortality .org. Data were downloaded on November 8, 2004.

Appendix 2

1. A. Newsholme, *The Prevention of Tuberculosis*. London: Methuen & Co., 1908. See also L.G. Wilson, "The historical decline of tuberculosis in Europe and America: its causes and significance." *Journal of the History of Medicine and Allied Sciences*, 45: 366–396, 1990.

2. Newsholme, *The Prevention of Tuberculosis*, p. 256.

3. Newsholme, *The Prevention of Tuberculosis*, pp. 270–271.

4. Newsholme, *The Prevention of Tuberculosis*, p. 273.

5. Newsholme, *The Prevention of Tuberculosis*, p. 313.

6. G. Cronje, "Tuberculosis and mortality decline in England and Wales, 1851–1910." In R. Woods and J. Woodward, eds., *Urban Disease and Mortality in Nineteenth-Century England*. London: Batsford Academic and Educational, 1984, pp. 81–82.

7. B. Bates, *Bargaining for Life: A Social History of Tuberculosis, 1876–1938*. Philadelphia: University of Pennsylvania Press, 1992, p. 318.

8. R. Catalano and J. Frank, "Detecting the effect of medical care on mortality." *Journal of Clinical Epidemiology* 54: 830–836, 2001.

9. L. Wilson, "The historical decline of tuberculosis in Europe and America: its

causes and significance." *Journal of the History of Medicine and Allied Sciences* 45: 366–396, 1990, and "The rise and fall of tuberculosis in Minnesota: the role of infection." *Bulletin of the History of Medicine* 66: 16–52, 1992.

10. P.D.O. Davies and J.M. Grange, "Factors affecting susceptibility and resistance to tuberculosis." *Thorax* 56 (Supplement II), ii23-ii29, 2001. R.P.O. Davies, K. Tocque, M.A. Bellis, T. Rimmington, and P.D.O. Davies, "Historical declines in tuberculosis in England and Wales: improving social conditions or natural selection?" *International Journal of Tuberculosis and Lung Diseases* 3: 1051–1054, 1999. See also J.M. Grange, M. Gandy, P. Farmer, and Z. Zumla, "Historical declines in tuberculosis: nature, nurture and the biosocial model." *International Journal of Tuberculosis and Lung Diseases* 5: 208–212, 2001. Swedish and Finnish data show an increase in death rates due to tuberculosis during the first half of the nineteenth century, but this may reflect the recession of competing risks as epidemic diseases waned and the chronic infectious diseases became more visible. See B. Puranen, "Tuberculosis and the decline of mortality in Sweden." In R. Schofield, D. Reher, and A. Bideau, eds., *The Decline of Mortality in Europe*. Oxford: Oxford University Press, 1991.

11. In a study of 687 skeletons from a medieval cemetery in Yorkshire, nine showed evidence of tuberculosis. DNA analyses of the lesions revealed that they were caused by human, not bovine, tuberculosis. In the pre-antibiotic era, 5% to 7% of active cases of tuberculosis showed bone changes. Applying these figures to the skeletal remains suggests that perhaps 130 to 180 of them would have had active tuberculosis at some point in their lives. In the twentieth century prior to antibiotics, active cases generally represented about 10% of tuberculin-positive reactors (that is, people who harbor the bacillus). Because only those who were resident in the parish could be buried in the churchyard, this suggests a very high level of infection and, indeed, of active disease. S. Mays, G.M. Taylor, A.J. Legge, D.B. Young, and G. Turner-Walker, "Paleopathological and biomolecular study of tuberculosis in a medieval skeletal collection from England." *American Journal of Physical Anthropology* 114: 298–311, 2001.

12. Bates, *Bargaining for Life*, op. cit., p. 325.

13. H.T. Waaler, "Height, weight and mortality: the Norwegian experience." *Acta Medica Scandinavica*, Supplementum 679, 1984, p. 47.

14. L.J. Reed and A.G. Love, "Biometric studies on U.S. Army officers—somatological norms in disease." *Human Biology* 5: 61–93, 1933. E. Long and S. Jablon, *Tuberculosis in the Army of the United States in World War II*. VA Medical Monograph. Washington, D.C.: U.S. Government Printing Office, 1955. C.E. Palmer, S. Jablon, and P.Q. Edwards, "Tuberculosis morbidity of young men in relation to tuberculin sensitivity and body build." *The American Review of Tuberculosis and Pulmonary Diseases* 76: 517–539, 1957. L.B. Edwards, V.T. Livesay, F.A. Acquaviva, and C.E. Palmer, "Height, weight, tuberculous infection, and tuberculous disease." *Archives of Environmental Health* 22: 106–113, 1971. D.E. Snider, "Tuberculosis and body build." *Journal of the American Medical Association* 258: 3299, 1987.

15. J.C. Riley, "Height, nutrition and mortality risk reconsidered." *Journal of Interdisciplinary History* 24: 465–492, 1994.

16. R. Floud, *Height, Weight, and Body Mass of the British Population Since 1820*. NBER Historical Working Paper No. 108. Cambridge, Mass..: National Bureau of Economic Research, 1998.

17. D.R. Weir, "Economic welfare and physical well-being in France, 1750–1990." In R. Steckel and R. Floud, *Health and Welfare during Industrialization*. S.H. Preston and E. van de Walle, "Urban French mortality in the nineteenth century." *Population Studies*

32: 275–297, 1978. A. Mitchell, "An inexact science: the statistics of tuberculosis in late nineteenth-century France." *Social History of Medicine* 3: 387–403, 1990. D.S. Barnes, "The rise and fall of tuberculosis in belle-epoque France: a reply to Alan Mitchell." *Social History of Medicine* 5: 279–290, 1992. A. Mitchell, "Tuberculosis statistics and the McKeown thesis: a rebuttal to David Barnes." *Social History of Medicine* 5: 291–296, 1992. B. Puranen, "Tuberculosis and the decline of mortality in Sweden," op. cit.

18. D.E. Snider, "Tuberculosis and body build," op. cit.

19. P.D.O. Davies and J.M. Grange, "Factors affecting susceptibility and resistance to tuberculosis," p. ii25.

20. A.J. Mercer, "Relative trends in mortality from related respiratory and airborne infectious diseases." *Population Studies* 40: 129–145, 1986. See also A.J. Mercer, *Disease, Mortality, and Population in Transition*. Leicester: Leicester University Press, 1990.

21. Hardy, *The Epidemic Streets*, p. 126.

22. P. Baldwin, *Contagion and the State in Europe 1830–1930*. Cambridge: Cambridge University Press, 1999, p. 266.

23. J. Weis Bentzon, "The effect of certain infectious diseases on tuberculin allergy." *Tubercle* 34: 34–41, 1953. I am grateful to Professors Caroline B. Hall, William Hall, and George Comstock for discussion of this issue, and to Professor Comstock for the reference to the paper by Weis Bentzon.

24. G. Davey Smith and J. Lynch, "Social capital, social epidemiology and disease aetiology." *International Journal of Epidemiology* 33: 691–700, 2004.

25. R. Woods, *The Demography of Victorian England and Wales*, pp. 272–273.

26. D.L. Blackwell, M.D. Hayward, and E.M. Crimmins, "Does childhood health affect chronic morbidity in later life?" *Social Science and Medicine* 52: 1269–1284, 2001, p. 1275.

27. In addition, Blackwell et al., showed that self-reported serious sickness in childhood was not associated with adult height.

28. W.O. Kermack, A.G. McKendrick, and P.L. McKinlay, "Death-rates in Great Britain and Sweden: some general regularities and their significance." *The Lancet* March 31, 1934, pp. 698–703. Reprinted in *International Journal of Epidemiology* 30: 678–683, 2001. See also G. Davey Smith and D. Kuh, "Commentary: William Ogilvy Kermack and the childhood origins of adult health and disease." *International Journal of Epidemiology* 30: 696–703, 2001.

29. The data in Appendix Figure A-1 are from V.H. Springett, "An interpretation of statistical trends in tuberculosis." *The Lancet*, March 15, 1952, pp.521–524. I am grateful to George Davey Smith for calling this paper to my attention. See also the better-known paper using similar cohort analyses of data from Massachusetts: W.H. Frost, "Age selection of mortality from tuberculosis in successive decades." *The American Journal of Hygiene* 30: 91–96, 1939.

30. G. Davey Smith and J. Lynch, "Social capital, social epidemiology and disease aetiology," op. cit.

31. E.M. Medlar, D.M. Spain, and R.W. Holliday, "Disregarded seedbed of the tubercle bacillus." *Archives of Internal Medicine* 81: 501–517, 1948.

32. E. Vynnycky and P.E.M. Fine, "Interpreting the decline in tuberculosis: the role of secular trends in effective contact." *International Journal of Epidemiology* 28: 327–334, 1999. Much of the following discussion on the dynamics of infection is based upon this article.

33. D.J. Dow and W.E. Lloyd, "The incidence of tuberculous infection and its relation to contagion in children under 15." *British Medical Journal* 2: 183–186, 1931.

34. F.B. Smith, *The Retreat of Tuberculosis, 1850–1950*. London: Croom Helm, 1988, p. 18.

35. Newsholme, *The Prevention of Tuberculosis*, p. 336.

36. Vynnycky and Fine, "Interpreting the decline in tuberculosis," op. cit., p. 333.

37. C. Lienhardt, "From exposure to disease: the role of environmental factors in susceptibility to and development of tuberculosis." *Epidemiologic Reviews* 23: 288–301, 2001, p. 291.

38. P.W. Ewald, "The evolution of virulence." *Scientific American* April, 1993, pp. 86–93.

Appendix 3

1. A.R. Dyer, J. Stamler, D.B. Garside, and P. Greenland, "Long-term consequences of body mass index for cardiovascular mortality." *Annals of Epidemiology* 14: 101–108, 2003.

2. U.A. Ajani, P.A. Loturfo, J.M. Gaziano, I-M Lee, A. Speslberg, J.E. Buring, W.C. Willett, and J.E. Manson, "Body mass index and mortality among US male physicians." *Annals of Epidemiology* 14: 731–739, 2004.

3. A. Engeland, T. Bjorge, R.M. Selmer, and A. Tverdal, "Height and body mass index in relation to total mortality." *Epidemiology* 14: 293–299, 2003.

4. V. Hosegood and O.M.R. Campbell, "Body mass index, height, weight, arm circumference, and mortality in rural Bangladeshi women: a 19-y longitudinal study." *American Journal of Clinical Nutrition* 77: 341–347, 2003. C.J. Crespo, M.R. Garcia Palmieri, R. Perez Perdomo, D.L. McGee, E. Smit, C.T. Sempos, I-M Lee, and P.D. Sorlie, "The relationship of physical activity and body weight with all-cause mortality: results from the Puerto Rico Heart Health Program." *Annals of Epidemiology* 12: 543–552, 2002. S.Kuriyama, K. Ohmori, C. Miura, Y. Suzuki, N. Nakaya, K. Fujita, Y. Sato, Y. Tsubono, I. Tsujy, A. Fukao, and S. Hisamichi, "Body mass index and mortality in Japan: the Miyagi cohort study." *Journal of Epidemiology* 14 [Supplement], S-33-S38, 2004.

Appendix 4

1. D.A. Griffith and L. J. Layne. *A Casebook for Spatial Statistical Data Analysis: A compilation of analyses of thematic data sets*. New York: Oxford University Press, 1999.

2. The Gini coefficients for 2000 are calculated as weighted averages of the Gini coefficients for counties within each state. The county values were supplied by Drs. John Lynch and Sam Harper. Mortality data are from: United States Department of Health and Human Services (US DHHS), Centers for Disease Control and Prevention (CDC), National Center for Health Statistics (NCHS), Compressed Mortality File (CMF) compiled from CMF 1968–1988, Series 20, No. 2A 2000, CMF 1989–1998, Series 20, No. 2E 2003 and CMF 1999–2002, Series 20, No. 2H 2004 on CDC WONDER On-line Database.

3. Caliper Corporation, Newton, MA

4. ESRI Inc., Redlands, CA.

5. SAS Institute Inc., Cary, NC.

6. R Development Core Team (2005). R: A language and environment for statistical computing. R Foundation for Statistical Computing, Vienna, Austria. ISBN 3-900051-07-0, URL http://www.R-project.org.

7. SAS Institute Inc. 2004. SAS OnlineDoc® 9.1.3. Cary, NC: SAS Institute Inc.

8. This will be examined further in the future using Anselin's local, Moran's I, and Getis-Ord statistics for local spatial autocorrelation, but also see the following paragraph.

9. It is not clear why a spatial autocorrelation value of −1 was found at the region level but may be due to a problem with the algorithm, small sample size, or an interaction between the two. The problem is not further investigated here.

10. For an interesting example of how the economies and cultures of states matter, in this case for the association between voting patterns and income, see A. Gelman, B. Shor, J. Bufumi, and D. Park, "Rich state, poor state, red state, blue state: What's the matter with Connecticut." Departments of Statistics and Political Science, Columbia University, New York City, NY. November 30, 2005.

Appendix 5

1. The homicide rates are from the United States Department of Health and Human Services, (US DHHS), Centers for Disease Control and Prevention (CDC), National Center for health Statistics (NCHS), Compressed Mortality File (CMF) compiled from CMF 1999–2002, Series 20, No. 2H 2004 on CDC WONDER On-line Database, ICD 10 codes X85-X99.9 and Y00-Y87.1. The Gini coefficients are calculated as weighted average of the Gini coefficients for counties within each state. The county values were supplied by Drs. John Lynch and Sam Harper.

Index

Page numbers followed by *f, t,* and *n* refer to figures, tables, and notes respectively.